Healing with water

MANCHESTER
1824
Manchester University Press

For Graham, with love

Healing with water

English spas and the water cure, 1840–1960

Jane M. Adams

Manchester University Press

Published by
Manchester University Press
Altrincham Street, Manchester M1 7JA
www.manchesteruniversitypress.co.uk

British Library Cataloguing-in-Publication Data
A catalogue record for this book is available from the British Library

Library of Congress Cataloging-in-Publication Data applied for

ISBN 978 0 7190 9569 6 hardback

First published 2015

Typeset
by Frances Hackeson Freelance Publishing Services, Brinscall, Lancs
Printed in Great Britain
by Lightning Source

Contents

Figures

Tables

Acknowledgements

This book would not have been written without the financial support of the Wellcome Trust for the project 'Healing cultures, medicine and the therapeutic uses of water in the English Midlands 1840–1948', carried out at the Centre for the History of Medicine, University of Warwick (Grant No. 077552/Z/05/Z/AW/HH) with Hilary Marland as principal investigator. My heartfelt thanks go to the Wellcome Trust for their generosity and to Hilary for her unceasing guidance and inspiration. This work has benefited enormously from her comments on various versions of the text. Thanks are also due to past and present staff and students at the Centre for the History of Medicine at Warwick for their encouragement, advice and many conversations and debates over the years. I am grateful for comments and feedback on papers delivered at conferences organised by the Society for the Social History of Medicine, the European Association for the History of Medicine and Health and at seminars and workshops at universities in Brest, Birmingham, Kent, Warwick, Wolverhampton and the Open University. I am indebted to the anonymous referees for their insightful comments and suggestions and to Manchester University Press for turning it all into a book. Any shortcomings remain my own.

One of the true joys of carrying out this research has been the opportunity to visit the English spas and hydropathic centres discussed in the text. I am grateful to staff and volunteers at many archives, libraries, museums and information centres who have shared their knowledge and enthusiasm for all things to do with spas and hydropathy, showed interest in this project, gone out of their way to help me with source material, introduced me to their collections and local buildings and guided me on walks around resorts. I would particularly like to thank those at Ashby De La Zouche Museum, Bath Central

Library, Bath Record Office, Buxton Art Gallery and Museum, Buxton Library, Cheltenham Art Gallery and Museum, Cheltenham Library, Derbyshire Record Office and Local Studies Collection, Droitwich Spa Heritage and Information Centre, Droitwich Spa Library, Harrogate Library, Royal Pump Room Museum, Harrogate, Leamington Spa Art Gallery and Museum, Leamington Spa Library, Malvern Library, Malvern Museum, Worcestershire Archive and Archeology Service and Woodhall Spa Cottage Museum. Thanks are also due to staff at the Wellcome Library, the British Library and the National Archives.

My deepest debt is due to my husband, Graham, for his support for my work over many years and for always being willing to take a look at another spa. Thanks too to family and friends who have been there as the project unfolded.

Abbreviations

Archives of Medical Hydrology	*AMH*
Balneological and Climatological section	B&CS
Bath General Infirmary	BGI
Birmingham Hospital Saturday Fund	BHSF
British Balneological and Climatological Society	SB&C
British Health Resorts Association	BHRA
British Medical Association	BMA
British Medical Journal	*BMJ*
British Spa Federation	BSF
Cotton Districts Convalescent Fund	CDCF
Derbyshire Record Office	DRO
Devonshire Royal Hospital	DRH
Flintshire Archive Service	FAS
International Society of Medical Hydrology	ISMH
Journal of Balneology and Climatology	*JB&C*
Journal of British and Foreign Health Resorts	*JBFHR*
Leamington Spa Art Gallery and Museum	LSAGM
Malvern Urban District Council	MUDC
Ministry of Health	MoH
National Health Insurance	NHI
National Health Service	NHS
North Yorkshire County Council	NYCC
Proceedings of the Royal Society of Medicine	*PRSM*
Provincial Medical and Surgical Association	PMSA
Provincial Medical and Surgical Journal	*PMSJ*
Royal Society of Medicine	RSM
The National Archives	TNA
Warwickshire County Record Office	Warwickshire CRO
Worcestershire Archive Service	WAS

Introduction

At the start of the twenty-first century, spa treatment and the water cure occupy a marginal place in British health care although interest in water applications among leisure consumers continues to be buoyant. The contemporary spa provides swimming, jacuzzis and steam rooms as an integral part of facilities aimed at satisfying a demand for 'wellness' that taps international demand for health, luxury and pleasure. The use of English mineral waters for either therapeutic or leisure purposes is at a low ebb although spa-goers can still immerse themselves in the mineral springs at Bath or imbibe the iron-rich waters of Trefriw Wells packaged in sachets containing the recommended daily dose.[1] British medicine does not recognise a separate specialty in water therapeutics but the activities of the International Society of Medical Hydrology and Climatology demonstrate that attitudes vary between countries. Although spa treatments have fallen out of favour with the medical establishment in Britain they continue to be endorsed in some other parts of Europe.[2] While some of the techniques of the water cure, notably hydrotherapy and massage, continue to be taught and practised in Britain, these treatments are considered to be part of physiotherapy rather than medicine and are no longer associated with natural waters. Despite this ambivalent endorsement by the National Health Service (NHS), some private developers are investing in spa centres focused on healing therapies as well as recreation. Plans to redevelop the crescent and natural baths at the once flourishing spa at Buxton will reinstate a thermal spa along with a visitor centre.[3]

This study was inspired by an assessment that earlier work on English spas in the nineteenth and twentieth centuries remains substantially incomplete despite being undertaken from a variety of historical perspectives. Early modern historians have investigated spas as the first example of resort towns, part of the urban renaissance associated with the rise of consumer society, increased interest in leisure and sociability and with the selling of 'diversion and pleasure'.[4] In these settings the practices associated with 'taking the waters' – either by bathing or drinking – are seen as part of formalised daily routines performed by the social elite in the public spaces of communal baths and pump- and assembly-rooms. Studies of resort development for the nineteenth century have focused on the expansion of the seaside towns and the popularisation of more informal leisure cultures adopted by the middle and working classes.[5] While the close relationship between health and leisure practices is recognised, it is the demand for the latter that is seen as the principal driver of demand. The single monograph on British spas and watering places from 1815 does recognise that their number and size grew over the course of the nineteenth century but places this in the context of relative decline in the face of competition from the seaside and foreign spas.[6] Yet a walk around several inland resorts reveals the traces of substantial investment in bathing complexes, pump rooms, hydropathic institutions and mineral water hospitals that indicate that treatment remained a concern of many visitors in the nineteenth and twentieth centuries. Medical historians have also given limited attention to the therapeutic application of water, focusing rather on the management and provision of water supplies in sanitary reform.[7] Research has been limited to hydropathy's association with alternative medical approaches in the mid-nineteenth century and discussion of the use of spa treatments in the campaign against rheumatism in the inter-war period.[8] This book sets out to understand the ideas and practices associated with healing with water in England between 1840 and 1960 and to assess the role of water therapeutics in the development of spas and hydropathic resorts.

The wider relevance of a study of English water cures is suggested by research highlighting significant variation in approaches to water therapeutics across Europe and North America. This body of work shows that support from orthodox and unorthodox practitioners, patients, entrepreneurs, the central state and welfare systems, are all influential. Henry Sigerist first drew attention to these international variations in 1942, noting that by the mid-twentieth century the medical use of hydrotherapeutics was stronger in Germany than in North America or Great Britain.[9] He hypothesised that the strength of the medical specialty and the size of the spa industry are important variables in understanding these differences. George Weisz concurred, arguing that close ties between the French Academy of Medicine, hydrologists and promoters of spas encouraged state endorsement of therapeutic springs, access to capital funds and later support from social insurance.[10] Thomas Maretzki's work also emphasised the importance of support from the emerging welfare system in consolidating the reputation of water therapeutics in Germany. In addition he drew attention to sustained support for water cures from unorthodox practitioners arguing that this also contributed to the popularity of these approaches.[11] Attitudes towards spa therapies are therefore shaped by a mix of social, medical and cultural factors. This study considers the English context and asks why water therapies were or were not supported by the medical profession, unorthodox practitioners, patients, investors, central and local government bodies and the NHS.

Ideas about the therapeutic potential of water's chemical and physical properties shifted in this period as did the ways developed to harness this power in treatment applications. This area of practice was notable for continuous innovation in therapeutic approaches as well as the range of chronic health conditions to which they were applied which included cardiac problems, neurasthenia and rheumatism as well as general health maintenance. This study explores similarities and differences between spa medicine and hydropathy and the extent to which they overlapped in theory and practice. Whereas previous studies have placed spa medicine and hydropathy on the margins of orthodox practice there is substantial evidence to show that many of the techniques of hydropathy were adopted and endorsed by members of the medical profession by the last quarter of the nineteenth century. The specialty of balneology and hydrotherapeutics that developed from the 1880s engaged with new cultures of scientific analysis and systematic investigation within medicine using chemistry and physiology to assess and measure the healing potential of waters. Many of the principles and practices of the hydropathic system continued to be endorsed by unorthodox practitioners too and were incorporated into naturopathy in the early twentieth century.[12] Important principles underpinning hydropathy – notably self-reliance and natural methods – were linked to broader health reform movements in North America and England.[13] Several adherents of the system were also active supporters of food reform and anti-vaccination campaigns and saw the perceived 'natural' methods of water therapeutics as being in tune with these causes. Hydropathy and hygienic practices were propagated through a wide variety of magazines and domestic advice manuals from the mid-nineteenth century. By the early decades of the twentieth century the value of diet, exercise and hygienic practices – including hydrotherapy – were being actively marketed in Britain under the banner of naturopathy.[14] In the late nineteenth century the central state and the orthodox profession also began to promote healthy living and preventive medicine for all classes. These measures were given further impetus after the First World War with the introduction of the Ministry of Health (MoH). Growing interest in the potential of hydrotherapeutics to treat rheumatism shaped attitudes towards the inclusion of facilities in the NHS.[15]

Case studies

This study considers spas and hydropathic centres in England from 1840 to 1960, a period marked by sustained industrialisation and urbanisation that transformed economic, social and cultural life. The word 'spa' has been in use since at least 1560 and has retained an association with both health and leisure throughout this period. However the complex set of ideas and practices the term refers to have taken varied forms and had multiple meanings in different historical contexts. Spas have long been perceived as places of retreat from the business of everyday life, offering a mix of opportunities for healing, recreation and social intercourse. The balance between these functions has changed over time and also varied between individual spas.[16] The origin of settlements which developed around water sources is often apparent in the suffix 'Spa', 'Bath' or 'Wells'; for example Matlock Bath, Malvern Wells and Cheltenham Spa. These words denote more than the existence of a natural water source implying instead a place where waters were used for curative and social purposes. They signal the availability of facilities providing access to the waters and a service industry to support visitors.

In the early nineteenth century the healing properties of spa waters were attributed to their mineral content or natural heat. In Britain there are numerous naturally occurring waters with a significant mineral content as well as many pure springs, although relatively few of these are warm. The most famous thermal, mineral-rich springs rise at Bath. Other thermal waters include those at Buxton and Matlock which have a lower mineral content and cooler temperature. At some spas, including Malvern, it was the purity of the water that was accorded healing power.

In contrast, hydropathy, the 'cold water cure' introduced to England in the early 1840s, asserted that water's power acted by encouraging the body to heal itself by stimulating the *vis mediatrix naturae*. Although cold spring water was valued, any clean water could be successfully used. In the mid-nineteenth century a small number of inland centres – notably Malvern, Ilkley and Matlock Bank – became renowned as hydropathic resorts. Treatment was also available at stand-alone institutions established in a number of locations, including many spas and seaside towns. Hydropathic practitioners developed techniques to apply water at a variety of temperatures in many different applications, including showers, wraps and enemas. In the mid-nineteenth century the term water cure was associated with hydropathy and its wider regime. Both spa and hydropathic treatment emphasised diet and exercise as well as bathing and drinking, with treatment tailored to the needs of individual patients. This holistic approach and the profusion of methods used by specialists working in these fields means there is no simple definition of water therapeutics. The multiple terms used to refer to healing with water, called variously spa medicine, hydropathy, balneology, hydrotherapy and medical hydrology, point to fluid boundaries that shifted over time.[17] The approach taken in this study is an inclusive one and while particular attention is given to water therapies a wider range of auxiliary treatments and techniques are also discussed. In general the word spa is used to refer to approaches using natural waters and hydropathy to approaches using any water. The terms water cures and hydrotherapy are used to refer to the variety of therapeutic approaches that developed to encompass elements of spa medicine and hydropathy.

The map at Figure 0.1 shows the resorts discussed in the text. These include the seven spa towns of Bath, Buxton, Cheltenham, Droitwich, Harrogate, Leamington and Woodhall which became members of the British Spa Federation (BSF). The appellation 'spa' became closely associated with health practices and by the inter-war period was restricted to fewer than a dozen resorts across Britain which met the criteria set by the BSF. In addition to the seven English resorts, the Scottish spas at Strathpeffer and Bridge of Allan and the Welsh spas at Trefriw Wells and Llandrindod Wells became members by the 1930s.[18] Resorts were required to demonstrate adequate medical expertise and treatment facilities as well as access to natural mineral waters with an established reputation for therapeutic use. The three leading English hydropathic resorts at Malvern, Ilkley and Matlock Bank are also discussed in this

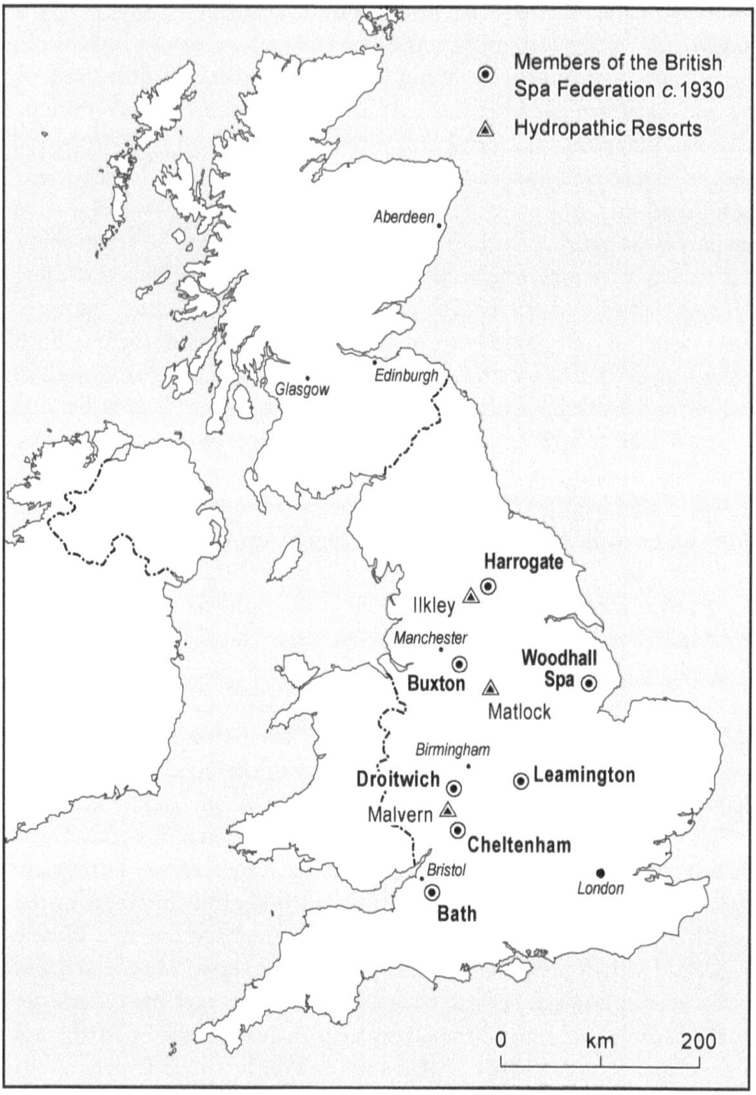

Figure 0.1: English spas and hydropathic resorts.

book. The development of all-inclusive hydropathic establishments and elaborate bathing institutions from the 1840s onwards meant that specialist facilities for water therapies were no longer limited to places where there were natural springs. While the BSF only included resorts with natural waters, the British Health Resorts Association (BHRA) actively marketed a wider group of health resorts which had good facilities for invalids, including some seaside towns.[19] This study has a thematic rather than chronological or geographic structure to develop analysis that builds on the histories of individual resorts and the surveys of British spas by Phyllis Hembry.[20] Individual case studies show that the timing and pattern of development varied between resorts according to local factors, including land ownership and entrepreneurial interest as well as the development of the railway system. While the importance of these local factors justifies use of a number of case studies the detailed examples considered have been balanced with analysis of broader trends.

Research questions and sources used

Chapter 1 explores two related research questions; the changing theories put forward to explain water's therapeutic effect and how it was applied in practical treatments. The discussion offers a unique perspective by considering both spa medicine and hydropathy and the relationship between them from the early nineteenth to the mid-twentieth century. Books and specialist journals authored by practitioners are crucial in developing an understanding of the theoretical frameworks underlying water therapeutics and the ways in which it was used to treat patients. Numerous printed works discussing the medical and chemical properties of mineral waters were produced from the seventeenth century onwards.[21] Frequently authored by medical practitioners these invariably provided a chemical analysis of the waters and gave general directions for their use. Some also included individual case histories in order to demonstrate the range of conditions that could benefit from treatment with water. Usually dealing with the waters of one locality and often revised or re-published when facilities were refurbished or extended, it is important to recognise that the primary aim of these guides was to promote a particular spa to potential patients. Despite this commercial angle they do provide evidence for ideas underpinning the practice of water therapeutics. From the 1840s an extensive and varied literature on hydropathy emerged, mainly written by hydropathists outlining their approach and publicising their businesses.[22] Although much of this was addressed to a lay audience most publications also dealt with the principles underlying hydropathic treatment and gave detailed descriptions of methods used as well as including case studies of successful cures. From the 1870s a number of publications on hydrotherapeutics, balneology, hydrology and climatology were published. These subjects were also included in compendium volumes on therapeutics as well as treatises and books on specific diseases. Hermann Weber, for example, authored works on balneology and climatology and edited translations of seminal German publications on hydrotherapeutics and the use of mineral springs.[23] He contributed to general medical textbooks and produced an English guide to spas and mineral waters in Britain and Europe.[24] The first comprehensive medical guide dedicated to the British spas and health resorts was *The Climates and Baths of Great Britain*, compiled under the aegis of a committee of the Royal Medical and Chirurgical Society and published in two volumes in 1895 and 1902.[25] *The Journal of Balneology and Climatology* (*JB&C*), later incorporated into the *Proceedings of the Royal Society of Medicine* (*PRSM*) is important in assessing the development of this emerging specialty at the end of the nineteenth century. Robert Fortescue Fox became the best-known British writer on medical hydrology in the inter-war period and authored the first textbook on medical hydrology for medical students.[26] This body of material includes studies aimed at three distinct audiences, the medical specialist, the general practitioner and the informed patient. It had a variety of functions; to disseminate changing ideas about water's effectiveness, knowledge about the treatment of various diseases and practical information on facilities at resorts. In the twentieth century these were supplemented by publications by the BSF and the Spa Practitioners' Group of the British Medical Association (BMA).[27]

This chapter challenges the established view that water was of marginal importance to medical practice in the nineteenth and early twentieth centuries, demonstrating that this field engaged with the approaches of the new scientific medicine as well as clinical experience and was an expanding area of therapeutic innovation. The expertise of other specialists, including chemists and medical practitioners working in other countries, influenced views of the composition of water and theories about how it stimulated healing responses. Despite the acrimonious relationship between orthodox and unorthodox practitioners in the 1840s, from around 1870 medical opposition to hydropathy declined as water-based therapeutics shifted from a fringe treatment to an accepted specialism within orthodox medicine. Although hydropathy was presented as a radical new system by both its adherents and opponents this masked continuities with established spa and hygienic practices and the broad range of opinion about its potential among the medical profession. Clinical experience and individual skill had long been used to substantiate water's healing powers. The extravagant claims made for hydropathy as a natural alternative to 'physic's' reliance on drugs and heroic treatments lent added urgency to providing a scientific explanation for water's healing powers to justify its place as part of the new rational therapeutics of orthodox medicine. Dissemination of the work of an international cohort of balneologists was key to changing perceptions among the British profession. Although efforts to find a definitive explanation of how water worked were inconclusive and understanding of its potential remained conjectural, therapies continued to proliferate. Far from fading away over the course of the nineteenth century, water cures were central to a growing range of therapeutic applications offering treatment for a number of conditions.

Having established that water therapeutics continued to attract support from the medical profession, Chapter 2 considers the extent to which the appeal of facilities for health and therapeutics contributed to the growth of spas and hydropathic resorts. There is significant evidence of investment in facilities to exploit mineral and pure water springs and thus increase their commercial potential to meet rising demand from middle- and working-class populations. How much emphasis was given to waters and treatment methods in publicity material? What role did new municipal authorities play in the management and expansion of facilities for treatment and broader strategies for resort development? Key sources used to investigate these questions are the numerous guidebooks for resort towns produced from the eighteenth century onwards. By 1815 this genre was well-established, catering for tourists interested in antiquarianism, topography and local history.[28] These publications were intended to assert the value and interest of a town to a wider public and aimed to create a specific image of a place that would be attractive to potential visitors. They provide valuable evidence of facilities deemed to appeal to consumers. While guides to individual resorts continued to proliferate, volumes providing comparative information on the expanding number of spa and seaside resorts were also produced from the early nineteenth century. An influential work of two volumes was authored by A. B. Granville, published in 1841, the year before hydropathy became widely known in England.[29] Guides covering British or a wider range of European and international resorts with a particular focus on water cures were published up to the 1930s.[30] Another new departure in the nineteenth century was the launch of specialist magazines aimed at the potential patient, for example *Health Resort*. Material from national newspapers including *The Times* and lay periodicals such as *Queen* featuring the water cure or resorts has also been drawn on. These sources are particularly valuable in tracing trends in facilities and resort development and in the marketing of the water cure. Analysis of this material, much of which was produced for publicity purposes, allows engagement with both historical reality and its representations, an approach used to good effect by Peter Borsay in his investigation of how the 'image' of Georgian Bath has come to dominate perceptions of that city's past.[31] Once again the analysis presented has benefited greatly from a number of studies of individual resorts.[32]

The importance of spa towns in the growth of provincial and urban culture in the pre-industrial period has been highlighted by historians. Their success, most notable in Bath, was based on their appeal to the social elite as places where a complex mix of medical and social activities offered opportunities for consumption and display while fulfilling expectations of propriety.[33] The history of spas in the nineteenth and twentieth centuries has received less attention with research focused on the rise of industrial towns and cities and the new form of coastal leisure resorts.[34] Current historiography sees a relative decline in the importance of spas in England due to a shift in patterns of demand away from health-related activities towards new forms of leisure along with a sense of dwindling confidence in the efficacy of water cures encouraged by the rise of scientific medicine.[35] This study challenges these assumptions and argues that ideas and practices associated with health continued to be an important draw for visitors and patients. The attraction of therapeutics and health was integral to the economic and social development of numerous resorts and the ways they were represented in guidebooks and promotional material. The number of specialist spas and water cure resorts expanded in size and number as paying patients drawn from the middle and upper classes took advantage of the services they provided.

Chapter 3 assesses a range of evidence to examine the extent to which spas and hydropathic institutions provided specialist treatments. The claims made in town guides are tested against a variety of other sources, including records of businesses, hospitals, charities, mutual associations and friendly societies. These also provide an insight into how provision of the cure was organised and delivered. This has been supplemented with use of material from census enumerators' books, trade directories and local newspapers. Fragmentary business records survive, for example some for Smedley's hydro and the Buxton estate owned by the Duke of Devonshire. From the mid-nineteenth century local authorities became major investors in facilities and their records also provide evidence for investment and financial returns for this later period. Most of these established a sub-committee dealing with the spa and wells and several also ran a medical advisory committee. While it is recognised that evidence from each of these sources is limited, for example entries in trade directories may be incomplete or biased towards the interests of those responsible for their compilation, together they are of value in assessing trends in the numbers and categories of practitioners and facilities.[36] As is well established, any assessment of visitor numbers to resorts is fraught with difficulties with no reliable long-term data for Britain available. These difficulties are compounded by the problem of distinguishing between those whose main purpose was treatment and those who visited a town for leisure purposes. Patients were frequently accompanied by family members or friends who may or may not have taken treatment while at the resort. Once again little more than an assessment of trends can be attempted through an examination of indicators such as the development of facilities.

A case study of Smedley's hydro at Matlock Bank is used to investigate the plethora of new treatment techniques introduced to hydropathy from mid-century and to explore how these were organised and provided. The rigorous regimes developed from the 1840s required skilled personnel, both men and women, to provide a wide range of physical treatments to a broad clientele, male and female, young and old. What facilities were provided at the new inpatient hydropathic institutions, constructed from the 1840s onwards? What evidence is there that skilled personnel were employed to deliver the personalised treatment regimes advertised? Institutional records and census details as well as prospectuses and the published guides by John and Caroline Smedley outlining their system are used to investigate these questions.[37]

Bathing institutions at spas were modified to provide facilities for the newly popular hydropathic treatments. In addition to the sources cited, newspaper reports and records of municipal authorities are useful in charting investment in the refurbishment and expansion of treatment facilities and in identifying an increase in male and female practitioners working in this field. What skills were bath attendants, hydropathists, medical rubbers and medical electricians expected to have and what evidence is there to show how they acquired these? Research on hydropathy in Scotland has shown that the emphasis on intensive therapeutic regimes characteristic of mid-century practice had declined to be replaced by more leisurely routines by the last decades of the nineteenth century.[38] The evidence for the English centres is assessed to see if a similar trend is apparent or whether renewed interest in hydrotherapeutics along with the introduction of treatments first developed at European spas meant that investors continued to provide specialist facilities for patients from the 1880s.

The chapter goes on to assess the social and medical functions of the growing number of specialist hospitals that developed at spas from the mid-nineteenth century.[39] Until the 1820s the only bathing hospital was at Bath but by the 1880s charitable institutions were operating at all the English spas. These institutions had complex functions including managing access to treatment facilities by the poorer classes, promoting the prestige of resorts and the therapeutic reputation of the natural waters and providing a basis for greater collaboration among local practitioners. A case study of the Devonshire Royal Hospital (DRH) at Buxton which opened in 1856 and became the largest of the English specialist bathing hospitals is used to investigate a number of research questions.[40] Why did inpatient institutions come to be preferred to the earlier model of free outpatient treatment? To what extent did the hospital become a centre treating industrial workers from the surrounding area? The discussion is supplemented with evidence from other spa hospitals as well as selected charitable and mutual organisations including the Cotton Districts Convalescent Fund (CDCF) and the Birmingham Hospital Saturday Fund (BHSF). These provide evidence for the ways in which bathing hospitals became integrated into wider medical and welfare networks.

Chapter 4 examines the relationship between water cures and wider cultures of healthy living to explore their particular appeal to patients and practitioners. The rise of hydropathy coincided with rapid growth in the publishing industry with the 'invalid narrative' becoming a distinct genre produced in both book form and in periodical literature in the middle decades of the nineteenth century.[41] The earliest such work relating to hydropathy in England was Edward Bulwer Lytton's account of his experiences in Malvern published in 1845.[42] This, along with a number of other volumes, was produced for a commercial market, with some drawing on satire and humour in their descriptions.[43] Considered together, they provide insights into the attraction of the water cure and perceptions of its relevance to those experiencing the rapid and fundamental social and cultural shifts of the mid-Victorian period. A published journal by F. C. Foster providing a rare account of treatment at Smedley's Matlock Bank Hydro is discussed in detail. It gives a personal perspective on the health concerns of patients and their attitudes to treatment.[44] Regimes at both spas and hydropathics emphasised the importance of lifestyle in maintaining and recovering good health with advice on diet and exercise integral to treatment plans. These approaches also addressed concerns about the impact of lifestyle changes forced by rapid economic and social change on health. The effects of dirty noisy environments, sedentary employment, new occupations requiring 'brain work' and the stresses associated with the disintegration and formation of communities and ways of living are among the factors referred to in these sources. From the last quarter of the nineteenth century the culture of invalidism gave way to greater interest in health and fitness for both men and women.[45] Sport and exercise became popular leisure activities for all social classes. The discussion assesses the extent to which practices implemented at spas and hydropathic institutions from the 1850s onwards contributed to shaping changing ideas about what constituted a healthy lifestyle.

Although the benefits of a healthy regimen remained influential in orthodox medical ideas, the importance of the 'rules of living' were also stressed by many advocating a more radical agenda of self-help and domestic care.[46] Several hydropathists, describing themselves as health missionaries, stressed that effective treatments required active participation from their patients, and offered their clients the opportunity to contribute to their own recovery and health maintenance.[47] Some, including John and Caroline Smedley, demonstrated their zeal further by publishing self-help guides to the water cure. The links between hydropathy and broader reform movements have received some analysis.[48] This discussion extends this to explore how ideals of self-help and health maintenance, as well as the attractions of holistic approaches, continued to be influential into the late nineteenth and early twentieth centuries. Mary Gove and Thomas Low Nichols promoted hydropathy as part of a wider agenda of healthy living, which included vegetarianism and temperance.[49] By the start of the twentieth century the adoption of natural healing methods was being promoted under the banner of naturopathy. By the inter-war period practitioners were asserting an identity separate from orthodox medicine and propagating their ideas through practice, health hydros and magazines.[50]

The close relationship between therapeutics, hygiene and leisure pursuits is explored in Chapter 5. The nineteenth century saw a marked transformation in the commodification of water as well as in the cultural norms relating to its use for bathing and drinking.[51] For a growing proportion of the population clean water ceased to be a scarce luxury and became a commonplace commodity considered essential to healthy living, the focus of public health projects and the reform of domestic habits as well as leisure uses.[52] Developments initiated at spas and hydropathics were instrumental in shaping diverse bathing cultures incorporating hygiene and leisure as well as medical treatment. At Leamington, the new municipal authority was crucial to the development of a range of facilities encompassing slipper, Turkish, medical and swimming baths designed to meet the needs of both residents and visitors.[53] Evidence from selected towns is assessed to examine the extent to which bathing institutions offering a variety of facilities became available outside spas and how medical bathing shaped broader leisure cultures. A case study of Malvern illustrates how growing domestic demand for water as well as the needs of commercial bottling operations led to pressure for improved harvesting and management of limited water resources. This example highlights the real difficulties faced in safeguarding a reliable, clean and safe water supply and the importance placed on this in health resorts. Evidence from Holywell in Flintshire serves to further underscore the competing demands made on water sources and the variety of purposes to which it was put which could range from industrial to religious uses.[54]

Chapter 2 demonstrated how rising incomes and improved transport infrastructure supported the expansion of a variety of resorts catering to middle-class tastes. Recreation and relaxation had always been an integral part of spa life. In the eighteenth century this was closely associated with the values and interests of a pre-industrial elite class. How did the growth of a predominantly middle-class clientele influence social life and recreational activities at water resorts? How did spas and hydropathic resorts meet the growing preference for rational amusements including parks, libraries and music concerts characteristic of the Victorian period? What effect did new attitudes towards privacy and sobriety have on earlier forms of social life formulated around extravagant public display and formality? How distinctive was the social life at English spas compared to that found at seaside resorts? The English spas retained a reputation as specialist resorts offering relaxation, recuperation and facilities for invalids. They also provided a range of attractions for a wider group of visitors that embraced a growing interest in sport, fitness and the outdoors. This chapter also investigates perceptions of English centres in the context of the expansion of European resorts.[55] What evidence is there that a proportion of British consumers preferred to travel to European spas and what explanations for this were put forward by contemporaries? Despite a lack of comprehensive data on numbers of visitors evidence suggests that British visitors were an important group of consumers at some European spas up to the outbreak of the First World War, attracted by better facilities, the reputation of skilled personnel and a cachet of exclusiveness.

English spas and resorts developed through a mix of private, local authority and charitable investment throughout the nineteenth century. Chapter 6 assesses the impact of the growing influence of the central state though National Health Insurance (NHI), the policies of the MoH and the introduction of the NHS in 1948. The discussion starts with an investigation of how facilities at spas and hydros contributed to the national effort during the First World War. To what extent were British resorts able to take advantage of restrictions on foreign travel to attract patients to visit home spas, a choice promoted as a patriotic duty in several national newspapers? Were spa facilities used in the emergency and, if so, how were treatments adapted to target new priorities such as amputated limbs? To what extent were they integrated with wider rehabilitation services? How did these factors influence perceptions of spa treatment by the medical profession and the MoH? Evidence from government circulars, medical journals and information collated and published in the *Archives of Medical Hydrology* (*AMH*), the journal of the International Society of Medical Hydrology (ISMH), are used to assess these questions. The value of hydrotherapeutic treatment in rehabilitation was widely recognised, particularly when applied within a framework of intensive physical therapy which also included massage and exercise regimes. The *AMH* also provided a comparative international perspective on support for hydrological methods in the inter-war period. A series of articles offered assessments of the strength of spa industries and the emphasis given to medical hydrology in teaching which demonstrated that support and funding for spas and hydrological methods varied markedly across Europe.

The introduction of NHI provided a potential mechanism for state funding for spa treatment to treat rheumatism among the working class and thus contribute to national well-being and economic success.[56] Archive records of meetings between the BSF and the MoH are used to explore representations made by the British spas for support from central government. These sources are supplemented with evidence from individual spas to explore a series of related questions. What were the aims of the BSF lobby campaign and how successful were they? To what extent did established strategies for the development of local networks and support continue? What influenced decisions about whether or not spa treatment should be incorporated into the NHS and how did arrangements for funding and management differ from the pre-NHS system? What evidence is there to explain why support for treatment at the specialist spa hospitals was being withdrawn by NHS bodies from the 1960s? Support for spa treatment in England is compared to that in France and Germany where research has shown that national and regional authorities provided greater support after the Second World War.[57] The long-established collaborative networks that had served to develop and maintain institutions and resorts in England had drawn on the combined efforts of local authorities, an entrepreneurial medical profession, charitable institutions, generous benefactors and private investors to adapt to changing ideas about therapeutics and the preferences of paying patients. The rapid shift to central funding and management of facilities within a dedicated health service introduced in 1948 brought about a reduction in the influence of local authorities, patients and lay supporters. There was a corresponding increase in the decision-making power of practitioners in the medical specialities of rheumatism and physical medicine and managers with responsibilities for geographic areas wider than individual resorts. The impact of these changes is explored.

This study demonstrates the complexity of factors which shaped the development of practices at English spas and hydropathic resorts between 1840 and 1960. These included changing medical ideas and practices, cultural attitudes towards health and recreation and increasing demand from the middle class. It is clear that the withdrawal of funding by the NHS has not marked the end of the English spa. From the late twentieth century spa practices have moved out of designated medical spheres, integrated with the NHS, into privately run organisations focused on recreation. Their association with well-being and leisure continue to be emphasised and celebrated. While systematic analysis of these more recent trends is beyond the scope of this book, it is evident that the principles that underpinned the water cure, which encouraged a healthy lifestyle including relaxation, exercise and dietary advice, continue to be valued for their contribution to good health.

Notes

1 www.thermaebathspa.com, accessed 17 February 2014. Water from Trefriw Wells is marketed as Spatone, see www.nelsonsnaturalworld.com, accessed 17 February 2014.

2 www.ismh-direct.net, accessed 17 February 2014.

3 www.visitbuxton.co.uk, accessed 17 February 2014. The Buxton Crescent and Thermal Spa project is a major restoration initiative developed through a public–private partnership including High Peak Borough Council and Derbyshire County Council with funding from the Heritage Lottery fund.

4 Peter Borsay, *The English urban renaissance: culture and society in the provincial town, 1660–1770* (Oxford: Oxford University Press, 1989), p. 33.

5 John K. Walton, *The English seaside resort: a social history 1750–1914* (Leicester: Leicester University Press, 1983); John F. Travis, *The rise of the Devon seaside resorts 1750–1900* (Exeter: University of Exeter Press, 1993).

6 Phyllis Hembry, *British spas from 1815 to the present*, edited and completed by L. W. Cowie and E. E. Cowie (Madison, NJ: Fairleigh Dickinson University Press, 1997), p. 7.

7 See for example, Christopher Hamlin, *Public health and social justice in the age of Chadwick: Britain 1800–1854* (Cambridge: Cambridge University Press, 1997) and Anne Hardy, *The epidemic streets: infectious disease and the rise of preventive medicine, 1856–1900* (Oxford: Clarendon Press, 1993).

8 James Bradley, Marguerite Dupree and Alastair Durie, 'Taking the water-cure: the hydropathic movement in Scotland, 1840–1940', *Business and Economic History*, 26 (1997), 426–37; James Bradley, 'Medicine on the margins? Hydropathy and orthodoxy in Britain, 1840–60', in Waltraud Ernst (ed.), *Plural medicine, tradition and modernity, 1800–2000* (London: Routledge, 2002), 19–39; James Bradley and Marguerite Dupree, 'Opportunity on the edge of orthodoxy: medically qualified hydropathists in the era of reform, 1840–60',

Social History of Medicine, 14 (2001), 417–37; James Bradley and Marguerite Dupree, 'A shadow of orthodoxy? An epistemology of British hydropathy, 1840–1858', *Medical History*, 47 (2003), 173–94; Robin Price, 'Hydropathy in England 1840–70', *Medical History*, 25 (1981), 269–80; Kelvin Rees, 'Water as a commodity: hydropathy in Matlock', in Roger Cooter (ed.), *Studies in the history of alternative medicine* (Basingstoke: Macmillan, 1988), 28–45; David Cantor, 'The contradictions of specialization: rheumatism and the decline of the spa in inter-war Britain', in Roy Porter (ed.), *The medical history of waters and spas, Medical History*, Supp. No. 10 (London: Wellcome Institute for the History of Medicine, 1990), 127–44; David Cantor, 'The aches of industry: philanthropy and rheumatism in inter-war Britain', in Jonathan Barry and Colin Jones (eds), *Medicine and charity before the welfare state* (London: Routledge, 1991), 225–45.

9 Henry E. Sigerist, 'American spas in historical perspective', *Bulletin of the History of Medicine*, 11 (1942), 133–47. I am grateful to an anonymous referee for drawing my attention to the importance of Sigerist's work.

10 George Weisz, 'Water cures and science: the French Academy of medicine and mineral waters in the nineteenth century', *Bulletin of the History of Medicine*, 64 (1990), 393–416; George Weisz, 'Spas, mineral waters and hydrological science in twentieth-century France', *Isis*, 92 (2001), 451–83.

11 Thomas W. Maretzki, and Eduard Seidler, 'Biomedicine and naturopathic healing in West Germany: a historical and ethnomedical view of a stormy relationship', *Culture, Medicine and Psychiatry*, 9 (1985), 383–421; Thomas W. Maretzki, 'The *kur* in West Germany as an interface between naturopathic and allopathic ideologies', *Social Science and Medicine*, 24 (1987), 1061–8; Thomas W. Maretzki, 'Cultural variation in biomedicine: the *kur* in West Germany', *Medical Anthropology Quarterly*, 3 (1989), 22–35.

12 James C. Whorton, *Nature cures: the history of alternative medicine in America* (Oxford: Oxford University Press, 2002).

13 Susan E. Cayleff, *Wash and be healed; the water cure movement and women's health* (Philadelphia: Temple University Press, 1987); Jane B. Donegan, *'Hydropathic highway to health': women and water-cure in antebellum America* (New York: Greenwood Press, 1986).

14 Jane M. Adams, 'Developing naturopathy in interwar Britain', in Nicola K. Gale and Jean V. McHale (eds), *Routledge handbook of complementary and alternative medicine: perspectives from social sciences and law* (Routledge: forthcoming 2015).

15 Jane M. Adams, 'Healthy places and healthy regimens: British spas 1918–50', in Virginia Berridge and Martin Gorsky (eds), *Environment, health and history* (Basingstoke: Palgrave Macmillan, 2012), 113–32.

16 Phyllis Hembry, *The English spa 1560–1815* (London: Athlone, 1990); Hembry, *British spas from 1815*. In addition to the volumes by Hembry see William Addison, *English spas* (London: Batsford, 1951); E. S. Turner, *Taking the cure* (London: Michael Joseph, 1967); Peter J. Neville Havins, *The spas of England* (London: Robert Hale, 1976); William A. R. Thomson, *Spas that heal* (London:

Adam and Charles Black, 1978); J. A. Patmore, 'The spa towns of Britain', in R. P. Beckinsale and J. M. Houston (eds), *Urbanization and its problems: essays in honour of E. W. Gilbert* (Oxford: Basil Blackwood, 1968), 47–69.

17 The terms adopted emphasised a variety of principles; spa medicine, in use before 1840, referred to the use of natural waters used in conjunction with a wider regimen, hydropathy, introduced in the early 1840s, to applications of pure water; balneology or the science of baths came into use in the 1870s; hydrotherapy also used from around 1870, referred to the mechanical application of water in therapeutics. The term medical hydrology, adopted in the early twentieth century encompassed both the science of waters and baths and practical therapeutics.

18 British Spa Federation (BSF), *The spas of Great Britain* (Bath, Pitman Press, n.d. but c. 1931). This organisation was sometimes called the British Spas Federation and sometimes the British Spa Federation, this book uses the latter throughout with the abbreviation BSF.

19 British Health Resorts Association (BHRA), *British health resorts: spa, seaside, inland, including the British dominions and colonies* (London: BHRA, 1939).

20 Hembry, *English spa 1560–1815*; Hembry, *British spas from 1815*.

21 Christopher Hamlin notes there are literally thousands of these most dealing with individual spas. Christopher Hamlin, 'Chemistry, medicine and the legitimization of English Spas, 1740–1840', in Porter (ed.), *Medical history of waters and spas*, 67–81, footnote 3 on p. 67.

22 Examples of this genre are Richard T. Claridge, *Hydropathy or the water cure as practised by Vincent Preissnitz*, 5th edn (London: James Madden & Co., 1843); James Wilson, *The water-cure: stomach complaints and drug diseases* (London: J. Churchill, 1843); J. Weiss, *The handbook of hydropathy: for professional and domestic use: with an appendix on the best mode of forming hydropathic establishments* (London: James Madden and Co., 1844); James Manby Gully, *The water cure in chronic disease*, 4th edn (London: John Churchill, 1851); John Smedley, *Practical hydropathy* (London: John Kendrick, 1858); Caroline Smedley, *Ladies' manual of practical hydropathy* (London: W. S. Partridge, 1861); Mary S. Gove Nichols, *A woman's work in water cure and sanitary education* (London: Longmans, Green, and Co., 1868).

23 For example Julius Braun, *On the curative effects of baths and waters being a handbook to the spas of Europe*, an abridged translation with notes edited by Hermann Weber (London: Smith, Elder & Co., 1875).

24 Hermann Weber and F. Parkes Weber 'Hydrotherapy and balneotherapy', in Thomas Clifford Allbutt and Humphrey Davy Rolleston (eds), A *system of medicine by many writers* Vol. 1 (London: Macmillan, 1905), 342–81; Hermann Weber and F. Parkes Weber, ed. F. Parkes Weber, *Climatotherapy and balneotherapy: the climates and mineral water health resorts (spas) of Europe and North Africa* (London: Smith, Elder and Co., 1907).

25 W. M. Ord and A. E. Garrod (eds), *The climates and baths of Great Britain*, Vol. 1, *The climates of the south of England, and the chief medicinal springs of*

Great Britain (London: Macmillan and Co, 1895); C. Theodore Williams and P. Horton-Smith (eds), *The climates and baths of Great Britain*, Vol. 2, *The climate of London and the central and northern portions of England, together with those of Wales and of Ireland* (London: Macmillan, 1902).

26 R. Fortescue Fox, *The principles and practice of medical hydrology: being the science of treatment by waters and baths* (London: London University Press, 1913).

27 BSF, *The spas of Britain: the official handbook of the BSF* (Bath: Pitman Press, n.d. but after 1923); British Medical Association (BMA), *The spa in medical practice* (London: BMA, 1951).

28 Rosemary Sweet, *The writing of urban histories in eighteenth-century England* (Clarendon Press: Oxford, 1997), pp. 100–7.

29 A. B. Granville, *Spas of England and principal sea-bathing places*, Vol. 1, *Northern spas*, Vol. 2, *Midland and southern spas* (London, Henry Colburn, 1841).

30 For example, Edwin Lee, *The mineral springs of England* (London: Whittaker and Co., 1841), republished as *The watering places of England*, 3rd edn (London: J. Churchill, 1854); John Macpherson, *The baths and wells of Europe*, 3rd edn (London: Edward Stanford, 1888); I. Burney Yeo, *The therapeutics of mineral springs and climates* (London: Cassell, 1904); Neville Wood (ed.) *Health resorts of the British Islands* (London: London University Press, 1912); M. G. Foster, *Baths and medicinal waters of Britain and Europe* (London: Simpkin Marshall, 1933).

31 Peter Borsay, *The image of Georgian Bath* (Oxford: Oxford University Press, 2000).

32 These include E. G. Baxter, 'The social life of visitors to Leamington Spa in the first half of the nineteenth century; part I', *Warwickshire History*, 3.1 (1975) 15–37 and 'part II', *Warwickshire History*, 3.2 (1975) 46–70; Janet Browne, 'Spas and sensibilities: Darwin at Malvern', in Porter (ed.), *Medical history of waters and spas*, 102–13; Mike Dixon and Gregory Radick, *Darwin in Ilkley* (Stroud: History Press, 2009); John Winsor Harcup, *The Malvern water-cure* (Malvern: Winsor Fox Photos, 1992); Gwen Hart, *A history of Cheltenham* (Stroud: Alan Sutton, 1981); Bernard Jennings (ed.), *A history of Harrogate and Knaresborough* (Huddersfield: Advertiser Press, 1970); Mike Langham, *Buxton: a people's history* (Lancaster: Carnegie Publishing Ltd, 2001) and Cora Weaver, *The healing baths of Droitwich Spa* (Malvern: Cora Weaver, 1999).

33 Borsay, *English urban renaissance*; Peter Borsay, 'Health and leisure resorts 1700–1840', in P. Clark (ed), *The Cambridge urban history of Britain*, 3 Vols, Vol. 2, *1700–1840* (Cambridge: Cambridge University Press, 2000), 775–803; R. S. Neale, *Bath: a social history 1680–1850* (London: Routledge and Kegan Paul, 1981); Sylvia McIntyre, 'Bath: the rise of a resort town, 1660–1800', in Peter Clark (ed.), *Country towns in pre-industrial England* (Leicester: Leicester University Press, 1981),197–249; Hembry, *English spa 1560–1815*.

34 Walton, *English seaside resort*; John K. Walton, *The British seaside: holidays and resorts in the twentieth century* (Manchester: Manchester University Press, 2000).

35 Hembry, *British spas from 1815*, pp. 241–2.

36 For the difficulties inherent in interpreting early town directories see P. J. Corfield with Serena Kelly, '"Giving directions to the town": the early town directories', *Urban History Yearbook* (1984), 22–34.

37 John Smedley, *Practical hydropathy*; Caroline Smedley, *Ladies' manual*.

38 Alastair Durie, *Water is best: the hydros and health tourism in Scotland 1840–1940* (Edinburgh: John Donald, 2009).

39 Jane Adams, 'Accommodating the poor: the role of the voluntary hospital in nineteenth-century English spas', in Annic Cossic and Patrick Galliou (eds), *Spas in Britain and in France in the eighteenth and nineteenth centuries* (Newcastle: Cambridge Scholars Press, 2006), 161–91.

40 The Devonshire Hospital was renamed the Devonshire Royal Hospital in 1934. The abbreviations DRH are used throughout this text. Mike Langham and Colin Wells, *A history of the Devonshire Royal Hospital at Buxton and the Buxton Bath Charity* (Leek: Churnet Valley Books, 2003), p. 95.

41 Maria Frawley, *Invalidism and identity in nineteenth-century Britain* (London: University of Chicago Press, 2004).

42 Edward Bulwer Lytton, 'Confessions and observations of a water patient', *New Monthly Magazine* (1845), 1–16, later republished as *Confessions of a water-patient* (London: Henry Colburn, 1845).

43 See for example R. J. Lane, *Life at the water cure: facts and fancies noted down during a month at Malvern* (London: Henry Bohn, 1846).

44 F. C. Foster, *Journal kept by F. C. Foster whilst residing at the hydropathic establishment, Matlock Bank, Derbyshire, and undergoing treatment there, from August 15th to October 25th 1860* (Bridgewater: W. H. Prosser, 1877).

45 Ina Zweiniger-Bargielowska, *Managing the body: beauty, health, and fitness in Britain, 1880–1939* (Oxford: Oxford University Press, 2010).

46 J. F. C. Harrison, 'Early Victorian radicals and the medical fringe', in W. F. Bynum and Roy Porter (eds), *Medical fringe and medical orthodoxy* (London: Croom Helm, 1987), 198–215; Alastair Durie, 'Almost twins by birth: hydropathy, temperance and the Scottish churches 1840–1914', paper given to the Scottish Church History Society on 27 November 2001, www.schs.org.uk/samplepaper.htm, accessed 26 June 2006.

47 Hilary Marland and Jane Adams 'Hydropathy at home: the water cure and domestic healing in mid-nineteenth-century Britain', *Bulletin of the History of Medicine*, 83 (2009), 499–529.

48 Kathryn Gleadle, '"The age of physiological reformers": rethinking gender and domesticity in the age of reform', in Arthur Burns and Joanna Innes (eds), *Rethinking the age of reform: Britain 1780–1850* (Cambridge: Cambridge University Press, 2003), 200–19.

49 Bernard Aspinwall, 'Social Catholicism and health: Dr. and Mrs Low Nichols in Britain', in W. J. Sheils (ed.), *The Church and healing* (Oxford: Basil Blackwood, 1982), 249–70.

50 Adams, 'Developing naturopathy'.

51 Jean-Pierre Goubert, *The conquest of water: the advent of health in the industrial age*, trans. Andrew Wilson (Princeton: Princeton University Press, 1989).

52 See for example Hamlin, *Public health and social justice*; Mark S. R. Jenner, 'From conduit community to commercial network? Water in London 1500–1720', in Paul Griffiths and Mark S. R. Jenner (eds), *Londinopolis* (Manchester: Manchester University Press, 2000), 250–72; Sally Sheard, 'Profit is a dirty word: the development of public baths and wash-houses in Britain 1847–1915', *Social History of Medicine*, 13 (2000), 63–85.

53 Slipper baths were used for hygienic bathing in wash houses. The standard design was shaped like a slipper with a high back.

54 T. W. Pritchard, *St Winefride, her holy well and the Jesuit mission, c.650–1930* (Wrexham: Bridge Books, 2009).

55 See for example, David Blackbourn, '"Taking the waters": meeting places of the fashionable world', in Martin H. Geyer and Johannes Paulmann (eds), *The mechanics of internationalism: culture, society and politics from the 1840s to the First World War* (Oxford: Oxford University Press, 2001), 435–57; Douglas Peter Mackaman, *Leisure settings: bourgeois culture, medicine, and the spa in modern France* (London: University of Chicago Press, 1998); Jill Steward, 'The spa towns of the Austro-Hungarian Empire and the growth of tourist culture: 1860–1914', in Peter Borsay, Gunter Hirschfelder, Ruth-E. Mohrmann (eds), *New directions in urban history: aspects of European art, health, tourism and leisure since the Enlightenment* (Munster: Waxmann, 2000), 87–125.

56 Cantor, 'Contradictions of specialisation' and 'Aches of industry'.

57 Weisz, 'Spas, mineral waters and hydrological science'; Maretzki, 'Cultural variation in biomedicine; Jackie L. Bennett-Ruete, 'A social history of Bad Ems; spa culture and the welfare state in Germany' (PhD dissertation, University of Warwick, 1988).

1

The theory and practice of the water cure

> A distinction should always be drawn between a treatment or art of any sort and the science or orderly knowledge that may or may not substantiate it. The art must be practised though it rest only on the experience and wisdom of the physician. If it runs counter to no ascertained facts it must be admitted and allowed to wait its scientific justifications hereafter. But the sick man cannot wait.[1]

> Pure water, pure air, proper diet, and regulated exercise, are the great agents in effecting the cure of disease by aiding the natural efforts of the body, through the instrumentality of the nervous system.[2]

Introduction

This chapter investigates the theory and practice of the water cure in England between 1840 and 1960, examining ideas about how water worked and the ways it was used. It challenges the view that water was of only marginal importance to the therapeutic armoury arguing instead that the period was notable for new and innovative methods developed to harness its potential curative properties. These incorporated both early nineteenth-century spa therapy which used naturally occurring mineral or thermal waters, and the myriad of hydropathic techniques introduced from the 1840s that applied pure water both internally and externally. The quotations above highlight two important issues. The first emphasises an ongoing conundrum; although many people believed water had important healing properties, these were not easy to explain. Despite improvements in analytical techniques, the way water worked remained a mystery. Although some advocates of water were content that experience of its curative effects was sufficient to justify its use, others felt that reliance on empiricism alone undermined claims that it was an important healing resource. The second quotation emphasises that the water cure comprised much more than the use of water. It was rooted in a holistic approach that affected many aspects of a patient's lifestyle, incorporating diet, fresh air, exercise and mental rest in addition to water treatments. Later innovations to the auxiliary methods included in treatment regimes included medical gymnastics and massage in the 1860s and the development of baths incorporating other media including mud, air, electricity and light in the late nineteenth and early twentieth centuries. Despite an increasing focus on technique and technology, water cures continued to be practised within a wider holistic framework.

The existing historiography has presented a partial and distorted view of the water cure in England between 1840 and 1960, primarily because spa medicine and hydropathy have been considered separately. Much of the research on hydropathy is limited to the period between 1840 and 1870, exploring claims that it was an alternative to allopathic treatment and investigating radical aspects of its theory and practice.[3] Along with homeopathy, mesmerism and herbal medicine, hydropathy has been considered as one of several popular unorthodox health systems in the mid-nineteenth century. This approach presents hydropathy as innovative and alternative.[4] However as Bradley and Dupree have shown, it was also taken up by orthodox practitioners holding conventional views of disease causation.[5] Although their work has somewhat tempered the earlier view of hydropathy as dissident it does not explore its relationship to orthodox practice after 1870 when, as this study shows, hydropathic techniques were embraced by the emerging new specialty of balneology and hydrotherapy. Although the water cure in Scotland and the north of England has been studied over a longer time frame, these studies have given attention to the importance of leisure and tourism rather than the interface with healing practices.[6] With the exception of several papers in an edited volume by Roy Porter, spa medicine in nineteenth-century England has been largely ignored by medical historians and for the twentieth century research is limited to its contribution to the fight against rheumatism.[7] This has fostered the view that tensions and difficulties in the inter-war period were part of a slow decline from the eighteenth century onwards.[8] The research presented in this chapter demonstrates that this presents a misleading picture of the interest in spa therapies from the mid-nineteenth century to the 1960s.

This chapter adopts a chronological approach to highlight continuity and change in the theory and practice of the water cure. The first section examines the practice of spa medicine in the mid-nineteenth century, drawing principally on evidence from Buxton, Leamington, Cheltenham and Malvern. It includes discussion of the use of mineral-rich, pure and thermal waters for bathing and drinking and the importance of both clinical experience and science, particularly chemistry, in explaining its curative power. The discussion moves on to examine the practices introduced by hydropathy, placing this in the context of established uses of pure water and exploring continuities as well as innovation. Evidence from Malvern and Matlock is used to demonstrate the variety of forms of hydropathy that emerged in England as well as changing perceptions of the system as alternative or orthodox. The third section explores how and why opposition from the medical profession declined from about 1870 as hydropathy and spa medicine merged into a new specialty of balneology and shifted from a fringe treatment to an accepted specialism within medicine. It is argued that new research methods developed by Wilhelm Winternitz in Vienna as well as support by some members of the London medical elite for treatments developed at European spas were important factors in rescuing English water cures from the opprobrium of empiricism. The use of spa therapy to treat wounded soldiers during the First World War brought further recognition of the contribution specialist bathing and hospital facilities could make to national priorities. However it also fostered the view that water treatments were part of a wider group of physical therapies including massage and electrical applications. This undermined the view of hydrology as a separate medical specialty despite international efforts to assert its distinctive attributes.

Early nineteenth-century spa practice

Spa cures in the early nineteenth century used naturally occurring waters for healing taken either internally by drinking or applied externally through bathing. The most renowned natural thermal waters in Britain are at Bath and Buxton both of which have been used for therapeutic bathing since at least Roman times. The waters at Bath are the warmest, ranging from 117°–120°F (47°–49°C), while the Buxton waters, often described as tepid, are 82°F (28°C). Cold waters at various other spas were in medical use by the seventeenth century.[9] The temperature of most cold springs, such as those at Malvern, is around 54°F (12°C) although some other water sources have a higher temperature, for example the spring at Matlock Bath which is 68° F (21°C).The healing properties of waters were attributed to their temperature and mineral content and these factors determined the ways in which they were used in internal and external applications.[10] Mineral waters were considered to form part of *materia medica* and were used as part of the therapeutic repertoire of regular medical practitioners, for example as a purge acting to clear the bowels or induce vomiting.[11]

In the seventeenth century chemical analysis of mineral waters was based on investigation of the solids remaining after evaporation. Techniques were also developed that allowed mineral waters to be reconstituted from this dried residue as with Epsom salts.[12] Although these evaporation techniques only allowed investigation of solid components, by the early eighteenth century it was recognised that water contained other substances as well. For example in a 1734 guide to Scarborough Spa, Peter Shaw identified earths, sulphurs and fumes or spirits in addition to mineral salts and, although unsuccessful, he tried to analyse these volatile elements too.[13] Later in the eighteenth century the distinctive chemical attributes of various dissolved gases was recognised and investigated. However improved methods of chemical analysis did not lead directly to any clearer understanding of the therapeutic effects of waters.[14] For some, continuing uncertainty about the active agent in mineral waters did not undermine belief in their efficacy. As John Wall remarked of the Malvern waters,'(B)ut whether by any Experiments we can discover the principal Contents of this Water or not, so long as it is found to produce such Extraordinary Effects, we may therefore rest satisfied.'[15] Thomas Jameson from Cheltenham was among those who argued that rather than focusing on detailed chemical analysis, clinicians would do better to examine the effect of waters on the body and thus 'distinguish them by their medical properties; as diluent, cathartic, tonic, diaphoretic and astringent'.[16] After all, an understanding of the effects of the waters and the ability to harness them for the benefit of patients was of paramount importance to the spa physician, whose reputation and livelihood was based on expertise in the application of the particular waters with which he worked.

An important tool in articulating and promoting this personal knowledge were the published guides which proliferated from the eighteenth century for every watering place. By the early nineteenth century, a typical example, such as Jameson's, would include discussion of the chemical composition of the waters and a commentary on the conditions deemed to benefit from taking them. Jameson believed the Cheltenham waters, with their high volume of Glauber salts, were particularly useful for the treatment of bilious disorders and he estimated that half the patients visiting the spa suffered from these complaints, marked by inflammation of the liver or digestive system. Many patients visiting the spa were assessed as having had their health ruined by long residence in the colonies due either 'to intemperance in eating and drinking' or the 'burning heat of climate'.[17] The purging waters, normally drunk in the early morning in doses of between one and three pints, were celebrated for their effective but gentle action in increasing the activity of the bowels: 'though it purges powerfully, the operation is lenient, and effected with the greatest ease to the drinker; being never attended with griping, tenesmus, nausea, languor, or any other painful consequences'.[18] Not all patients suffered from these digestive complaints; it was claimed that a course of Cheltenham waters could also benefit those suffering from skin complaints, inflamed eyes or ulcers, kidney stones, female diseases and some stages of rheumatism or gout. Whether waters had specific actions only useful for particular diseases or whether a course of the waters could benefit everyone was a point of some contention. While it was commercially beneficial to appeal to as great a number of patients as possible, designation as a cure-all could open the way to allegations of quackery. In pondering this point, Jameson referred to Cullen's observation, made some thirty-three years earlier, that as chalybeate, sulphurous and saline waters had all been found to have a beneficial effect on scrofula, perhaps it was 'the elementary water that is the chief part of the remedy'.[19] This action of water as a diluent might explain how simple waters with very low mineral content, such as those from Matlock, Malvern, Buxton and Bristol could have a beneficial effect.[20]

Another example of this extensive literature on mineral waters is the short pamphlet 'designed for every pocket' written in 1847 by William Robertson, physician to the Buxton Bath Charity.[21] Buxton's tepid spa water had a low mineral content and was used for both drinking and bathing. Robertson's advice to patients was to spend their first day or two in the resort taking aperients to open the bowels, and resting the mind and body. In general, bathing for medical benefits was limited to three or four times a week, less for healthy visitors, and normally took place before breakfast or two to three hours afterwards, allowing time for the meal to digest. Baths were taken in the natural tepid waters in a large communal pool with the length of time spent in the water increased by a minute or two each session to between four and eleven minutes. Before bathing, patients were advised to exercise to warm the body and on first entering the bath to splash their heads with a few handfuls of water before immersing themselves fully. During the bath patients were instructed to move about in the water and to rub themselves to generate a full 'reaction'.[22] Sometimes a water jet was directed at specific parts of the body, a technique known as 'pumping'.[23] After bathing patients were advised to rest without sleeping for an hour or two, after which further exercise or visits to the natural or chalybeate drinking wells might be prescribed.[24]

In many respects this bathing regime incorporating immersion in natural waters in communal pools, sometimes combined with the use of pumping with water jets, was similar to that followed at Bath in the seventeenth century.[25] However, by the end of the eighteenth century, the sexes normally bathed separately. A ladies' bath is first recorded at Buxton in 1784.[26] The bathing facilities built at Cheltenham and Leamington, the premier spas to develop at the end of the eighteenth century, reflect this preference for bathing in smaller baths in private rooms rather than in a larger communal pool. The wider availability of coal supplies and developments in heating technologies meant that these private baths could also be provided at a variety of temperatures; cold, warm or hot, depending on medical advice or patient choice. In contrast to Bath and Buxton which both had monopolistic provision of spa facilities, by the Corporation and the Duke of Devonshire respectively, Cheltenham and Leamington were developed by a number of private investors. By 1816 Leamington had seven spa centres which operated in competition with each other, the largest of which was the Pump Rooms.[27] This provided seventeen hot and three cold baths, separated into bathing suites for male and female patients. There was a plentiful supply of water in the town and patients could expect to have a freshly drawn bath. This was not necessarily the case in Cheltenham, where spring water was in shorter supply. In 1802 Jameson noted that the spring at the Lower Old Well had more than once been 'drunk dry in the space of an hour and a half'.[28] Jameson was actively involved in the search for new springs in the town in the winter of 1802–03 in order to ensure a sufficient supply to satisfy the growing demand from visitors. In a new edition of his guide, published in 1814, he described a new baths complex recently opened opposite the Cambray spa which had six baths providing cold, tepid and hot baths as well as facilities for a shower bath. Four of the baths were over four feet deep and large enough to swim in. They were 'emptied every two or three days … by which means the water is always fresh and pure'.[29] In 1818 the communal baths at Buxton were supplemented with limited facilities for hot baths, including showers and spray pumps.[30] However, for many, the natural tepid waters remained the main attraction. Granville, who visited the town in 1841, was of the opinion that the beneficial effect of Buxton's water 'is to be ascribed entirely to that very temperature' and he took the waters in the tepid spring-water 'generalizing plunging' bath.[31]

Patients suffering from rheumatic and joint pain formed a large part of the clientele at many spas, including Bath and Buxton. Roy Porter and George Rousseau's discussion of gout shows that spa treatment was used as one strand in complex and eclectic treatment plans used to manage a chronic health condition over many years.[32] In addition to dietary advice, the wide repertoire of treatments for the disease routinely included patent medicines and various preparations of colchicum, several of which had severe side effects. There were many more exotic and complex treatments too and water played a part in several of those recorded. In 1752 the benefits of the Indian sweat box were advertised, a treatment which comprised of sweating in a heated room interspersed with dips in a cold river that was described as having similarities with the Finnish sauna.[33] In the early nineteenth century Dr Kinglake recommended his refrigeration treatment based on soaking the affected limb in cold water as a means of pain relief.[34] While a complete cure at a spa was unlikely, patients could benefit from relief from bothersome symptoms. For example, some thought that the Bath treatment might precipitate a short-term crisis or aggravation of gout but took the view that this 'clearing of the system' would yield benefits in a lengthy remission from the ravages of the disease.[35] Some alleviation of pain or improved mobility was all that was reasonably expected.

Thus by the middle of the nineteenth century, English spas offered a range of treatments to benefit a variety of conditions including digestive problems, skin diseases, hepatic ailments, nervous diseases and rheumatic and joint complaints. Waters were taken either internally by drinking or externally through bathing. Bathing generally involved full immersion of the body and while communal baths were still in use, notably at Buxton and Bath, private bathrooms with facilities for individual patients to bathe at a variety of temperatures were becoming more commonplace. Friction rubbing, douches and shower baths might also be included in bathing regimes. Although chemical analysis was used to produce detailed analyses of mineral waters this did not provide a simple explanation for their therapeutic effects. Clinical experience was also accorded importance in establishing the healing claims of waters, publicised through descriptions of cases included in the various medical guides to individual spas. While the mineral content and temperature of the various springs were believed to contribute to their healing properties, similarities in the effects of different mineral waters led some, such as Jameson, to suggest that the therapeutic benefits were due to some more generic property of water. Spa treatment also included a wider regimen described, for example, by James M'Cabe in 1823. 'It not only refers to the diet ... but also embraces air, exercise, society, or seclusion from society; and thus connects the physical necessities of the body with the moral influence of the mind'.[36] The spa cure therefore involved far more than water treatments, being grounded in a holistic regime including advice on other aspects of lifestyle.

Hydropathy: change and continuity in the water cure

In the 1840s the pre-eminence of spa medicine in the English water cure was challenged by hydropathy which used pure cold water, remarkable for the absence rather than presence of any special minerals. The system's advocates claimed that by drinking or applying water externally, the body was encouraged to heal itself, through stimulating the *vis mediatrix naturae*.[37] Developed in Silesia by Vincent Preissnitz the system was first actively promoted in England in 1842 by Richard Claridge through a lecture tour and book describing his personal experience of treatment.[38] Preissnitz was renowned as a gifted though unqualified healer whose system used cold water in an extensive range of external applications, including a variety of wraps and packs as well as baths and douches in addition to recommending the benefits of drinking plenty of water. Claridge's description of the rigorous and intensive regime he followed became very well known, with similar descriptions repeated by several later authors.[39] The daily routine started early at around 4 a.m.

with a wet pack applied while the patient was still in bed followed by immersion in a cold plunge bath and a walk in the hills to drink water from various springs. A douche, foot bath and sitz bath were taken in the morning and repeated in the afternoon, before Claridge retired to bed at 9.30 p.m. with his feet and legs wrapped in bandages. In his words 'I continued this treatment for three months, and, during that time, I drank about 1,500 tumblers of water, perspired 200 hours, took 900 baths of different sorts, and walked 1,000 miles.'[40] This suggests an average of ten water treatments a day including two hours in a pack, walking eleven miles and drinking sixteen tumblers of water. The beneficial effects of this intensive treatment were very apparent to him, as he declared 'I enjoyed more robust health than I had ever done before ... It is to these bandages, the perspirations, and the baths, that I am indebted for the total departure of my rheumatism, indigestion, headaches, &c.'[41]

Preissnitz's cold water cure was presented by Claridge and others as wholly innovative, but not all agreed, pointing to continuities with earlier uses of water and the wider spa regime particularly with regard to the emphasis given to diet, fresh air and exercise. Sir Charles Scudamore, an established specialist on gout and rheumatism who practised at Buxton, visited Gräfenburg in 1843 to assess the hydropathic system for himself. He concluded that while the techniques used were not new in themselves they could nevertheless be considered as innovative because of the systematic way in which they were applied.[42] A review of spa guides and other medical literature provides considerable evidence of earlier uses of pure cold water in healing. For example John Wall describes the use of bandages and wet poultices to treat skin diseases and sores at Malvern in the eighteenth century. Among the numerous cases he cited was that of Mrs Blondel from Worcester treated for 'a violent scorbutic eruption' who 'lay every night with her Limbs wrapt up in wet Linen; and yet never received the least Cold from it. The painful Itching is relieved by nothing so soon or so effectually as by this Application.'[43] Fortescue Fox, writing some sixty years after the introduction of hydropathy also highlighted continuities with earlier practices, citing John Floyer's works published in the late seventeenth and early eighteenth centuries as the first to seriously promote the use of water in cold, tepid and sweating baths and as part of recommended healthy regimens. He also notes the importance of the work of John

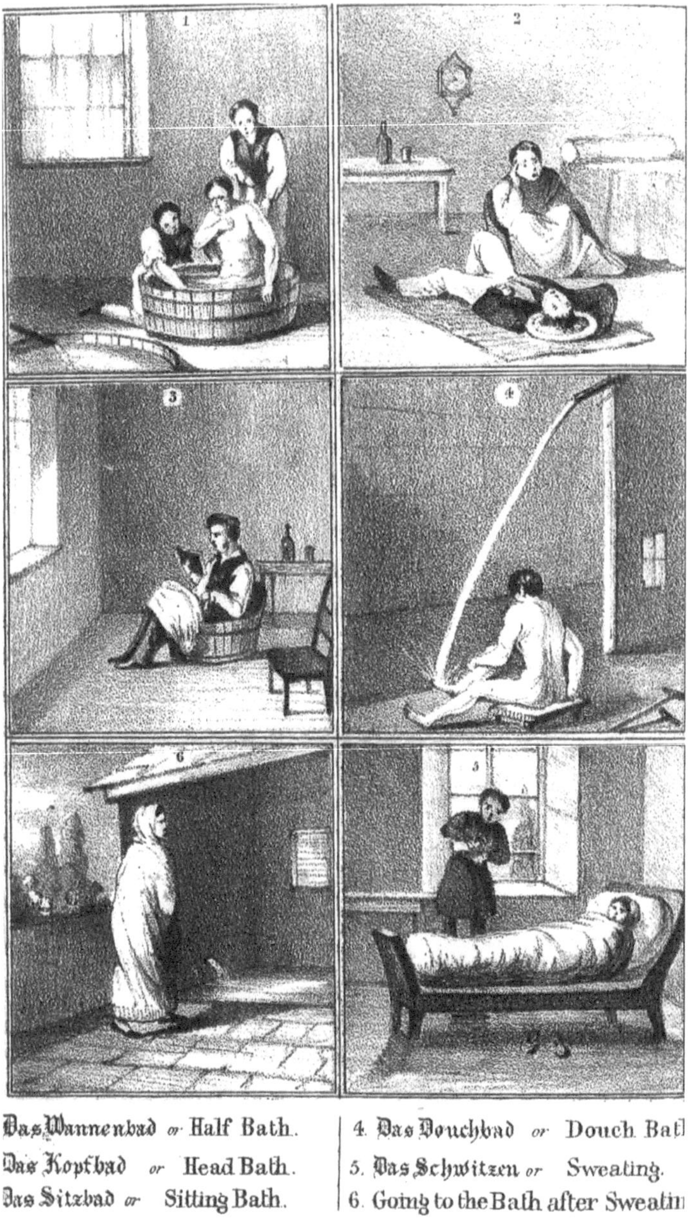

Figure 1.1: Frontispiece to R. T. Claridge, *Hydropathy; or the cold water cure.*

Hancock, William Wright and James Currie on fever and John Wesley on domestic medicine, commenting that lay writers such as Hancock and Wesley had played an important part in keeping these practices in use.[44] However, while recognising these earlier traditions, Fox also acknowledged Preissnitz had introduced significant new methods that had served to re-assert the important contribution to healing that pure water could make.

Scudamore, who suffered from poor health, found his own symptoms of rheumatic and nervous headache, noises and deafness in the left ear and a reliance on medication to keep the bowels moving were all relieved by Preissnitz's treatment regime. Based on this and observations of other patients he concluded that the system had much to offer and recommended it be adopted as part of the therapeutic armoury of regular physicians. He felt it was suitable for treating many but not all illnesses and was especially useful in the alleviation of chronic conditions and acute fevers and inflammations.[45] Although persuaded by Preissnitz's methods, Scudamore rejected what he described as his extreme humoural doctrine which believed all disease was due to the collection of morbid matter in the blood which the water cure helped the body to throw off.[46] Rejecting this 'one single theory of disease', Scudamore suggested that hydropathy worked through action on the whole body rather than on a single organ and put the benefits of the system down to its effect on 'vital force and nervous energy'.[47] James Bradley has argued that many orthodox practitioners around 1850 still saw the body as an interconnected system with health determined by environment and constitution despite the rise in popularity of ideas about the local nature of disease rooted in the pathology of individual organs. Hydropathic practices, which aimed to stimulate the *vis mediatrix naturae* did not therefore challenge prevailing medical theory as the idea of using treatments to encourage the body's own healing powers remained central to British therapeutics.[48] This was also the case at Vienna, where although Wilhelm Winternitz and his colleagues accepted Virchow's ideas of cellular pathology which established the local nature of disease, they still endorsed the importance of the *vis mediatrix*. As Winternitz put it, 'Nature alone can cure; this is the highest law of practical medicine, and the one to which we must adhere even when we have discovered a principle of cure second to it'.[49]

The emphasis given to the body's ability to heal itself was due in part to widespread and profound scepticism about the efficacy of many of the treatments and concoctions prescribed by doctors or available in the marketplace. While the early English hydropathists were castigated for their rejection of 'physic', effective remedies were few in number. W. F. Bynum notes that several doctors of the progressive Paris school, including Laennec and Corvisart, were not 'aggressive therapists', remaining sceptical of medicine's ability to heal.[50] For the American context, John Harley Warner has noted a decline in the use of heroic treatments, based on purging and the prescription of heavy metallic compounds from the 1830s, due in part to greater recognition that much ill health was self-limiting and patients would recover with a minimum of intervention. Physicians adopting this approach gave greater emphasis to palliation, or the relief of suffering, and to providing a healing environment in which natural processes of recovery could proceed.[51] As Erna Lesky has argued, this therapeutic nihilism, or reluctance to treat, by some members of the orthodox profession in the middle decades of the nineteenth century goes some way to explaining why patients were willing to try out therapies such as homeopathy and animal magnetism which promised some relief.[52] For the British context James Bradley and Marguerite Dupree have shown that although hydropathy has been defined as a heterodox practice by many historians, it was also supported by a number of medically qualified practitioners, notably James Wilson and James Gully, the early promoters of hydropathy at Malvern. They argue that these practitioners diverged from their orthodox colleagues on the basis of therapeutics rather than epistemology and that hydropathy's classification as a heterodox practice owed more to differences in the treatment regime and the behaviour of practitioners than to radical theories of disease or the body.[53]

Although there is evidence that some orthodox practitioners shared Scudamore's view that the medical profession should embrace the water cure in order to counter attempts by quacks and charlatans to claim ownership of its approaches, others disagreed.[54] As has been well documented, in the early years following its introduction, hydropathy attracted considerable opposition from the medical profession. The *Lancet* sought to ally it with the other mid-century alternative systems, objecting to its claim to be a cure-all and using satire to good effect to undermine its serious pretensions. 'Like mesmerism, the water-cure is omnipotent, and acts with a magical effect: the most malignant diseases, the most fatal organic changes, come but under the influence of a bath of cold water, and presto! – they are gone'.[55] Other articles stressed the potential dangers of the cure and reported the deaths of some patients or attacked hydropathists for their greed in profiteering from gullible invalids or engaging in unseemly behaviour in actively advertising their businesses.[56] However the contemporary debate was more nuanced than these polemical attacks in the *Lancet* suggest. Bradley argues that radical hydropathy 'as portrayed in the medical press was a rhetorical construct that bore little relationship to the actual theories and practices connected with it'.[57] The *Lancet* certainly published a wider selection of views on hydropathy than the historiography has suggested. In November 1842, for example, it published two consecutive articles; the first of which presented various case studies to illustrate the 'terrible power of that remedy which Preissnitz and his followers rudely and mistakenly wield, and indiscriminately apply'.[58] However the second, taken from a lecture to medical students, was more measured, and commented that 'one is amused with its pretensions, which are to overturn all other methods of cure', but noted that after the 'popular excitement has passed away, cold water will find its proper level; it will be known as a valuable expedient under certain circumstances, many of which are yet to be learned'.[59]

James Wilson felt that some of the hostility apparent in the national medical press was fuelled by an essentially local dispute arising from Charles Hastings' displeasure at competition at Malvern. Based in his father-in-law's successful practice at Worcester, Hastings developed an expertise in spa medicine first at Malvern and later at Droitwich where he invested in new baths established in the 1830s.[60] By 1835 he had also begun to attract a national reputation as a founder member of the Provincial Medical and Surgical Association (PMSA), the forerunner of the British Medical Association (BMA), which he had helped to launch at Worcester Infirmary in 1832. Hastings' active role in the PMSA and the national medical reform campaign was recognised with the award of a knighthood in 1850.[61] Wilson became the main butt of a campaign against hydropathy launched by Hastings in several articles in the *Provincial Medical and Surgical Journal* (*PMSJ*) in the autumn of 1842. These attacked the 'water-doctors' as quacks and hydropathy as a quack system. As Hastings earned useful fees from sending patients to Malvern he did not totally refute the idea that the waters there could be beneficial but suggested this was only 'as an *adjuvant* to other means'. In framing his attack against the claims by some hydropathists that the new system should replace orthodox medical approaches he argued 'I only repudiate the absurd notion, that it is the *only remedy* which providence has placed at our disposal for the alleviation of the pain and suffering of the human race'.[62] His remarks were hard hitting and aimed to destroy Wilson's personal reputation on charges of ineffective and dangerous treatment approaches that were at best useless and at worst fatal. Among the cases he cited in his attacks was that of Elizabeth Sherwood treated ineffectually by Wilson for chronic pain for five weeks who later sought treatment at Worcester Infirmary from Hastings and his colleagues.[63] Further allegations over the next two years included the cases of John Mills and Mr Probert who, he claimed, had died as a result of Wilson's ministrations after being treated for an abscess and gout respectively.[64]

Wilson's response was to vigorously refute these allegations, defend his position and attack Hastings' motives. Probert's case prompted him to reply to the *PMSJ* and he later appended two open letters addressed 'to Dr Hastings of Worcester' to the text of his second book published in 1843.[65] In addition to robust attacks on Hastings, alleging that his M.D. stood for 'Man of Drugs', Wilson included many patient testimonials supporting his claims to success. He proved himself an able publicist, engaging with Hastings' attacks and seeking to turn them to his advantage. He co-authored *The dangers of the water cure* with James Gully the same year.[66] Wilson's works were written for an audience of potential patients, several in conversational style, some adopting a question and answer format to simulate direct discussion between the expert hydropathist and the prospective patient that sought both to allay fears and encourage active participation in treatment.[67] The campaign by the medical establishment seems to have failed to deter potential customers as the number of patients choosing to try hydropathy continued to rise. However the public wrangling let to a long-lived association of hydropathy with quackery which lingered on to the end of the nineteenth century.

Consolidation within the orthodox profession

The figure credited with undertaking systematic investigation into the physiological effects of water on the body was Wilhelm Winternitz who claimed that his interest in the cold water cure had led him to Gräfenburg 'with the set purpose of putting the methods of Preissnitz upon a scientific footing'.[68] Research there and later on at his institute in Vienna was based on detailed experiments to measure the physiological effects of water at various temperatures on the human organism, studying the skin, respiration, heart, blood vessels and nerves. He concluded that water provided a powerful means of stimulating or sedating the body's systems and that its general effects were to do with helping the body to help itself. Water at various temperatures acted through the skin to promote healing, cold water acting as a powerful stimulant to various organs and systems while warm water acted by facilitating a healing response in the whole body. Winternitz's findings had implications for both hydropathy and spa medicine, as, in his view, 'common water brings about alterations in the living animal organism, firstly, by its temperature; secondly, by its aggregate form (mechanical actions); and thirdly, by its actions dependent upon its chemical constitution'.[69] His findings, published as the *Physiological and clinical basis of hydrotherapy* in Germany in 1879, with an English translation in 1886, were widely acclaimed as establishing a scientific explanation for the effects of water cures. As he triumphantly stated, through his scientific experiments 'that which medicine of the nineteenth century has struggled to attain since it awoke from the desperate period of absolute skepticism – namely, practical, prophylactic, and therapeutical action, based upon the results of theoretical research ... all this hydrotherapeutics is on the way to accomplish'.[70]

Winternitz's research explored the mechanical action of water as a generic substance and was therefore applicable to both pure and mineral water therapies. His comments on the use of waters accorded temperature greater importance than mineral content and thus provided an explanation of the effects of thermal waters with low mineral content as well as cold, mineral-rich ones. This new rational hydrotherapeutics was not synonomous with the use of mineral waters, by now called balneotherapeutics. Otto Leichenstein defined this as including hydrotherapy, the pharmaco-dynamic of gases, hygienic factors such as climate and diet and psychical aspects.[71] In order to distinguish themselves from charlatans and align themselves with the new rational therapeutics, balneologists espoused the doctrine of scientific enquiry. However they were forced to admit that, as yet, research had only served to undermine older established ideas justifying the efficacy of mineral-rich waters while failing to identify any new principles explaining their action. Research on the skin had raised doubts about its permeability and therefore the ability of the body to absorb the minerals in spa waters at all and it was now suggested that there were no grounds for believing that artificial mineral waters could not produce the same results as the natural water flowing from the source.[72] It was widely recognised that climate, diet and exercise were crucial influences on patients taking a mineral water cure which encouraged a view that 'the spring alone is no longer considered to be, in its various applications, the sole curative agent'.[73] The understanding of the mode of action of the spa cure had been transformed. The mineral content of the water was now accorded much less influence and while the temperature of water was considered to be an influential factor this was but one element in a much wider therapeutic regimen.

This shift away from a belief in the importance of the mineral elements in spa water occurred despite further progress made in analytical techniques. The development of the spectograph by Robert Bunsen and Gustav Kirchoff in 1857, which used light rather than the older evaporation techniques, enabled greater precision in analysing water. It came into common use from the 1860s and led to the discovery of new alkali metals including caesium and rubidium. Methods of creating artificial mineral waters were also improved and these became more widely available, further undermining the claims of spas to have unique healing resources.[74] Thus paradoxically, although scientific analyses were producing increasingly sophisticated knowledge about the constitution of mineral waters, research focused on their action on the body seemed to be undermining the importance placed on the unique action of specific waters, or even of water at all. Julius Braun placed baths at the end of a long list of therapeutic factors in the spa cure. 'These influences which concur in all cures effected by means of baths and springs are, travelling, country and mountain life, air, bodily exercise, altered diet, temporary relinquishment of all injurious habits of life, increased consumption of water, and lastly, its external application as the vehicle of moisture, warmth and cold'.[75] However, although science had as yet failed to provide an explanation of the healing action of water, spa physicians remained convinced by clinical observation and experience that the cures worked. The strategy proposed was to be open about the findings of scientific observations, to encourage further investigation and to recognise that at present justification for balneotherapeutics continued to be based on clinical observation and experience.

Braun's work, published in an English translation edited by Herman Weber in 1875, incorporated a review of the latest research findings and showed the extent to which hydropathic methods had become integrated with spa medicine. Water was routinely used at a variety of temperatures, including the use of steam in sweating or Turkish baths, within a wider treatment regime that included advice on diet, fresh air and exercise. Weber's stated intention as editor was to bring these new hydrotherapeutic approaches to the attention of the whole English profession and to promote the view 'that the treatment of diseases and morbid tendencies by waters and climate is only a branch of general medicine, that it rests on the same principles, and that it ought to go hand in hand with other measures of sound practice'.[76] In other words, to bring water cures back within the envelope of orthodox therapeutics. In his opinion, this was necessary in order to improve knowledge of the principles of hydrotherapy and balneology among the majority of orthodox practitioners who remained ignorant of their potential as, in Britain, 'so little intercommunication exists between general scientific medicine and hydrotherapeutic practice'. Patients' expectations also needed to be managed, as 'even in the highest classes of society, the ideas regarding baths and climate are often very curious, and the most marvellous effects are frequently expected with confidence'.[77] Weber referred obliquely to the bitter split that had occurred between hydropathists and the orthodox profession in the 1840s and argued that it was now time to heal these wounds. He suggested the fault may lie with 'our own profession, which seems afraid of connecting itself with a practice which formerly has been carried on in a rude empirical manner, and in opposition to so-called rational medicine'.[78] To demonstrate his own acceptance of the value of the water cure and encourage others to recommend the approach to their patients, Weber added information on some British establishments to the European spas described in Braun's text, endorsing hydropathic establishments at Malvern and Matlock in addition to those at Ilkley, Sudbrook Park and Crieff.[79] Weber, who was born in Bavaria in 1823, had come to London to take up a position at the German Hospital in 1851 and by the 1870s was becoming a leading specialist in climatotherapy. He acted as an important bridge between the developments in German medicine and the English medical establishment, contributing the chapter on climatotherapy to von Ziemssen's handbook of therapeutics in 1885 and going on to author several publications on climates and baths in English.[80]

The attitude of some members of the London medical elite was also influential in the transformation of the status of the water cure among the medical profession in the last decades of the nineteenth century. Several recommended spas as part of treatment regimes, particularly for upper-class patients, many of whom went to European spas on a regular basis.[81] One of these was Alfred Baring Garrod, a renowned gout specialist and active scientific researcher, whose work transformed understanding of the pathology of gout through investigation of the effect of kidney function on levels of uric acid in the blood.[82] Despite improved understanding of its disease pathology, gout remained a chronic disease that was impossible to cure. While mineral waters were no panacea, Garrod recommended their use along with advice on regimen including diet, exercise and fresh air as well as other remedies. Among the specific spas he recommended was Aix-les-Bains where a unique treatment had been developed which combined a douche with massage. Garrod's endorsement was reputed to have encouraged many thousands of British patients to visit Aix. His influence in promoting the spa was openly recognised by the authorities there who named a street after him.[83] In common with other signature treatments first developed at one spa using their unique mineral or thermal waters, the Aix douche was later taken up by other centres, either using the local water or an artificially reconstituted one. In Britain, the Aix douche was first introduced at Bath in a specially designed treatment suite built as part of the redevelopment of 1889 intended to re-launch the city as a premier spa destination. Within a few years the treatment was widely available at most leading British spas.[84]

The image reproduced at Figure 1.2 was used in publicity for the redevelopment. Experienced masseurs and masseuses from Aix were recruited to work in the new treatment suite. The specially designed rooms were fully tiled with decorative flooring and a wooden chair or stool for the patient to sit on. Typically, each patient was treated by two practitioners applying a douche spray through a hose to various parts of the body along with massage. The plumbing system visible in the image provided separate hot and cold water supplies with a mixing mechanism to allow the douche to be applied at the temperature and pressure required. Following the douche massage the patient took a needle bath in the circular shower shown in the corner of the bathroom before being wrapped in a blanket and cooling off in a separate rest room. This image, foregrounding both patient and workers, was typical of publicity material produced from the late nineteenth century which emphasised the intensive treatments and clean interiors of newly constructed bathhouses.

The example of the Aix douche illustrates that despite evidence of innovation in therapeutic practice at British watering places it was the leading European spas that were seen as being at the cutting-edge of research and development. Weber suggested that part of the explanation for this was stronger links between experts at water cure centres and the wider profession providing a bridge between research and clinical experience. In Britain there was a marked absence of any reliable, relevant and scientific comparative information on the natural waters and therapeutic methods available at the home resorts or guidance on cases likely to benefit from treatment. Understanding of the general use of climates and baths in the management of disease was poor with no provision made for this area in medical education on therapeutics. In 1889, in an effort to address these concerns, the Council of the Royal Medical and Chirurgical Society resolved that 'a scientific committee' be appointed to investigate the climatology and balneology of Great Britain with the aim of producing a comprehensive guide to British climatology and waters which carried the clear endorsement of the medical establishment. While a plethora of guide books were available on individual spas, and a number of guides to spas and health resorts had been published, these lacked any sort of official backing.[85] Unlike France, in Britain there was no national system of assessment and endorsement of mineral waters.[86] The first report covering the climate of the south of England and the chief medicinal springs was produced in 1895. This was followed by a second volume in 1902.[87] The survey was both an endorsement of the use of spas and climatic health resorts in medical practice and a plug for the facilities and expertise at the British resorts.

The paucity of readily available information was apparent in the method used to collate material for the volume. In the absence of any established source of systematic data the committee relied on the empirical knowledge and experience of medical practitioners at individual resorts who were asked to complete questionnaires supplying relevant information. This included details of the diseases treated successfully at the spa, any conditions for which application of the water was contra-indicated, details of the methods used for internal and external application and any auxiliary treatments used. Statistical data

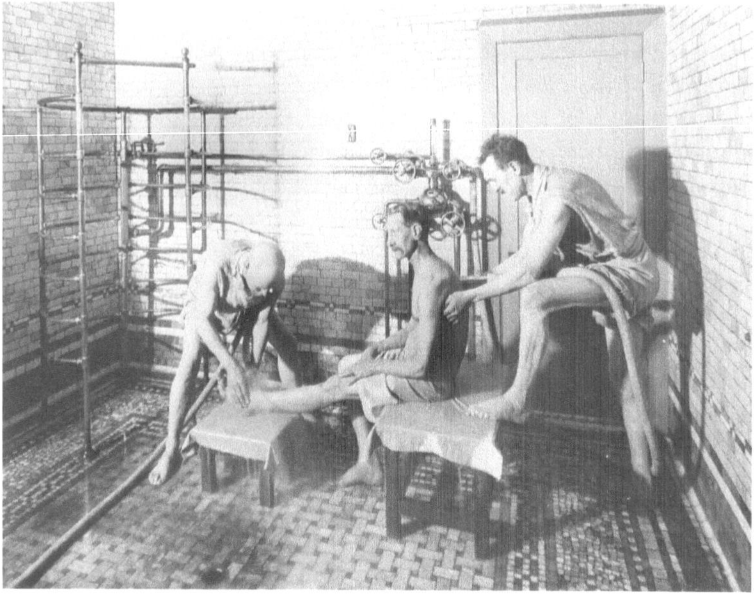

Figure 1.2: Aix douche, Royal Baths, Bath, after 1888.

from the Metereological Office and the Royal Metereological Society was drawn on in the sections on climatology.

The data collected demonstrated the variety of therapeutic approaches employed at spas which were by now far more elaborate than taking a simple immersion bath or drinking mineral water but incorporated hydropathic packs and wraps, massage, medical gymnastics and a variety of electrical treatments. However the report also highlighted that several of the broad categories of therapeutic waters available elsewhere in Europe were not present at the British spas. Notably there were no thermal waters also rich in minerals such as those found at Aix-les-Bains, strong chalybeate waters similar to those at Spa in Belgium, naturally effervescing waters akin to those found at Bad Nauheim or any alkaline waters comparable to springs at Vichy and Carlsbad. Nevertheless the report was able to commend the use of several spas deemed to be of 'first importance'. These included the thermal waters at Bath and Buxton, the sulphur waters at Harrogate, Llandrindod and Strathpeffer, the brine waters at Droitwich and the saline waters at Leamington, Cheltenham and Woodhall.[88]

Authors developed a variety of schemes for the classification of mineral waters designed to balance presentation of their valuable attributes while using the minimum of complicating categories. Table 1.1 draws on the method used by Burney Yeo in *The therapeutics of mineral springs and climates* published in 1904. Yeo used the term 'medicinal waters' to refer to water 'which either from its chemical composition or its thermality, or some other quality which experience has proved it to possess, is found useful in the treatment of disease'.[89] Table 1.1 serves to illustrate the comparative mineral properties of waters at the larger British spas and selected European resorts. As noted already, the survey edited by Ord and Garrod highlighted that Britain did not possess the full range of waters available in Europe. If emphasis was accorded to active therapeutic agents due to the natural thermal or mineral properties of water then the British spas as a group could not compete with all those in Europe. If on the other hand it was the mechanical action of any water or methods of application that were important then this could be addressed through investment in facilities and skilled staff.

The appeal of the latter approach to those interested in the commercial development of spas is apparent from growing convergence in the facilities and treatments available at spas in the last decades of the nineteenth century. Although the waters at Bath could not match the sulphur content of those at Aix-le-Bains, the plentiful supply of thermal waters offered many similar benefits and the Aix douche treatment was successfully introduced there. Plombières, where the waters had a low mineral content, developed a reputation for expertise in a variety of internal douches, including rectal, intestinal and vaginal applications. The Plombières douche used for the treatment of chronic diarrhoea was another specialist treatment later provided at many other spas including Harrogate and Buxton.[90] The natural resources of Carlsbad and Vichy, among the most prestigious spas in Europe, were harder to replicate. Both spas had alkaline waters high in sodium bicarbonate with well-established reputations for the treatment of a range of disorders including diabetes, gout and hepatic and renal disorders. There were some nineteen mineral springs at Carlsbad ranging in temperature from 48° F to 162°F all containing sodium sulphate and sodium bicarbonate. Vichy also possessed a number of springs of different temperatures. By the early nineteenth century the waters at both spas were employed both internally and at extensive and elaborate bathing establishments. The Carlsbad cure was well known for 'reducing corpulence' as the waters

Table 1.1: Classification of mineral waters at selected British and European spas showing main mode of treatment.

	British spas in BSF	*Minor British spas (selected)*	*Selected European spas*	*Main mode of treatment*
Simple or 'indifferent' thermal waters (low in minerals with temperature range 80° to 150°F).	Bath (hot), Buxton (indifferent)	Bakewell, Matlock Bath	Plombières, Wildbad	drinking (diuretic effect) bathing
Common salt waters (some with other salts)	Leamington	Ashby-de-la-Zouche	Baden Baden, Homburg, Kissingen	drinking (laxative effect) bathing
strong brines	Droitwich	Middlesborough, Middlewich, Nantwich, Stafford, Saltburn-by-the-Sea	Ischl	bathing
with carbonic acid			Bad Nauheim (hot)	bathing
with iodides and bromides	Woodhall Spa		Kreuzenach	bathing
Simple alkaline (with sodium bi-carbonate)			Vichy	drinking (diuretic effect)
Alkaline and common salt			Bad Ems	drinking
Alkaline and sodium sulphate			Carlsbad	drinking (purgative effect)
Bitter waters (magnesium and sodium sulphates)	Cheltenham, Leamington	Epsom, Melksham, Purton Spa, Scarborough	Brides-Salins, Pullna	drinking (purgative effect)
Iron or chalybeate waters	Buxton, Cheltenham, Harrogate, Llandrindod, Strathpeffer	Trefriw, Tunbridge Wells	Pyrmont, Schwalbach, Spa	drinking (tonic effect)
Arsenical waters			La Bourboule, Mont Dore	drinking/bathing
Sulphur waters (English all with salt)	Harrogate, Llandrindod, Strathpeffer	Askern	Aix-les-Bains (warm), Aix-la-Chappelle (Aachen) (hot)	drinking (stimulates intestines), bathing
Earthy or calcareous waters	Bath		Contrexville, Vittel	drinking

Source: I. Burney Yeo, *The therapeutics of mineral springs and climates* (London: Cassell and Company, 1904).

acted as 'great and powerful purifiers of the body, great eliminators' and the spa doctors insisted on a strict dietary plan and gave emphasis to exercise.[91] Although natural waters similar to those at Carlsbad or Vichy could not be found in Britain, a modified cure could be taken at home. A comprehensive, personalised regime tailored to include appropriate diet, exercise, baths and douches in water heated to various temperatures and incorporating commercially bottled water and reconstituted salts went some way to providing an alternative.

The formation of the British Balneological and Climatological Society (SB&C) in 1895 was a further step in consolidating water therapies within orthodox medicine and in asserting the specialist knowledge of those working in this field. The new society provided opportunities both for dissemination of research findings into balneological and climatological methods and practices and the promotion of their use among the wider medical profession. The main vehicle for this was the quarterly *Journal of Balneology and Climatology* (*JB&C*) published from 1897. Clifford Albutt summarised the aims of the journal as a 'record of progress, a nurse of research, and an invalid's guide'.[92] A regular publication would allow for the dissemination of research findings among a like-minded community and promote cooperation. A look back at the early years of the Society's life emphasised the importance of establishing a regular series of meetings in London where those practising at spas and seaside resorts could meet with colleagues able to travel to a central venue.[93] The interests of the new society were demonstrated in the first years of publication with articles on the principles and practice of hydrological and climatic treatment and their potential usefulness in treating specific diseases including pthisis, gout and uterine tumours.[94] Contributing authors included some with a national reputation, such as Hermann Weber, along with practitioners from spas and seaside towns. Although some articles did promote the advantages of specific resorts the focus was on developing an awareness of the broad scope of current practice. One way this was addressed was through editions focusing on a particular disease or treatment method offering a number of related articles. For example the April 1898 issue focused on the treatment of cardiac problems with contributions from Samuel Hyde of Buxton, Ernest Samson based in London and George Oliver practising at Harrogate.[95]

A list of fellows printed in 1900 recorded just over 370 members of the Society. Of these 292 were based in England, twenty-eight in Scotland, fourteen in Wales, nine in Ireland and twenty-eight elsewhere.

Of those in England seventy-one were recorded in spas or inland resorts, 102 from seaside places, eighty-nine in London and thirty from across the rest of the country. Therefore 59 per cent were recorded as based in resorts and 41 per cent elsewhere. This geographic spread confirms that information about balneology and climatology was not only relevant to medical professionals practising in resorts but also to those who might refer patients for treatment at a spa or climatic station.[96] In 1909 the Society of Balneology and Climatology (SB&C) was dissolved to become the Balneological and Climatological section (B&CS) of the Royal Society of Medicine (RSM), a further step in demonstrating the integration of the specialty within orthodox medicine.[97] The transactions of the section were incorporated into the *Proceedings of the Royal Society of Medicine* (*PRSM*), a move which led to wider circulation of their activities among the profession. While debate continued about the way that water worked and the efficacy or otherwise of various applications these discussions were now aired within the medical community as part of wider consideration of therapeutics and medical practice. By the 1890s the mainstream medical journals including the *Lancet* and the *BMJ* accepted articles on hydrological methods, for example on the development of treatment for cardiac disease at Bad Nauheim.[98]

In 1913 Robert Fortescue Fox published *The principles and practice of medical hydrology*, the first British work to attempt a comprehensive outline of work in this specialist area.[99] Based in part on a series of lectures first delivered at section meetings at the RSM, this provided a summary of the latest approaches and methods used and was intended for use by the wider profession as well as medical students.[100] The title of the work was carefully selected, highlighting use of a new term, 'medical hydrology' that Fox proposed be adopted to distinguish the modern twentieth-century specialism from its antecedents, and to meet his criteria of distinctiveness, comprehensiveness and conformity with international usage. He proposed adoption of a definition of medical hydrology as 'the science of waters, vapours, and mineral or organic deposits in connection with waters, as used in medicine, both by internal administration and in the form of baths and applications'.[101] This new terminology was important to signal the bringing together of the two 'great branches' of nineteenth-century water medicine, hydropathy which used pure water and spa medicine which used natural thermal or mineral springs. The nomenclature gave appropriate emphasis to both theory and therapy and asserted the value of specialist medical knowledge over lay experience. The new term clearly implied that water therapies and their practitioners were now firmly back in the orthodox camp. The legacy of charlatanism rooted in the disputes between the emergent profession and hydropathists between the 1840s and 1860s had faded and water cures were now integrated into the new 'rational medicine' based on scientific therapeutics. The shift in attitude of the British medical profession towards water cures is illustrated by the publication of a series of articles on British spas published in the *Lancet* in 1914 and 1915.[102] Although undoubtedly partly influenced by patriotic fervour, the articles asserted that the British spas together offered a range of mineral waters and treatment methods comparable to their continental rivals. The message was to urge patients who had previously patronised European centres to visit the home resorts during the current international crisis. Similar sentiments were endorsed in *The Times*: 'there are waters in Great Britain quite as good as any waters in Germany or Austria, and appliances for treatment quite as elaborate'.[103]

A commitment to scientific investigation of the therapeutic agent in water and its effects continued to be emphasised into the twentieth century. Following the discovery of radium by Pierre and Marie Curie, attention turned to the possible effects of radiation. In 1903 small quantities of radium were found in the mineral deposits from conduits feeding the baths at Bath and in 1912 the presence of a radioactive gas released in relatively large quantities at the spring heads was detected. The B&CS held a discussion on the subject led by T. Pagan Lowe from Bath later that year.[104] By the 1920s the radium content of the Bath water was being actively marketed and a radium inhalatorium established at the new Queen's Bath.[105] The Research Society at the DRH in Buxton also pursued this avenue and gave serious consideration to the effect of radon. Their booklet, *The natural thermal and chalybeate waters of Buxton: a brief account of their action and uses*, published in 1929, provided an up-to-date statement of the constituents of the thermal waters together with a commentary on their physiological effects and the scientific research undertaken to demonstrate these.

The stated aim of the Buxton Research Society was to provide evidence that would be accepted as 'laboratory proof' of the effects of drinking the waters. Although the current focus of interest was on the properties of radiation, the booklet also printed all eleven of the well-known analyses of the Buxton water dating back to the sixteenth century. The 'observations' of William Turner in 1572, Dr Short in

1734 and Dr Hunter in 1768 were noted together with the chemical analysis undertaken by Dr Pearson in 1784 and four further analyses in the nineteenth century. The radio-activity of the spring had been investigated between 1911 and 1912 by Dr Makower with a further analysis carried out by Beaumont Hart in 1920. In the year of the booklet's publication a spectrographic examination and analysis based on the latest techniques had been completed which distinguished between substances found dissolved in the water at ordinary pressure, the gas given off at the mouth of the spring and the content of mud found at the source. Buxton's natural tepid water was now described as 'thermal radioactive water' and the report suggested 'that radium emanation plays an important part in the action of the waters of which it is a constituent'.[106] However, detailed references to earlier analyses and the emphasis given to the long tradition of use of the Buxton waters provided a context that continued to give due consideration to clinical experience and established practices as well as the current theoretical suppositions which remained conjectural.

An article written by Alois Strasser, Winternitz's successor as professor of hydrotherapeutics at Vienna, recognised the continued reliance of medical hydrology on empirical results to justify therapeutic interventions. While applauding Winternitz's contribution in illustrating the physiological effects of water treatments Strasser acknowledged that they did not fully explain how this promoted the curative process. His own opinion was that the thermo-mechanical effects of water worked on several of the key processes of the body, including the circulatory system, metabolism and elimination but he hypothesised that full explanation of water's effects would only become more complicated as understanding of biological processes deepened.[107] Although several disciplines, including physiology and chemistry, contributed to debates about how water worked as a healing agent any clear understanding of its therapeutic powers continued to be elusive. The close association of water cures with holistic regimens including diet, exercise and climate further complicated scientific assessment of the effects of treatment. The words of Fortescue Fox, written in 1913, still held true in the mid-twentieth century.

> The latest scientific discovery is that science is everywhere rounded by the unknown. So in regard to the medicinal spring it has been shown that it does not depart in any way from the ordinary laws of Nature; but it has also been shown that its operation, like that of

any other natural agency, can be followed and scrutinised to a certain point, beyond which lies the ultimate and baffling analysis.[108]

For those who remained convinced of water's healing potential this dilemma was reconciled by recognising the limits of scientific knowledge. Clinical experience was used to justify its value in a range of therapeutic applications that continued to expand. In this context it is important to recognise that the failure to achieve convergence between scientific observation and research findings and clinical applications was not limited to water therapeutics. As noted by W. F. Bynum, although orthodox medicine became more closely associated with scientific method in the nineteenth century, with the exception of surgical applications this had only limited impact on daily clinical practice.[109]

Within a few months of the outbreak of the First World War, the B&CS were debating the contribution that hydrological methods could make to the treatment of wounded soldiers.[110] A booklet published in 1915 emphasised their use in treating a wide range of chronic conditions through their stimulating or sedative effect on circulation and nerve centres. In addition to the conditions for which baths were already an established treatment, such as chronic rheumatism, circulatory disorders, digestive complaints and skin diseases, their contribution to treating trauma and nervous disorders was also promoted. After surgery they could be used to improve mobility in joints, aid the healing of wounds and provide relief from pain and muscular spasms. Hydrological treatment could also be helpful for treating nervous disorders, including neurasthenia and depression.[111] Although new water treatments were developed during the war, notably the effervescent whirlpool bath to treat damaged limbs, the section was soon calling for investment by the authorities in 'combined physical therapy'. This approach was influenced by work at the Grand Palais in Paris where an intensive programme of rehabilitation had been developed.[112] The committee continued to press for the expansion of centres providing 'physical treatment consisting of hydrotherapy, electrotherapy (including radiotherapy), mechanical treatment, medical gymnastics, and massage' to treat disabled soldiers.[113] This was the start of a long-running campaign to provide physical treatment centres to tackle disability from war injuries and chronic rheumatism that continued throughout the inter-war period.[114] The interest in intensive treatment for rehabilitation highlighted the extent to which the field of physical therapy had expanded. Although members of the B&CS may have presented massage, actinotherapy and electrical treatments as an adjunct to spa therapy, for others these were emerging new specialties in their own right. For those taking a wider view, water was one medium among several options through which to apply heat or deliver physical therapies. As less emphasis was given to the mineral content of water the options for the geographical siting of new centres was no longer limited by the presence of natural springs. In addition, the availability of commercially developed bespoke equipment such as the Dowsing Radiant Heat and Light machine offered up-to-date treatment applications without the need for significant investment in bathing infrastructure.

From the early 1920s medical hydrologists sought to counter this trend by promoting links with colleagues in Europe, Australasia and North America through the International Society of Medical Hydrology (ISMH). Inaugurated in 1921, the Society's aims were to develop international cooperation, to encourage research into 'clinical and experimental study' and to promote the use of baths and waters among medical colleagues, principally through the publication of the *Archives of Medical Hydrology* (*AMH*).[115] The Society drew on the collaboration established between the allies during the war and was largely an Anglo-French collaboration with German colleagues excluded. The first generation of medical hydrologists were ageing, the first volume of the *AMH* included obituaries of 'three pioneers' with international reputations: Wilhelm Winternitz, Felix Garrigou 'the creator of medical hydrology in France' and Simon Baruch, chair in hydrotherapy at Columbia University.[116] In addition to these, Hermann Weber had died in 1918. Early issues of the journal provided comparative information on the strength of the specialty in various countries which indicated this was greatest in France and Austria.[117] The main weakness in Britain was identified as lack of integration with medical education. Based on a questionnaire sent to thirty-seven medical schools, the report concluded that although most institutions included hydrology in general courses on therapeutics and physiology some gave no instruction in its methods at all.[118] The SB&C and the B&C section had worked actively for the inclusion of hydrology within the medical curriculum from 1898 but their achievements had been modest.[119] Although the Hyde lectureship had been established with the support of the RSM in 1909 and Fortescue Fox had published a volume designed to teach the basics of the specialty in 1913 much remained to be done.[120] Better integration with medical education systems became a continuing focus of activity as without adequate inclusion in medical training it was unlikely that younger practitioners would be attracted to take up the specialty or that hydrology would become more fully integrated with general therapeutics. These two issues, the degree to which medical hydrology could assert an identity separate from physical medicine and the provision of teaching for undergraduate and postgraduate medical students were understood to be crucial to the future success of the specialty. The discussion returns to these in Chapter 6.

Conclusion

The principal argument presented in this chapter is that the use of water for healing expanded substantially in the period from the 1840s to the mid-twentieth century and that by the 1870s it was orthodox medical practitioners who led research into water's physiological effects and its treatment applications. This substantially modifies earlier historiography which associates spa treatments with a period before the advent of the 'rational therapeutics' of the nineteenth century based on scientific research and observation. In contrast to earlier work which has focused on hydropathy as a heterodox medical approach popular in the middle decades of the nineteenth century, this analysis has investigated how and why its methods were incorporated into scientific medical hydrology from the last quarter of the nineteenth century. The discussion has drawn on a selection of texts from an extensive published literature dealing with analyses of water and its therapeutic applications to trace the theory and practice of the water cure in England. It has explored changing ideas about its properties and the way it was used in curative treatments. Prior to the 1840s spa medicine, which harnessed mineral content and natural heat, dominated approaches to curing with water in English medicine although, as demonstrated through selective use of earlier sources, an established tradition of using pure cold water is also evident. With the introduction of hydropathy the focus shifted towards exploiting the properties of pure water in varied internal and external applications. Hydropathy's origin as the genius offspring of an untrained peasant, Vincent Preissnitz, together with his claim that it was a complete medical system, generated vituperative opposition from the orthodox medical profession during the middle decades of the nineteenth century. However this opposition was not sustained. Influenced by developments in Europe where systematic scientific research was carried out to explain water's physiological effects on the body, hydropathy and spa medicine later converged and achieved recognition as a rational therapeutic approach from the orthodox profession. In Britain the SB&C, founded in 1895, promoted the professional interests of those working in this area and were instrumental in it becoming recognised as a separate specialist section, the B&CS, within the RSM. From the late nineteenth century to the 1950s the activities and concerns of this group of practitioners were represented in mainstream medical journals including the *BMJ* and the *Lancet*. Discussion of the potential uses of water was therefore integrated within the normal vehicles for communication and debate for the orthodox profession. This chapter has established that water was considered to be a valuable healing resource from the early nineteenth to the mid-twentieth century and was used to treat a variety of complaints. Chapter 2 assesses the role of therapeutics in the growth and development of specialist water cure resorts.

Notes

1 Fortescue Fox, *Principles and practice*, p. 250.

2 Gully, *Water cure in chronic disease*, 4th edn, p. 452.

3 Price, 'Hydropathy'; Rees, 'Water as a commodity'.

4 Logie Barrow, 'Why were most medical heretics at their most confident around the 1840s? (The other side of mid-Victorian medicine)', in Roger French and Andrew Wear (eds), *British medicine in the age of reform* (London: Routledge, 1991), 165–85; Susan Kinder, 'The struggle for legitimacy in Victorian alternative medicine: the case of hydropathy and mesmerism' (PhD dissertation, University of London, 2005).

5 Bradley and Dupree, 'Opportunity on the edge of orthodoxy'; Bradley and Dupree, 'Shadow of orthodoxy?'; Bradley, 'Medicine on the margins?'

6 Bradley, Dupree and Durie, 'Taking the water-cure'; Alastair J. Durie, 'The business of hydropathy in the north of England, c. 1850–1930', *Northern History*, 39 (2002), 37–58; Durie, *Water is best*.

7 David Harley, 'A sword in a madman's hand: professional opposition to popular consumption in the waters literature of southern England and the Midlands, 1570–1870', in Porter (ed.), *Medical history of waters and spas*, 48–55; Noel G. Coley, 'Physicians, chemists and the analysis of mineral waters: "the most difficult part of chemistry"', in Porter (ed.), *Medical history of waters and spas*, 56–66; Hamlin, 'Chemistry, medicine and legitimization'; Cantor, 'Contradictions of specialization'; Cantor, 'Aches of industry'.

8 See, for example, Cantor, 'Contradictions of specialization', pp. 129–30.
9 The most comprehensive account of British spas are the two volumes by Hembry, *English spa 1560–1815* and *British spas from 1815*.
10 Coley, 'Physicians, chemists and the analysis of mineral waters'.
11 For example mineral waters are included in Alfred Baring Garrod, *The essentials of materia medica, therapeutics and the pharmacopoeias* (London: Walton and Mabberly, 1855).
12 Epsom salts were manufactured from the 1680s. Coley, 'Physicians, chemists and the analysis of mineral waters', p. 66.
13 Peter Shaw, *An enquiry into the contents, virtues and uses of the Scarborough and Spaw waters, with the method of examining any other mineral water* (London, printed for the author, 1734), cited in Coley, 'Physicians, chemists and the analysis of mineral waters', pp. 58–9.
14 Coley, 'Physicians, chemists and the analysis of mineral waters', pp. 61–6.
15 Martin Wall, *Medical tracts of the late John Wall of Worcester collected and republished by Martin Wall* (Oxford: Prince and Cooke, 1780), pp. 119–20.
16 Thomas Jameson, *A treatise on the Cheltenham waters & bilious diseases* (Ruff: Cheltenham, 1803) pp. xv–xvi.
17 Jameson, *Cheltenham waters*, p. 74.
18 J. Ridley, *The Cheltenham guide* (London: J. Ridley, 1781), p. 45. Tenesmus is defined as straining to pass either urine or a stool.
19 Jameson, *Cheltenham waters*, pp. xxvii–viii.
20 Jameson, *Cheltenham waters*, pp. xxv and xxxi–ii.
21 William Henry Robertson, *A guide to the use of the Buxton waters* (London: John Churchill, 1847), pp. 12–16.
22 This was described in the 1830s by Page as 'a glow, relating to the surface and the extremities; the feeling of weight and oppression about the head and chest is almost immediately relieved, and every vital function is carried on with increased activity and vigour'. T. J. Page, *Brief observations on the Buxton waters; with a few general directions for their use* (Bakewell: John Goodwin, 1832), p. 14.
23 The force of these jets was controlled to produce a gentle effect if projected through water as a wet douche or a more rigorous spray if used directly onto the patient's body as a dry douche.
24 A chalybeate water is one containing iron.
25 A contemporary description is provided by Celia Fiennes. See C. Morris (ed.), *The journeys of Celia Fiennes* (London: Cresset Press, 1949), pp. 17–20 and R. A. L. Smith, *Bath* (London: Batsford, 1944), pp. 47–51.
26 G. Pearson, *Observations and experiments for investigating the chymical history of the tepid springs of Buxton*, Vol. 1 (London: 1784), quoted in Mike Langham and Colin Wells, *The baths at Buxton Spa* (Leek: Churnet Valley Books, 1997), p. 33.
27 Hembry, *British spas from 1815*, p. 9.
28 Jameson, *Cheltenham waters*, p. viii.
29 Thomas Jameson, *Cheltenham waters: a treatise on the biliary diseases*, 3rd edn (Cheltenham: J. K. and S. Griffith, 1814), pp. 99–100.

30 Langham and Wells, *History of the baths at Buxton*, pp. 45–6.
31 Granville, *Midland and southern spas*, pp. 33 and 35.
32 Roy Porter and G. S. Rousseau, *Gout: the patrician malady* (London: Yale University Press, 1998), pp. 125–6.
33 *Gentleman's Magazine*, January 1752 cited in Porter and Rousseau, *Gout*, p. 129.
34 Robert Kinglake, *A dissertation on gout* (London, J. Murray, 1804) quoted in Porter and Rousseau, *Gout*, p. 139.
35 Porter and Rousseau, *Gout*, p. 126.
36 James M'Cabe, *Directions for drinking the Cheltenham waters* (Cheltenham: G. A. Williams, 1823), p. 17.
37 For a recent summary of the early years of hydropathy in Britain see Durie, *Water is best*, pp. 1–21.
38 Claridge, *Hydropathy*.
39 For example, Lane, *Life at the water cure*; Bulwer Lytton, 'Confessions of a water patient'.
40 Claridge, *Hydropathy*, p. 25.
41 Claridge, *Hydropathy*, p. 26.
42 Charles Scudamore, *A medical visit to Gräfenberg, in April and May 1843 for the purpose of investigating the merits of the water-cure treatment* (London: John Churchill, 1843), pp. 3–4.
43 Wall, *Medical tracts by the late John Wall*, p. 138.
44 Fortescue Fox, *Principles and practice*, pp. 22–6. Fox cites John Floyer, *An enquiry into the right use and abuse of the hot, cold and temperate baths in England* (London: R. Clavel, 1697) and *History of cold bathing, both ancient and modern* (London: W. and J. Innys, 1722); John Hancock, *Febrifugium magnum, or common water the best cure for fevers* (London: the author, 1723); John Wesley, *Primitive physick, or an easy and natural method of curing most diseases* (London, the author, 1747) and James Currie, *Medical reports on the effect of water, cold and warm, as a remedy in fever and other diseases* (Liverpool: Cadell and Davies, 1797).
45 Scudamore, *Medical visit*, p. 89. Among the conditions he listed as not benefiting from hydropathic treatment were consumption, epilepsy, cancer and cases of severe scrophula or debility.
46 Scudamore, *Medical visit*, p. 5.
47 Scudamore, *Medical visit*, pp. 5 and 91.
48 Bradley, 'Medicine on the margins?', p. 28.
49 Wilhelm Winternitz, 'Hydrotherapeutics', in H. von Ziemssen, *Handbook of general therapeutics in seven vols*, Vol. 5 (London: Smith, Elder & Co. 1886), 273–606, p. 348. Winternitz is quoting Deitl, an earlier professor at Vienna.
50 W. F. Bynum, *Science and the practice of medicine* (Cambridge: Cambridge University Press, 1994), p. 44.
51 John Harley Warner, *The therapeutic perspective: medical practice, knowledge, and identity in America, 1820–1885* (Cambridge: Harvard University Press, 1986), p. 97.

52 E. Lesky, *The Vienna medical school of the nineteenth century* (Baltimore and London: Johns Hopkins University Press, 1976), pp. 30–1; Winternitz, 'Hydrotherapeutics', p. 348.
53 Bradley and Dupree, 'Opportunity on the edge of orthodoxy', p. 419.
54 Edward Johnson also recommended that hydropathy be embraced by the medical profession. Edward Johnson, letter to the editor, 'Allegations respecting the cure of disease by water', *Lancet*, 1021 (25 March 1843), 934.
55 'Hydropathy', *Lancet*, 981 (18 June 1842), 429–30, p. 429 quoted in Kinder, 'Struggle for legitimacy', p. 131.
56 Kinder, 'Struggle for legitimacy', pp. 128 and 143–58.
57 Bradley, 'Medicine on the margins?', p. 34.
58 Robert Dick, letter to the editor 'The treatment and the maltreatment of disease, by water, hot and cold', *Lancet*, 1002 (12 November 1842), 241–4, p. 242.
59 'Some truths in medicine that may be allied to heresies: homeopathy and hydropathy', *Lancet*, 1002 (12 November 1842), 244–5, pp. 244 and 245.
60 Hastings' interest in promoting the development of spas in Worcestershire is discussed in Chapter 2.
61 P. W. J. Bartripp, 'Hastings, Sir Charles (1794–1866)', *Oxford dictionary of national biography* (Oxford: Oxford University Press, 2004) accessed online 9 May 2007. The PMSA was renamed the BMA in 1855 and in 1857 its weekly journal, *The Provincial Medical and Surgical Journal* (*PMSJ*) was renamed the *British Medical Journal* (*BMJ*).
62 Charles Hastings, 'Further illustrations of the water-cure as practised at Malvern', *PMSJ*, 3 (October 1842), 73–5, p. 75. Italics are as in the original.
63 Charles Hastings, 'Additional Illustrations of the water-cure as practised at Malvern', *PMSJ*, 3 (November 1842), 149–50, p. 150.
64 Charles Hastings, 'Illustrations of the water cure', *PMSJ*, 4 (January 1843), 328–9; Charles Hastings, 'A case of gout, in which the water cure was followed by diseased heart, dropsy and death', *PMSJ*, 4 (July 1843), 345–7.
65 James Wilson, 'The water-cure at Malvern', *PMSJ*, 4 (September 1843), 541–2; Wilson, *Water-cure: stomach complaints and drug diseases*; James Wilson, *The practice of the water cure with authenticated evidence of its efficacy and safety* (London: H. Bailliere, 1844).
66 James Wilson and James Manby Gully, *The dangers of the water cure* (London: J. Churchill, 1843).
67 James Wilson, *Principles and practice of the water cure*, 4th edn (London: J. Churchill, 1858).
68 Fortescue Fox, *Principles and practice*, p. 27.
69 Winternitz, 'Hydrotherapeutics' p. 373.
70 Winternitz, 'Hydrotherapeutics', pp. 371–2.
71 Otto Leichenstein, 'Balneotherapeutics', in von Ziemssen, *General therapeutics* Vol. 4 (1886), 243–472, p. 244.
72 Leichenstein, 'Balneotherapeutics', pp. 243–52.

73 Leichenstein, 'Balneotherapeutics', p. 244.
74 Coley, 'Physicians, chemists and the analysis of mineral waters', pp. 63–6.
75 Braun, *Curative effects*, p. 10.
76 Braun, *Curative effects*, p. vi.
77 Braun, *Curative effects*, pp. 122 and vi.
78 Braun, *Curative effects*, p. 122.
79 Braun, *Curative effects*, p. 122.
80 Hermann Weber, 'The treatment of disease by climate', in von Ziemssen, *General therapeutics*, Vol. 4 (1886), 3–239. See for example, Hermann Weber and F. Parkes Weber, 'Hydrotherapy and balneotherapy', in Thomas Clifford Allbutt and Humphrey Davy Rolleston (eds), A *system of medicine by many writers* Vol. 1 (London: Macmillan, 1905), 342–81; Hermann Weber and F. Parkes Weber (eds), *Climatotherapy and balneotherapy: the climates and mineral water health resorts (spas) of Europe and North Africa*, being a third edition of *The mineral waters and health resorts of Europe much enlarged with respect to medical climatology* (London: Smith, Elder & Co., 1907). Weber became the best-known English author on spas, hydrotherapy and climatology at the end of the nineteenth century and was knighted in 1899.
81 For the growth in British visitors to European spas see for example, Jill Steward, 'Representations of spa culture in the nineteenth-century British media: publicity, the press and the *ville d'eaux* 1800–1914', in Cossic and Galliou, *Spas in Britain and France*, 375–410.
82 Alfred Baring Garrod, *A Treatise on Gout and Rheumatic Gout*, 3rd edn (London: Longmans, Green, 1876).
83 Garrod, *Gout*, pp. 405–31. Sir James Kingston Fowler, *Aix-les-Bains and Mont Revard: the douche massage treatment of arthritis and fibrositis* (London: William Heinemann, 1926), p. 7.
84 Facilities for hydrotherapeutic treatment are discussed in Chapter 3.
85 Guides to health resorts are discussed in Chapter 2.
86 Weisz, 'Water cures and science'.
87 Ord and Garrod (eds), *Climates and baths*, Vol. 1 and Williams and Horton-Smith (eds), *Climates and Baths*, Vol. 2. The author A. E. (Archibald) Garrod was the son of Alfred Baring Garrod, the gout specialist discussed above.
88 W. M. Ord, 'Introductory remarks on the medicinal springs of Great Britain', in Ord and Garrod, *Climates and baths*, Vol. 1, 507–14. These nine spas all became members of the BSF in the inter-war period.
89 Burney Yeo, *Therapeutics of mineral springs*, p. 3.
90 Burney Yeo, *Therapeutics of mineral springs*, pp. 285–6.
91 Burney Yeo, *Therapeutics of mineral springs*, p. 137.
92 Clifford Allbutt, 'Preface', *Journal of Balneology and Climatology (JB&C)*, 1 (1897), 1–3, p. 2.
93 R. Fortescue Fox, 'Outlines of Medical Hydrology, Lecture 1, Analysis and Definitions', Balneological and Climatological Section (B&CS), *Proceedings of the Royal Society of Medicine (PRSM)*, 4 (1911), 63–80, pp. 65–8.

94 For example Edward H. Sieveking, 'Climatology and balneology, old and new', *JB&C*, 1 (1897), 2–6; Leonard Williams, 'The dietetic factor in climatic treatment', *JB&C*, 1 (1897), 133–8; Hermann Weber, 'A survey of the climatic health resorts of the United Kingdom compared with those of the Continent', *JB&C*, 3 (1899) 185–200; R. Fortescue Fox , 'On the gout in women', *JB&C*, 1 (1897), 139–52; Robert Cuffe, 'Notes on cases of uterine tumours treated by the bromo-iodine water of Woodhall Spa, and by electrolysis', *JB&C*, 1 (1897), 152–69.

95 Samuel Hyde, 'The treatment of cardiac disease by baths, exercises and climate', *JB&C*, 2 (1898), 119–36; George Oliver, 'On the physiological effects of baths and exercises in the treatment of cardiac disease', *JB&C*, 2 (1898), 136–49 and A. Ernest Sansom, 'On the treatment of affections of the heart and the circulation by baths, exercises and climate', *JB&C*, 2 (1898), 150–80.

96 'Names of towns where Fellows reside', *JB&C*, 4 (1900), 226–32.

97 'Valedictory', *JB&C*, 13 (1909), 203–6.

98 See for example, Theodor Schott, 'The treatment of chronic diseases of the heart by means of baths and gymnastics', *Lancet*, 3534 (23 May 1891), 1143–4 and *Lancet*, 3535 (30 May 1891), 1199–200; W. Bezley Thorne, 'The treatment of chronic diseases of the heart by baths and exercises according to the methods of Drs Schott', *Lancet*, 3688 (5 May 1894), 1117–20.

99 Fortescue Fox, *Principles and practice*.

100 Fortescue Fox delivered three lectures in a series 'Outlines of medical hydrology' in May 1911, 'Lecture 1, Analysis and definitions', 'Lecture 2, Modern hydrotherapeutics: a résumé and appreciation' and 'Lecture 3: The medicinal spring: the teaching of medical hydrology', B&CS, *PRSM*, 4 (1911), 63–118.

101 Fortescue Fox, *Principles and practice*, p. 259.

102 'The claims of British spas: I. Cheltenham', *Lancet*, 4752 (26 September 1914), 804; 'II. Buxton', 4753 (3 October 1914), 862–3; 'III. Harrogate', *Lancet*, 4755 (17 October 1914), 957–8; 'IV. Droitwich ', *Lancet*, 4756 (24 October 1914), 1009; 'V. Bath', *Lancet*, 4758 (7 November 1914), 1,111–12; 'VI. Leamington, VII. Strathpeffer', *Lancet*, 4762 (5 December 1914), 1322–3; 'VIII. Woodhall Spa, IX. Peebles, X. XI. XII. Three Welsh spas', *Lancet*, 4768 (16 January 1915), 145–6.

103 'England in time of war, xxix. The English Spas – Buxton', *The Times* (6 March 1915, p. 11.

104 T. Pagan Lowe, 'Radium emanation in mineral waters. An address introductory to a discussion on the subject', B&CS, *PRSM*, 5 (1912), 29–48.

105 J. Hatton, *The radium waters of Bath* (Bath: n. d.) cited in Roger Rolls, *The hospital of the nation: the story of spa medicine and the mineral water hospital at Bath* (Bath: Bird, 1988), p. 117, n. 9.

106 Research Society of the Devonshire Hospital, *The natural thermal and chalybeate waters of Buxton: a brief account of their action and uses* (Buxton: Derbyshire Printing Co. Ltd., 1929), pp. 10 and 16.

107 Alois Strasser, 'The scientific foundations of hydrotherapeutics', *Archives Medical Hydrology* (*AMH*), 1.1 (May 1922), 16–22.
108 Fortescue Fox, *Principles and practice*, p. 95.
109 Bynum, *Science and the practice of medicine*, pp. 220–2.
110 'Discussion on the value of medical baths for invalid soldiers', B&CS, *PRSM*, 8 (1915), 47–66.
111 Committee of the council of the section of balneology and climatology of the RSM, *Notes on hydrological treatment for wounded and invalid soldiers and sailors with a list of the British spas and health resorts and of the disorders which they benefit* (London: Adlard and Son, 1915).
112 'Report of committee of council: "A combined physical treatment"', B&CS, *PRSM*, 9 (1916), 45–52.
113 'Physical treatment for disabled soldiers', *Lancet*, 4879 (3 March 1917), 348–9.
114 R. Fortescue Fox, 'Physical treatment: the case for autonomous clinics', *Lancet*, 6096 (June 29, 1940), 175–6; Cantor, 'Contradictions of specialisation' and Cantor, 'Aches of industry'. The campaign against rheumatism is considered in more detail in Chapter 6.
115 'Introductory notes', *AMH*, 1 (1922), p. 6.
116 'Three pioneers: an appreciation', *AMH*, 1 (1922), 39–41.
117 By May 1924 the Society had members from twenty-two countries. A series of articles described aspects of the organisation and scope of medical hydrology in member countries under the same title. 'The present state of medical hydrology in the countries represented', *AMH*, 1 (1922), 8–12; *AMH*, 1 (1923), 48–52; *AMH*, 1 (1923), 109-10; *AMH*, 1 (1924), 138–9.
118 Domenico Barduzzi, Alois Strasser, Jean Billard *et al.*, 'The teaching of medical hydrology', *AMH*, 1 (1923), 104–8.
119 'Report of the committee on the proposal to establish chairs of medical balneology, climatology and geography', *JB&C*, 2 (1898), 273–6.
120 'Valedictory', *JB&C*, 13 (1909), p. 204.

2

The development and marketing of specialist water cure resorts

Introduction

While the English spas have been accorded an influential role in shaping elite social life in the seventeenth and eighteenth centuries, their importance to nineteenth-century society and culture is perceived to have waned. As a result there has been little systematic investigation of their growth and development after 1815.[1] Spas are considered to be the pre-eminent example of a new category of town – the health and leisure resort – that emerged as part of a broad expansion in diverse types of urban settlement across Britain from the seventeenth century.[2] However the rapid expansion in the number of seaside towns after 1750, some of which – including Scarborough and Brighton – also had mineral springs, is held to have undermined the appeal of the inland centres. An influential theme in the historiography has been a shift in patterns of demand away from health-related activities towards leisure and holidays.[3] It has been argued that seaside resorts and associated cultures emphasising informality and recreation came to supplant the public, social life characteristic of spas in an earlier period. The development of more integrated transport infrastructure comprising coaching and railway networks along with changing patterns of leisure associated with new working patterns further consolidated this trend. Although Pimlott noted as long ago as 1947 that by the last quarter of the nineteenth century spas were better known 'for cures than for pleasure', this aspect of their history has not been examined in detail.[4] This chapter considers case studies of inland resorts with a reputation as 'watering places' in the nineteenth and twentieth centuries to investigate their pattern of development and the ways they were marketed to visitors. As demonstrated in Chapter 1 the ideas and practices associated with healing with water continued to be reexamined and refined from the mid-nineteenth to the mid-twentieth century. The argument presented here is that resorts offering water cures did not simply stagnate as visitors shifted allegiance to the seaside but came to be increasingly associated with the specialist expertise and more elaborate treatment facilities characteristic of the new trends in water cure – hydropathy, balneology and hydrotherapy and medical hydrology. In a period marked by rapid industrialisation and urbanisation the economic success of individual centres fluctuated but despite this some broader trends are apparent.

The English resorts operated in a competitive market for health and leisure services and there is a wealth of printed material charting their development and setting out their particular attractions. These guides offer a valuable source through which to investigate the marketing of these centres. The attraction of a particular place was based on a mix of environmental factors, principally their waters but also climate and topography, along with man-made facilities including bath houses, assembly rooms, walks, parks and woodlands. Although the unique features of each health resort were given emphasis there was also a growing homogeneity in the facilities and amenities expected by visitors. The ideal of *rus in urbe* providing all that was best of both urban and rural environments continued to be referred to as useful shorthand for the mix of desirable amenities expected although the constituents of this model shifted over time.[5] As the larger spas grew into sizeable towns and their economies diversified, the construction of designated resort areas ensured that sites for consumption and production were kept separate to a large degree. Eighteenth-century spas have been assessed as being at the top of the leisure hierarchy of resort towns.[6] The degree to which this was sustained into the nineteenth century is investigated and evidence presented to show that a small number of them continued to be marketed as elite health resorts. The term 'spa' came to be reserved for centres providing services for treatment and the preservation of health in contrast to pleasure resorts where more emphasis was given to the provision of leisure facilities and amenities for holiday makers. The concept of the health resort was further refined with the introduction of measurement and classification of climate along with assessment of its potential therapeutic effects.

The analysis draws on case studies of mineral water spas at Bath, Buxton, Cheltenham, Droitwich, Harrogate, Leamington and Woodhall – which all became members of the British Spa Federation (BSF) in the twentieth century – and the hydropathic resorts at Malvern, Ilkley and Matlock. Selected examples of smaller places actively marketed as water cure resorts at various times, including Ashby-de-la-Zouche and Tenbury Wells, are also referred to. Table 2.1, which shows population growth at selected English resorts over the course of the nineteenth century, indicates the complexity of their pattern of expansion. The discussion is framed around three broad periods; the period to 1840 marked by buoyant interest in the exploitation of mineral waters, the rise of hydropathic resorts between 1840 and 1870 and the emergence of an elite group of mineral water spas from 1870 onwards. In 1801 Bath was by far the largest of the English spas with a population of over 30,000, almost ten times greater than that of Cheltenham. However Bath's popularity as a spa was in decline as first Cheltenham and then Leamington became fashionable. Both towns were among the fastest growing urban centres of the period with expansion funded by entrepreneurs and speculative investors. Although their initial growth

Table 2.1: Population of selected English spas and hydropathic resorts.

Place	*1801*	*1841*	*1871*	*1901*
Spas				
Bath	33,196	53,196	52,557	52,773
Buxton	816	1,569	3,717	10,181
Cheltenham	3,076	31,411	41,923	52,858
Droitwich	933	2,832	3,538	4,154
Harrogate	1,984	4,785	6,843	29,885
Leamington	315	12,864	20,917	26,888
Tunbridge Wells	c.1,000	8,302	19,410	33,373
Woodhall Spa	145	307	326	c.1,000
Hydropathic resorts				
Ilkley	462	778	2,511	7,455
Malvern	819	2,768	7, 606	16,449
Matlock	2,354	3,782	3,834	7,798

Source: Phyllis Hembry, *British Spas from 1815* (Madison, NJ: Farleigh Dickinson University Press, 1997), Appendix 1, p. 254 and census enumerators' reports all years for Droitwich and Ilkley, 1901 only for Matlock.

was based on services associated with the development of spa facilities, their economies later diversified to provide a broader range of services to meet the needs of a residential population as well as a seasonal influx of visitors. Investors were attracted to exploit several undeveloped springs into new spas – including those at Woodhall and Droitwich in addition to expanding facilities at Buxton and Harrogate. The most notable feature of the period 1840 to 1870 was the growth of inland hydropathic resorts exploiting pure water and unspoiled rural landscapes at Malvern, Ilkley and Matlock. These centres sought to distinguish themselves from spas by both therapeutic approach and methods. Their common characteristics included a culture that emphasised active medical treatment in secluded and often rural environments and the construction of the new institutional form of the hydropathic establishment offering inpatient treatment. Growth of mineral water resorts was more uneven and by the end of the century only a small number of centres had developed reputations as medical spas. Entry to this elite group required significant investment to create specialist facilities with provision for the latest treatment techniques. New building projects at Woodhall and Droitwich transformed these resorts with the development of new bathing and social amenities and a rapid expansion in accommodation for visitors. This renaissance in English spas was part of a wider boom across Europe with local investment influenced by the consolidation of medical hydrology as a medical specialism. Several resorts where facilities were not upgraded – for example at Ashby or Tenbury Wells – did not fulfil the criteria to be considered as a medical spa although some opportunities for taking the waters continued to be available. These trends are indicative of growing specialisation among resort towns as their numbers expanded.

Case studies of individual resorts illustrate the importance of local conditions to their success or failure at particular times despite the broad social and cultural trends that led to strong demand for health and leisure services. Several factors identified by John Walton as important in shaping the development of seaside resorts are relevant to the analysis; in particular the variety of investors involved in development schemes, the pattern of landholding, the timing of improved transport infrastructure and increased involvement of urban authorities in the ownership of facilities and the planning of resorts.[7] Particular emphasis is given to exploring the variety of roles played by medical personnel to demonstrate their contribution to shaping resort development – a topic underplayed in the existing historiography. Endorsement of the therapeutic benefits of waters and climate were an important element in promotional literature. Some medical practitioners were also entrepreneurs who invested in individual business ventures related to water cures. Several played wider roles serving as members of local boards and participating in advisory committees established to shape investment and operational policies adopted by the new municipal authorities. In addition they worked as honorary physicians and undertook management roles at charitable institutions including the bathing hospitals for the poor that made an important contribution to building a culture of curing at these resorts.

Trends in the marketing of these centres are examined to explore how they were represented to potential consumers. As the number of resorts expanded competition encouraged differentiation and targeting of segmented markets including the chronically ill and those seeking to improve their health. Guidebooks distinguished between broad categories of 'pleasure' and 'health' resorts using the terms spa, climatic or seaside to highlight the dominant attributes of individual places. Spas and the new hydropathic resorts fell within the broader category of 'health resorts' that emphasised healthy, natural settings and good facilities for invalids. All watering places were advertised as healing environments offering a contrast to polluted, unhealthy urban and industrial places. Despite pressure towards homogeneity in facilities offered, each resort sought to develop a distinctive character and appeal. The English watering places offered a variety of micro-environments ranging from the subdued pleasures of genteel, urban Leamington and Cheltenham to the untamed natural backdrops of Malvern and Ilkley; from the sedative climate of Bath to the bracing altitudes of Buxton and Harrogate.

From the 1850s onwards new municipal authorities became key players in the coordination, management and promotion of medical and leisure bathing facilities.[8] By the twentieth century many town councils took the lead in producing promotional material too. In addition to publicity for individual centres, a variety of specialist publications aimed at the public also promoted the generic brand of the health resort. By the 1840s there were a number of guidebooks which provided comparative information on treatment methods and facilities at resorts in Britain, Europe and in some cases even further afield. These attest to the size and competitive nature of the growing international market in health resorts.

Railway companies also influenced the development of advertising material and from 1918 the BSF produced promotional material aimed at both medical practitioners and the public which emphasised the benefits of British rather than European spas. Under the BSF spas were marketed as elite resorts with well-developed medical facilities. In 1939 the International Society of Medical Hydrology (ISMH) recommended a definition of a 'spa' for discussion by its members that asserted their specialist expertise in therapeutics: 'A spa is a place where there occur mineral waters or natural deposits of medicinal value, where the local administration has provided suitable facilities for making use of these, and where the treatments are given under medical direction'.[9] Although spas were endorsed as places offering specialist medical expertise, the health benefits of a wider group of resorts was also promoted. The British Health Resorts Association (BHRA), formed in 1931, published an annual guide listing a mix of spa, seaside and inland resorts that was widely distributed among the medical profession and the general public as well as being promoted through annual conferences held at different venues around the country.[10] The BHRA was established by medical practitioners and focused on supplying information to both professional colleagues and the public. Their activities attest to the active role played by medical practitioners in resort promotion into the inter-war period.

The expansion of mineral spas 1800–40

Augustus Bozzi Granville's two-part guide to English spas, based on a tour undertaken in 1839 and 1840, provides a survey of their pattern of distribution and current state of development. His general conclusion that the popularity of the English spas was fading as 'mineral waters have, for the last thirty years, been growing out of fashion' was influenced by his assessment of the four largest English spas – Bath, Tunbridge Wells, Cheltenham and Leamington.[11] Although all four towns had experienced rapid population growth, shown in Table 2.1, Granville was not convinced that this was a useful measure of their success as spas, indeed rather to the contrary. In his opinion, Bath's 'vast increase and almost unparalleled success' as a town meant that despite having excellent facilities for recreation, invalids 'are unwilling to plunge, when looking after health and tranquillity, into the turmoil and confinement of a large city'.[12] Both Bath and Tunbridge Wells had flourished as spas since the seventeenth century, becoming part of the annual social calendar of the London-based elite. While the exploitation of mineral waters had been important in their early expansion, later growth relied on their attractions as residential towns or leisure resorts with broader-based appeal. Although financial returns from spa facilities had ceased to be central to their prosperity, the population and economy of both towns continued to grow. The social facilities, shopping and general disturbance and noise associated with this increased urbanisation posed a potential threat 'to the quiet enjoyment of the benefit of mineral water'.[13] Granville found the facilities at Bath in a poor condition and approved the Corporation's decision to make them available for a commercial rent in the hope that market pressures would prompt the owners to invest in desperately needed upgrading to their fabric and organisation.[14] At Tunbridge Wells he found the renowned chalybeate water was still available for 'bibbers' although not much in demand with part of the pump room leased to an upholsterer.[15] The process of rapid urban expansion and relative decline in economic importance of the mineral waters to the local economy that had taken over a century at Tunbridge Wells and Bath, had been compressed into a few decades at Cheltenham and, in Granville's opinion, already posed an incipient threat to Leamington's future as a spa.

Developments in the latter two resorts share several similarities. Cheltenham's population more than quadrupled from 3,076 in 1801 to over 12,388 in 1821 fuelled by speculative investment on the back of new spa developments.[16] By 1841 its population was over 30,000. Leamington's period of expansion came a short time later; still a small village of just over 500 in 1811 the population rose almost twelvefold to 6,269 in the twenty years to 1831 before doubling to 12,864 in the decade to 1841.[17] The initial growth of both towns was based on exploitation of mineral waters and associated service industries which tapped an established demand for a mix of health and leisure practices. The confidence of investors created highly competitive local economies which offered visitors a choice of facilities and services. In 1814 Jameson, a local doctor and investor in the Sherborne spa in Cheltenham produced a guide and map of the town which plotted eight springs that had been developed to provide facilities for taking the waters.[18] Early development had centred on the Old Well and the high street but the discovery of additional springs led to the laying out and construction of new urban areas. Between 1824 and 1830 Pearson Thompson developed the Montpellier and Landsdowne estates providing residential accommodation and services for visitors close to the remodelled Montpellier spa with its extensive grounds and gardens. Joseph Pitt speculated on a new district to the north of the existing town. The scale of his vision was impressive and planned to provide over 600 houses laid out in gracious squares and streets centred on a new pump room and gardens.[19] At Leamington early development occurred around the cluster of springs found in Mill Street and Clemens Street. The discovery of an additional water source on the other side of the river encouraged development of an upper town. Both Cheltenham and Leamington had several libraries and numerous hotels offering a choice of facilities for visitors. Visitor numbers rose and both spas continued to attract wealthy members of the aristocracy as well as a growing number from the middle classes. In 1825 an estimated 15,000 visited Cheltenham which was linked to the national transport network by some fifty-six coaching services.[20] By 1841 Granville assessed that despite falling out of favour as a spa, Cheltenham remained 'a town of great resort and importance' although he claimed that the 'very tip-top of society' were now going to Leamington.[21] At Leamington a winter season centred on hunting was fostered to try and maintain visitor numbers all year round and a strong education sector developed in both towns which provided some employment outside the short summer spa season. Resident populations became more important to their prosperity and by the late 1840s investment in spa facilities was no longer the draw for investors it had been. The Sherborne spa at Cheltenham was redeveloped at huge expense into the top-class Imperial Hotel.[22] The remaining centres struggled to remain financially viable with the Montpellier spa changing hands several times in the 1850s.[23] Despite reorganisation of the financial structure at the Pittville spa the company eventually passed into administration by the Court of Chancery due to failure to service mortgage debt.[24] In the 1890s Montpellier and Pittville were taken into municipal ownership but all the other spas in Cheltenham closed.[25] A similar pattern set in at Leamington; by 1860 the only bathing establishment still in business was the Royal Pump Rooms and this too was facing financial difficulties. The threat of sale and demolition led to a local campaign to purchase the building. Ownership was later transferred to the Board of Health and then to the new municipal authority which redeveloped the centre to provide a range of health and leisure services.

Figure 2.1 shows the parade and Pump Rooms at Leamington in 1857. The Greek style colonnade of the Pump Rooms, built in 1814, is

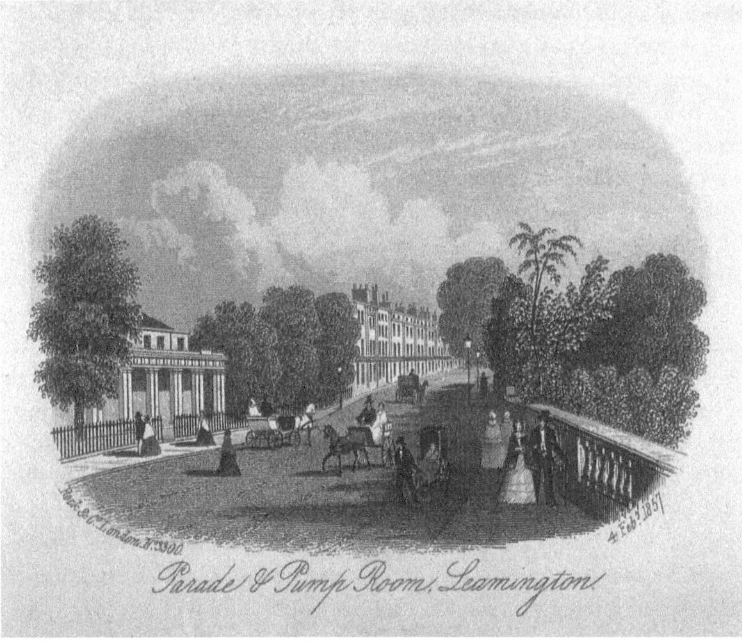

Figure 2.1: Parade and Pump Rooms, Leamington Spa, steel engraving, Rock and Co., 1857.

shown on the left of the image, adjacent to the spa gardens, beyond which is the parade marking the edge of the upper town. Opposite are the leafy fronds of the Jephson Gardens laid out as a formal park in 1846.[26] The Pump Rooms were strategically situated at the main river crossing between the old and new areas of town. By 1857 railway development had substantially altered the face of the old town leading to the destruction of several of the earlier hotels and bath houses. This view presents an image of ordered gentility – the lighting, architecture and wide paved streets show off the town's infrastructure. The streets are shown as not too busy with space for carriages to pass easily and wide pavements allowing visitors to enjoy the urban area on foot or perhaps in a bath chair. The Pump Rooms and open spaces of the riverside gardens, which led onto the extensive open spaces of Newbold Common, remained at the centre of the resort into the twentieth century offering visitors the opportunity to walk and relax in the open air after visiting the Pump Rooms. A variety of recreational opportunities including archery, croquet and lawn tennis were provided at various times as well as band concerts. Although dated 1857 this image is typical of many prints of spa facilities from the 1820s onwards. Most of these were of outdoor scenes in ordered urban settings showing fashionably dressed clientele – mainly adults – strolling or sitting in a garden area close to an impressive pump room.

The rapid growth of Cheltenham and Leamington occurred within a broader trend of increased urbanisation that accelerated in the first half of the nineteenth century. The 1851 census recorded over half the population living in urban areas with seaside resorts and watering places identified as the fastest growing type of town.[27] For Granville the bustle and noise of these busy places mitigated against their appeal for visitors who were also patients. Although the therapeutic effect of specific waters was at the heart of spa therapy, as 'mineral waters ... are medicines', the benefit of the spa cure was maximised through quiet living with too much society and nightlife inimical to the cure.[28] However, despite Granville's misgivings about the deleterious effects of rapid urbanisation on spa life, the expansion of Cheltenham and Leamington offered tantilising examples of the potential to profit from mineral waters. These proved sufficient to attract a number of investors to consider financing new business developments based on exploitation of mineral springs across the country.

Hembry records the 1830s as the decade with most investment activity in spa facilities in the nineteenth century with twenty new developments and improvements at a further fourteen existing centres.[29] One eager investor was Charles Hastings, a founder member of the Provincial Medical and Surgical Association (PMSA) who was based in Worcester but also practised in Malvern.[30] By 1835 Hastings had identified at least sixteen salt springs in the county, several of which he considered to have potential for commercial exploitation.[31] The Cradley spring close to Dudley and the Hampton waters near Evesham were similar in mineral content to waters at Cheltenham and Leamington, while the Droitwich brine water offered a potential alternative to sea-bathing in a location accessible to the expanding population of the industrial towns in the Birmingham area. Hastings urged enterprising folk to come forward to develop the Worcestershire springs, alluding in particular to the potential for harnessing 'the medium of that all-powerful engine, the press' in future promotional efforts.[32]

Malvern was the largest spa in Worcestershire with numerous springs scattered over the hills. Most were undeveloped but there were small pump rooms at Holy Well and St Ann's Well. Visitors enjoyed hill walks, pure spring water and a quiet rural life. The spa's reputation had developed from the mid-eighteenth century, promoted by the practice and writings of Dr John Wall and his son Martin.[33] By 1822 Great Malvern offered visitors a range of comfortable hotel accommodation, facilities for warm baths and recreational amenities for reading, music and billiards at the Royal Library.[34] The other springs Hastings mentioned were less developed; although at Hampton, near Evesham, a well, pump room and baths had been built in 1821 to serve a local clientele and at Cradley Lord Dudley had set up simple bathing facilities. Hastings listed a number of factors, including poor transport infrastructure and the problems of industrialisation, that he believed mitigated against the likelihood of Dudley's further expansion as a spa, arguing 'the remote situation, the vicinity of collieries, badness of roads, and all deficiency of convenience will, for ever, prevent this being a fashionable place of resort'.[35]

Hastings had first-hand experience of the difficulties of developing spa facilities close to an industrial centre, gleaned from his involvement with the brine springs at Droitwich. The town had been an established centre for salt production since Anglo-Saxon times exploiting the strongest natural brine springs in the country. During the eighteenth century production had increased due to improved evaporation processes, the ability to access stronger brine reservoirs and the extension of the canal network.[36] The therapeutic potential of bathing in the brine is reputed to have first been noticed during the cholera epidemic of 1832 and by 1835 local businessmen had formed a joint stock company to promote the building of brine baths.[37] The Droitwich Saline Baths, which opened the following year, were situated away from the main salt works but even so the spa could not escape the town's industrial environment particularly the atmospheric pollution caused by smoke from the many coal chimneys which merged with the clouds of steam from the numerous evaporation vats. The new baths were advertised locally through the *Berrows Worcester Journal* and attracted some 800 bathers in the first year. However this early success was not sustained and by 1843 visitors were down to 200.[38] Hastings was among investors tempted to expand the spa in the 1850s with a planned development outside the town but the scheme failed to attract sufficient financial backing.[39] Whatever the potential therapeutic applications of the mineral waters the industrial aspect of the town was not attractive to a visiting public in search of restoration and relaxation. Droitwich remained a small brine spa based around facilities built in the 1830s, overshadowed by the success of hydropathy at nearby Malvern.

The difficulties of developing a spa centre in an industrial area were also faced in Leicestershire where the eventual solution adopted was to transport the mineral water several miles from the spring to a more suitable site. In 1812 brine springs had been found near Moira in an area being developed for iron works and collieries by the estate of the Marquis of Hastings. First thoughts were to exploit the saline water for the production of soda or soap and it was only when this venture failed that a spa centre was considered. A small set of baths opened in 1815 which attracted a local clientele but the proximity of the coalmines remained an impediment to further expansion.[40] Instead a new site was developed at Ashby-de-la-Zouche some three miles away despite the significant investment in infrastructure needed to transport mineral water by canal and store it in large reservoirs. Although Ashby had no natural mineral spring it offered other potential attractions for visitors, principally a castle with romantic associations to Walter Scott's popular novel *Ivanhoe*. The several-acre site chosen for the new bath and hotel complex afforded fine views of the hilltop castle and along with pump rooms and gardens provided an appropriate infrastructure for health and leisure. The Ivanhoe Baths, named after the title of Scott's novel, opened in 1822 along with visitor accommodation. The Hastings' estate's interest in developing a leisure resort as part of a wider investment portfolio followed the example of the Devonshire estate which included the spa complex at Buxton and the seaside resort of Eastbourne.[41] The ability to successfully undertake these projects reflects the wider culture of technological invention and innovative solutions characteristic of the early industrial period. Mineral waters were natural resources to be exploited for profit as any other. The estate secured the necessary funding to purchase land and finance the design and construction of a new resort area in Ashby as part of a wider portfolio of agricultural and industrial enterprises. Potential profit depended on attracting the local gentry and middle classes to the new bathing and recreational facilities.

New technology was also integral to the discovery and exploitation of the mineral waters at Woodhall which were discovered in an abandoned coal mining shaft sunk by a contractor attracted to

Lincolnshire to work on drainage schemes for the fens. Thomas Hotchkin, the local landowner, opened a pump room and baths in 1838 and the Victoria Hotel the following year. The surrounding landscape was also remodelled by large-scale projects to drain the marshy ground and develop extensive fir plantations. Despite only basic facilities an estimated 2,000 people visited the spa in the 1840 season. Granville had high hopes of Woodhall's potential for success as the water there had the highest concentrations of iodine and bromine of any in Britain and were endorsed as useful for treating a variety of conditions including 'scrofula ... disordered digestion ... symptomatic rheumatism, rheumatic gout, and gout itself'.[42] An up-to-date chemical analysis of the water commissioned from a reputable expert was used in publicity aimed at visitors and potential investors. Granville also endorsed the nascent spa at Tenbury Wells on the borders of Herefordshire and Shropshire where the spring water contained high levels of iodine.[43] As at Woodhall, experts in medicine and chemical analysis were found to endorse the attributes of the water and a temporary bathing suite was hastily built to ensure the spa opened in 1841 to take advantage of the publicity generated from the publication of Granville's guide.

The established spas at Buxton and Harrogate also prospered in the early decades of the nineteenth century, their success based on growing demand from middle-class patrons from the surrounding industrial and manufacturing areas. As industry and commerce grew in the northern mill towns and the mushrooming metropolis of Manchester both towns attracted increasing numbers drawn from those benefiting from rising incomes from manufacturing and trade.[44] At Harrogate Granville noted that the 'clothiers from Leeds and cutlers from Sheffield' were attracted by reduced prices in the early summer with 'better company' following on later in the season.[45] Significant new investment in the 1830s centred on the saline and sulphur-impregnated waters found in the Bogs Field in Lower Harrogate. New facilities in Harrogate at the Grecian-style pump room at Gordon's Cheltenham saline water spa, the expanded Montpellier Spa and baths and the new sulphur spa at the Victoria Room and Baths provided visitors with alternatives to complement the established chalybeate wells on the Stray in High Harrogate. The *Harrogate Advertiser*, launched in 1836 and a new guide book published in 1838 helped to publicise the town to potential visitors.[46] Granville estimated there were 20,586 visitors for the 1840 season based on numbers from registers kept by the *Harrogate Advertiser*.[47]

In contrast to the multiple spa sites at Harrogate, ownership of the waters and spa complex at Buxton were in the hands of the Duke of Devonshire. Facilities were grouped around the Crescent constructed between 1780 and 1805 to provide accommodation and a large assembly room as well as mineral water baths.[48] By the 1840s the bathing complex provided separate provision for men and women that included hot baths and showers in addition to the traditional communal tepid bath. There was also a separate bath for the use of charity patients.[49] The Devonshire estate consolidated its hold over Buxton's development with the purchase of various inns, shops and houses and the construction of Hall Bank and the Square. Attention was also given to laying out the wider resort area. In 1818 the hillside in front of the Crescent was landscaped to provide a series of terraced walks known as 'the slopes'. By 1833 the town boasted a new music room and theatre to complement the Assembly Rooms and Promenade, all in the compact area close to the Crescent and baths.[50] Medical expertise was extensively used in publicity for the town. A popular treatise on local mineral waters written by Charles Scudamore, a London-based physician who practised from Buxton in the season, was published in 1820 and reprinted several times into the 1830s.[51] By 1849 daily connecting coach and rail services linked the town to Manchester, London and Derby and confidence in the town's future attracted private investment in hotels and accommodation.[52] In the 1850s the bathing complex was substantially enlarged to provide two suites, the natural baths using the tepid Buxton water and new hot baths. This latter provision was housed in a landmark new iron and glass structure designed by Joseph Paxton, architect of the Crystal Palace. An up-to-date description of the medical benefits of the Buxton water and the attractions of the town and surrounding area was provided in *A handbook to the peak of Derbyshire or Buxton*. Written by a local physician, W. H. Robertson, this remained the definitive guide to the Buxton waters into the 1880s.[53] The character of the spa was also influenced by the decision taken in 1856 to convert the circular stables into accommodation for patients receiving treatment from the Buxton Bath Charity.

Figure 2.2 shows The Crescent and new hot baths at Buxton in the early 1850s. The eighteenth-century Crescent is shown flanked by the hot baths on the right with the lower roofline of the natural baths at the far end linking the Crescent to the Old Hall Hotel. This ensemble of

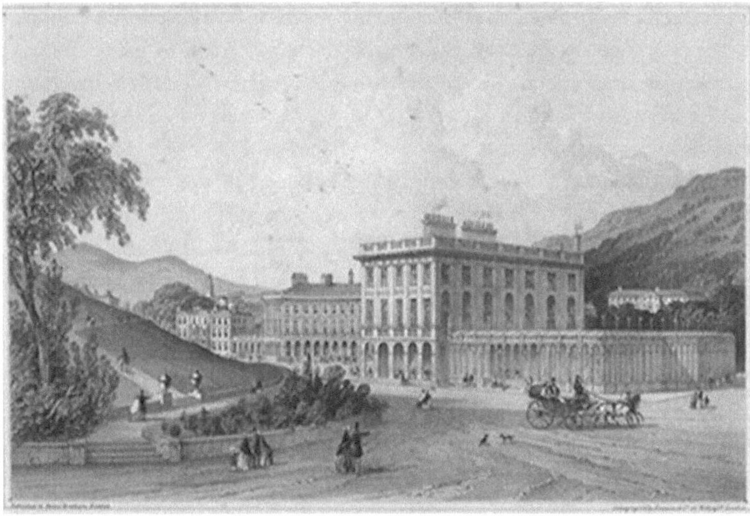

Figure 2.2: The Crescent, Buxton, and the new hot baths, lithograph c. 1853.

buildings formed a dedicated resort area close to the natural springs and away from the rest of the town developing at the top of the graduated hillside seen to the left of the image. The tower of St John's church, built in 1812, can be seen behind the Old Hall Hotel. Not visible is the small well house at the base of the slopes where mineral water was dispensed for drinking. The Crescent included several hotels, one of which had a large assembly room on an upper floor and was linked by covered walkways to the baths. In the background behind the hot baths are the stables, constructed at the same time as the Crescent, which were to be converted into hospital accommodation a few years later. The whole view is framed by the bowl of hills that surround the town, with some planting on the slopes on the right behind the stables softening the exposed hillsides of the upland areas. As visitor numbers grew in the nineteenth century the resort area expanded beyond the Old Hall Hotel with new gardens laid out alongside the River Wye. Several more large hotels and hydros were later constructed within walking distance of the Crescent complex. Separate baths for hospital patients were provided within the bathing suites until 1875 when a separate bath house was constructed to the rear of the Crescent, obviating the need for charity patients to enter the main resort precinct.

These case studies show that during the first half of the nineteenth century a range of investors continued to be attracted to invest in spa ventures in the expectation of a profitable return. While Cheltenham and Leamington sought to attract the wealthier classes, including the aristocracy, smaller centres targeted a more local clientele drawn from the growing middle class, many of them based in the new industrial towns and cities. Mineral waters were seen as natural resources to be exploited. Technological innovation in production and management techniques increased the ability to identify and access new springs or even to transport large quantities of water to a more suitable site as at Ashby. Among those investing in spas were aristocratic landowners including the Hastings estate at Ashby, the Devonshire family at Buxton and Lord Bertie Percy at Leamington as well as speculative builders such as Joseph Pitt and Pearson Thomson at Cheltenham. Some medical entrepreneurs including Davis at Tenbury, Jameson at Cheltenham and Charles Hastings at Droitwich took more active roles in a number of commercial ventures. The minimum requirements for the launch of a new spa were confirmation of the mineral content of its natural water by a competent chemist along with endorsement of its therapeutic value by a reputable medical expert. Basic facilities expected were a pump room, gardens, bathing suite and comfortable accommodation. However the wider environment was also crucial. Although Cheltenham and Leamington had developed into fashionable towns in the early decades of the nineteenth century, they were not immune to the widespread problems of rapid urbanisation including poor sanitary infrastructure and overcrowding. For some, including Granville, urban growth threatened their suitability as resorts for the chronically ill. The cholera epidemics of the 1830s and 1840s further increased awareness of the potential health hazards of crowded environments while industrial production methods and increasing use of coal meant that many districts were polluted and dirty. In this wider context, the concept of the spa as a place for relaxation and health became more closely associated with smaller, more rural environments. Part of the attraction of spas was the ideal of *rus in urbe*, the opportunity to access the pleasures of urban life such as theatres, libraries and luxury shops in a rural environment separate from the perils of production processes.[54] Developers at Droitwich clearly grappled with the problem of creating an attractive spa in an industrial town while at Ashby the problem was solved by transporting the water to a site deemed more suitable for treatment and recuperation. Granville endorsed two nascent spas in undeveloped small villages at Woodhall and Tenbury both free from associations with industrial production or urbanisation and yet accessible to the public due to improvements in transport infrastructure. Patterns of demand were shifting from an emphasis on the urban amenities of Bath, attractive in the pre-industrial era, towards smaller, more rural centres untainted by new industrial processes that offered respite from noisy towns and overcrowded streets. The growing appeal of quiet and healthy environments was given further impetus with the introduction of hydropathy which required pure water, fresh air and mountains.

Hydropathic resorts 1840–70

The rise of hydropathic centres in the middle decades of the nineteenth century demonstrates the trend towards specialisation as resort numbers grew. Within a few years of the introduction of the new system the reputations of Malvern and Ilkley had become closely associated with hydropathy although both resorts were already small spas. Malvern became known as the 'English Gräfenburg' while at Ilkley the magnificent Ben Rhydding hydropathic institution overshadowed the long-established cold water baths. Both resorts offered the perfect site for hydropathic practice; springs already well known for their purity, established centres linked to a transport infrastructure, accommodation and bathing facilities and access to open hills and unspoiled uplands where patrons could walk for hours in the fresh air. Malvern was within easy travelling distance of Cheltenham with its established transport routes from London and was also accessible from the Birmingham area, while Ilkley was close to the expanding industrial centres of Yorkshire and Lancashire. Hydropathy was introduced to Malvern by James Wilson and James Gully who both made personal fortunes from their practices there. Hamar Stansfield, a member of the Unitarian community in the Yorkshire area, who had been successfully treated by Preissnitz, was instrumental in setting up a consortium to finance the large and luxurious purpose-built hydropathic, Ben Rhydding, which opened at Ilkley in 1844.[55] The third specialist hydropathic resort to develop in England was at Matlock Bank, the creation of John Smedley, a wealthy retired mill owner, and his wife Caroline.[56] Their first small hydropathic enterprise, which opened in 1851, achieved remarkable commercial success which continued after their death. Smedley's at Matlock Bank became the largest of the English hydropathics and continued to operate until the 1950s when a compulsory purchase order was enforced. A sister company was established at Southport.

Preissnitz was an empiricist, who developed his extensive system over many years of practice but never committed the details to paper. Direct experience of his work was therefore essential to those wishing to acquire and demonstrate competency in the new treatment methods. James Wilson spent several months at Gräfenburg in 1841 where he met Richard Claridge and both men published books promoting hydropathy's benefits in 1842.[57] Knowledge about the system's approach and therapeutic techniques spread rapidly through these publications, Claridge's extensive lecture tours, discussion in the press and personal networks.[58] The reputation of Wilson and Gully attracted others wishing to learn about the system including William Macleod, who built up his skills and experience working at Malvern, before taking up a post at Ilkley in 1847. Within three years Wilson and Gully had each invested in purpose-built institutions with Wilson opening the Establishment in 1845 and Gully setting up Tudor House and Holyrood House. The town attracted other practitioners too and by the 1850s Edward Johnson, Leopold Stummes, Ralph Grindrod, Dr Marsden and Dr Ayerst all had separate practices in the town.[59] By the early 1860s it was claimed that the Malvern hydros treated some 6,000 patients a year.[60]

Figure 2.3 shows James Wilson's water cure establishment nestled at the foot of the Malvern Hills. A few scattered villas are shown along the wooded lower slopes but the upland areas are presented as open and untamed. Preissnitz's own institution at Gräfenburg was set in spectacular hills and fresh air and mountain walks were an important part of hydropathic treatment routines. Below the lowering hills sits the impressive purpose-built hydro, complete with smoking chimneys; asserting the substantial size of Wilson's enterprise. The institution is surrounded by a spacious, flat lawn laid out with paths with the central role of water symbolised by an ornate fountain in the foreground. Despite the scale of the hydro, emphasis is given to the natural surroundings providing a rural retreat in which patients would spend their time. The vision of nature untamed is offset by several substantial buildings providing the requisite amenities for genteel diversions; these include Great Malvern Priory, the library, Haywell Baths and the hotel where Wilson had first set up in practice. The decorously clad figures in

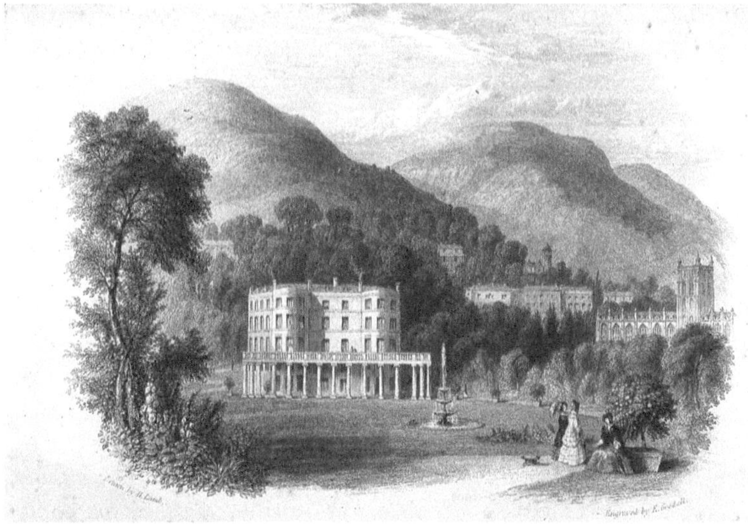

Figure 2.3: Dr Wilson's water cure establishment, Great Malvern, line engraving by E. Goodall after H. Lamb.

the foreground, along with the ancient priory, assert the moral tone of the resort. Several small centres developed around the hills first at Great Malvern and Holy Well with later expansion at West Malvern, Colwall and Malvern Link. The area retained a rural feel into the twentieth century despite a scattered population of over 16,000 by 1901.

Ilkley also proved to be a success with investors from Leeds opening a second hydro there in 1856.[61] This venture, Ilkley Wells House, provided luxurious and expensive facilities to match those of Ben Rhydding, but by the 1860s cheaper treatment was also available at more modest institutions linked to these two premier institutions. The smaller hydros offered board, lodgings, baths and medical attendance at two guineas a week, two-thirds of the price charged at the larger establishments although patients received medical attention from the same practitioners. Macleod provided medical supervision at Ben Rhydding and Craiglands while Dr Harrison oversaw treatment at Ilkley Wells House and Troutbeck.[62] Ilkley's development was further spurred by the arrival of the railway in 1865 with 'building mania' reported in the 1870s.[63] Another three hydros were built; Rockwood House, The Grove and Marlborough House, as well as additional visitor accommodation in hotels and apartments.[64]

In contrast to the early hydros in Malvern and Ikley which catered for the well-off, with charges of around £16 a month, John Smedley wished to provide hydropathy at a price affordable by 'the respectable rather than the affluent' and aimed to treat those from the lower middle classes.[65] His small enterprise at Matlock Bank, which opened in 1851 provided 'board, lodgings and treatment at 3s a day' or just one guinea a week.[66] By 1857 the enterprise had expanded to accommodate thirty and John and Caroline were treating around 600 patients a year.[67] The hydro was further enlarged in 1858 and by 1867 they were treating 2,000 patients annually.[68] Smedley always espoused a commitment to extending access to the water cure to a wider section of the population by offering basic accommodation and treatment at reasonable prices. However as the popularity of Matlock Bank grew and facilities there became more elaborate, prices rose and Smedley changed his policy to supporting selected ex-employees to set up in independent practice offering more modest accommodation with treatment still overseen by Smedley and his wife.[69] The *Derbyshire Post Office Directory* for 1864 listed eight hydros including Smedley's own and those of four of his ex-employees.[70] Census records, business directories and local guide books show that these practices were able not to only survive but to grow and develop as Matlock Bank became celebrated as a specialist hydropathic resort. Other investors attracted to the town developed high-class hydros with facilities to rival those at Smedley's. One of the most successful ventures was Rockfield Hydro later owned by the Goodwin family. After John Smedley's death in 1872 a private company re-launched his hydro under the brand name Smedley's.[71] The institution retained its formidable reputation as the premier specialist hydropathic in England, with medical practitioners employed to assess and oversee patients, until its premises were requisitioned at the outbreak of the Second World War.

Figure 2.4 shows a postcard of Smedley's hydropathic establishment in the 1920s, celebrating its substantial buildings and leisure amenities. The oldest part of the building, constructed in the 1850s, is to the right, but the hydro was extended several times on the same site to provide additional accommodation and luxurious public rooms in addition to substantial bathing facilities sited in the basement. Smedley's *Practical Hydropathy*, first published in 1858, included an exterior view of the

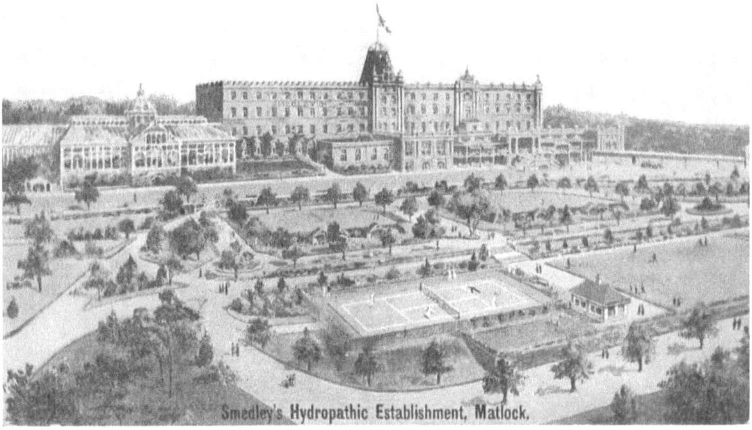

Figure 2.4: Smedley's Hydro, Matlock, postcard c. 1920s.

hydro which demonstrated its size and impact on the surrounding landscape. Other prints included in the volume showed the rural nature of Matlock – still a small hamlet – illustrating the picturesque views from the hydro over the Derwent valley towards Matlock Bath. Patients were depicted walking in the surrounding countryside or resting in the spacious lounges. This postcard disguises the steep slopes that characterise the town and the extent to which the hydro was by then hemmed in by other buildings, for example Rockfield Hydro higher up the hill is not shown. Instead Smedley's is portrayed standing alone within a rural setting with spacious, level grounds, well laid-out paths, bowling green and tennis court – a self-sufficient resort. The glazed winter gardens on the left, constructed after Smedley's death to extend indoor areas for recreation, were later used as a ballroom. In contrast to earlier images presenting respectable patients enjoying the salutary benefits of natural surroundings, this image gives little emphasis to the clientele who are reduced to indistinguishable figures engaged in popular sports and leisure activities, dwarfed by the hydro's buildings and facilities. Growing emphasis being given to physical activities and a continuing focus on integrating recreation into the hydropathic cure is discussed further in Chapter 5.

The success of the new hydropathic resorts in the 1840s was due to the popularity of the therapeutic approaches offered which were aimed at patients rather than leisure travellers and charged a premium price for the expertise and care they provided. Hydropathic institutions at these resorts offered an experience that was markedly distinct from that available at an established spa. Among the important differences were of course the new techniques and therapies but also closer supervision by a medical practitioner, even when the patient chose to live outside an inpatient institution, and an intensive daily regime that emphasised that the purpose of the patient's stay was to improve their health.[72] The reputations of individual hydropathists were crucial to their personal success but were also vital in launching and shaping these emerging resorts. John Smedley's wealth and personal influence guided development at Matlock Bank through his investment in his own and his ex-employees' hydros, but also through the force of his personality and status in the local community. His new home, Riber Castle, built on a rocky promontory, looked out over the valley and dominated the skyline from Matlock Bank. At Malvern James Gully took an active role in the development of the resort, serving as Chairman of the Town Commissioners between 1858 and 1866. He was also owner of a local newspaper, the *Malvern News*, invested in the Imperial – the town's premier luxury hotel – became a director of the Worcester and Wolverhampton Railway Company and supported the development of Malvern College as a public school for boys.[73]

James Nott considered that hydropathy was more or less a spent force in Malvern by the time Gully left the town in 1872. James Wilson had died in 1867 and several of the large hydropathics had been converted into schools or boarding houses.[74] Richard Metcalfe's assessment of the state of hydropathy in 1906 was also broadly pessimistic, describing it as a system that has 'not only stood still but lost much of the life that was formerly in it'.[75] Yet although he bemoans the lack of support for hydrotherapeutic methods by the general medical profession his detailed review indicates that the provision of treatment continued to be emphasised at almost thirty hydros in England. This is likely to be an underestimate as, for example, the institutions listed do not include Metcalfe's own hydro at Richmond. Table 2.2 lists the number of hydros Metcalfe noted as being primarily focused on the provision of treatment under medical supervision. Several hydros at Matlock and Ilkley were still flourishing. Smedley's had opened a sister venture at Southport where there were several other reputable institutions too, notably the Limes run by Samuel Kenworthy, as well as a hydropathic hospital for children.[76] The success of the first-class hydros at Buxton and Harrogate which complemented the opportunities for spa treatment using the mineral waters demonstrates the consolidation of balneology and hydrotherapeutic approaches at the major spas from the 1880s onwards. In his study of hydropathy in Scotland, Alastair Durie dates a change in culture at the hydros there to the 1870s, arguing that over the next decades they changed from 'being places where people went for a cure to being centres of rest and recreation' with emphasis shifting away from medical and towards social activities.[77] In contrast to Scotland therefore, it appears that treatment continued to be given emphasis at the premier English hydropathics into the early decades of the twentieth century.

Table 2.2: Hydros with medical supervision recommended by Metcalfe.

Resort	*Number of hydros*
Buxton	3
Harrogate	4
Ilkley	3
Malvern	1
Matlock	12
Southport	4
Total	27

Source: Richard Metcalfe, *The rise and progress of hydropathy in England and Scotland* (London: Simpkin, Marshall, Hamilton, Kent, 1906), pp. 91, 108, 119, 209, 213–14, 225.

The specialist hydros could cater for leisure visitors too as their facilities were designed to provide tailored regimes ranging from the intensively therapeutic to the recreational. However visitors were paying a premium for the availability of hydropathic treatment. A rare surviving bill for a one-week stay at Smedley's for Mr and Mrs Haworth in September 1878 shows they were charged a basic rate of £6 17s for board, lodging and medical attendance for two. They paid an additional one guinea for a special attendant and 6 shillings for galvanism.[78] T. D.

Luke's guide published in 1919 notes that specialist hydros were still operating in all the resorts listed by Metcalfe. Luke describes Matlock Bank as a resort specialising in hydropathy with between thirty and forty hydros in the town 'varying in size, catering for all classes of visitors'. Smedley's was singled out as an institution 'where treatment is extensively carried out, the proportion of invalids varies from 50 to 70 per cent'.[79]

The consolidation of the medical spa 1870–1914

Between 1870 and 1914 the major English spas also consolidated their reputation for medical expertise and treatment facilities. The formation of the Society of Balneology and Climatology (SB&C) discussed in Chapter 1 demonstrates the growing reputation of water therapeutics within the orthodox medical profession and the elite resorts became showcases for their skills. Rising incomes among the middle and professional classes and further expansion of the railway infrastructure contributed to a period of renewed prosperity for the English spas. Buxton expanded rapidly through continuing patronage from the Devonshire estate while Harrogate flourished under the management of the municipal authority which had begun to purchase the privately owned wells from the 1840s. At Droitwich, land ownership was increasingly consolidated in the hands of John Corbett, owner of the local salt works. He led the reshaping of this industrial town into an elite spa with first-class bathing facilities and accommodation. Rapid development at Woodhall was financed by an investment syndicate to create a purpose-built garden spa with baths, accommodation and shopping facilities. The resurgence of interest in spas by the medical profession and the public was also sufficient to encourage the municipal authorities to update facilities at Bath, Leamington and Cheltenham in the last decades of the nineteenth century.

Buxton's popularity as a spa expanded substantially in the second half of the nineteenth century, its reputation as a genteel resort for the middle and upper classes finally endorsed by a visit from King Edward VII and Queen Alexandra in 1905.[80] In 1863 both the London North Western and the Midland Railway Companies opened stations in the town further stimulating growth in visitor numbers. By 1876 four trains a day made the journey from London to Buxton in five to six hours, Manchester was within an hour and Derby could be reached in under two.[81] Among several new luxury hotels to open were the Railway and the Lee Wood in 1864 and the Palace in 1868. Measures were taken to develop the infrastructure of the town with a series of projects initiated by the Local Board to improve streets and sewers and introduce bylaws to regulate bath chairs and carriages.[82] The baths continued to be popular, bringing the Devonshire estate a good return that was sufficient to encourage further improvements in 1886.[83] Another prestigious project was the remodelling of the hospital building to construct a huge dome to cover the earlier open circus of the stables. The project, made possible by funds secured from the Cotton Districts Convalescent Fund (CDCF), increased bed numbers to 300 – making the DRH the largest of the English mineral water hospitals. The grand opening took place in 1881.[84] Parks and gardens were also improved, most notably the Pavilion Gardens laid out on land adjacent to the River Wye in 1871. These included a glass and iron winter garden, bandstand, paved terrace and grassy walks. By 1876 a concert hall and skating rink were also under construction.[85]

Buxton's 'indifferent' waters which were low in minerals and its established reputation for therapeutic bathing meant that the resort was ideally suited to amalgamate the new hydrotherapeutic approaches into established spa practice. James Shore, a protégé of John Smedley, opened Malvern House Hydro for forty patients in 1865.[86] Later renamed the Buxton House Hydro, this grew to accommodate 300 guests by 1906 with medical supervision provided on site. Samuel Hyde, who was instrumental in setting up the B&CS, was another entrepreneur who invested in hydropathy. His Peak Hydro expanded to accommodate 200 patients with further capacity at the Haddon Hall Hydro.[87] The Buxton hydropathics offered a combination of luxurious accommodation and treatment under medical supervision, providing an alternative to the Buxton Baths which continued to provide the only access to the natural tepid spring water.

At Harrogate, development was spearheaded by the new public authorities and from around 1868 'a great burst of municipal enterprise' redeveloped the urban area with projects including improvements to sewage works, the building of a market and the purchase of the Crescent estate and Victoria Baths in the lower part of the town. Almost £20,000 was spent on the new Victoria Baths project which included opening up new wells to ensure a sufficient supply of mineral water.[88] This large-scale urban development brought a real change to the feel of the town as the two separate areas of High and Low Harrogate merged and finally lost their raw rural look. The growing wealth of Lancashire and the West Riding as well as improved rail links to expanding regional centres, including Leeds and Bradford, contributed to Harrogate's increased popularity as a resort town.[89] Private investment in specialist facilities continued through the development of new hotels and hydropathic companies. The Swan Hotel operated by the Harrogate Hydropathic Company opened in 1878, the Connaught and Imperial in the 1880s and the Cairn and Harlow Manor in the 1890s.[90]

Figure 2.5 shows a view across Harrogate's Valley Gardens towards the Bath Hospital which was enlarged in 1889 in Scottish baronial style. The gardens were remodelled from 1886 from the 'Bogs field', the site of Harrogate's numerous sulphur water springs. Water was now piped from the springs to the Victoria Baths and Old Sulphur Well which were both close by. The view shows the ordered parkland that had been created, providing a place for patrons to walk and sit after drinking at the Sulphur or Magnesia wells. The gardens were one of several extensive open spaces created in Harrogate, laid out with flower beds and streams. Although the lower area of the park, shown here, was laid out as gardens, it extended to an area of pine woods and out onto Harlow Moor, offering easy access to long walks. In 1893 the compulsory purchase of the Stray which had become a centre for noisy and unruly behaviour, further regulated access to and use of urban spaces in the genteel resort.[91] Confidence was such that the corporation embarked on substantial investment in new bathing provision at the Royal Baths intended to place Harrogate in the first rank of European spas, to rival Baden-Baden and Aix-les-Bains. These opened in 1897. The extensive municipal investment in spa enterprises proved to be commercially viable; Jennings records a small surplus by 1913–14 despite significant interest payments.[92] This image was included in the lavishly illustrated guide produced by Harrogate Corporation from 1898 and is one of a series of views depicting a respectable clientele enjoying the specially designed open spaces for recreation within the growing town.

The last quarter of the nineteenth century saw the transformation of Droitwich from an industrial salt town into a spa with a Europe-wide reputation for its strong brine waters. This was largely due to the investment and vision of John Corbett, who made his fortune out of salt before determining to establish the town as an elite health resort. Corbett began to invest in accommodation to cater for the increasing

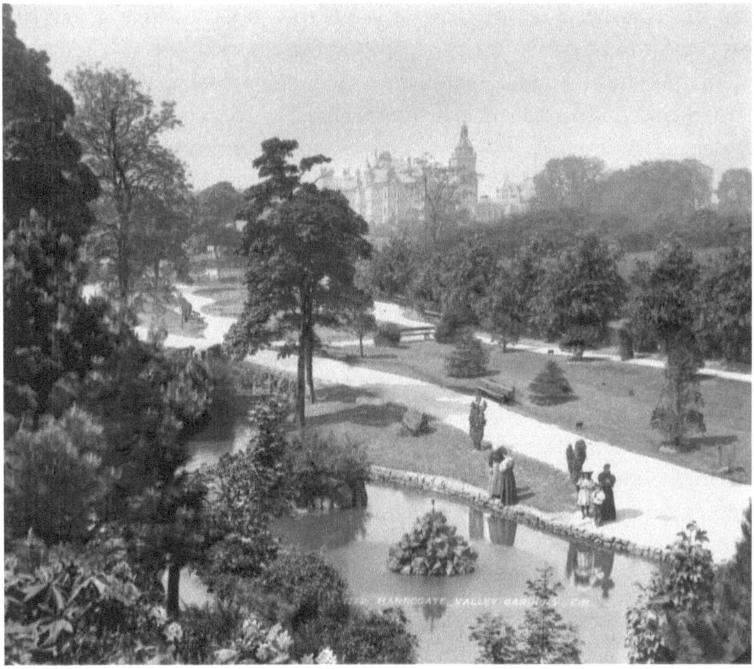

Figure 2.5: Valley Gardens and Bath Hospital, Harrogate.

number of visitors to the refurbished Royal Baths which now provided a full range of hydropathic treatments and a Turkish Bath as well as three classes of brine baths.[93] William Bainbrigge, the lessee, had published a new book setting out the therapeutic benefits of the brine in 1871.[94] In 1887 Corbett began to build the St Andrews Baths to provide elegant new first- and second-class facilities for a wealthy clientele and two years later acquired the Royal Baths and converted them into second-class baths offering treatment at a cheaper price. Among his other developments were luxurious accommodation at the Worcestershire Brine Baths Hotel which opened in 1891 and the redevelopment of the Royal Hotel in 1900.[95] Corbett's initiatives coincided with renewed interest in mineral waters by the medical profession. Although the top-end hotels provided luxurious accommodation and amenities for newly popular sports including tennis and golf, the brine baths remained the resort's key attraction. The medical reputation of the spa was further enhanced by the establishment of the St John's Brine Bath Hospital in

1881. The transfer of salt production out of town was an essential part of this project to refashion the town around the spa complex.

In 1885 a business syndicate, including several members of Parliament, developed an ambitious plan for the construction of a model resort town at Woodhall Spa capable of attracting aristocratic visitors from Britain and abroad. The spa's bromo-iodine waters which were unique in Britain were similar to those at Kreuznach, a popular German spa with a particular reputation for effective treatment of women's diseases.[96] Publicity for the venture promoted Woodhall as 'the English Kreuznach' thus emphasising its attractions to female patients, an important group of consumers. The syndicate paid a close eye to publicity in establishing the credentials of the new spa. The architect selected for the redevelopment had been responsible for the recently refurbished New Massage Baths at Bath. The decision to promote a new charitable hospital 'national in its character, open to all comers on the presentation of a subscriber's order' was a further strategy to assert the medical credentials of the spa.[97] The planned layout of the wider resort was influenced by the design concept of the garden city and comprised an integrated scheme for the high street that incorporated hotels, inns, shops and lodging houses. Fundamental to the success of the scheme was the development of better rail links, particularly with London.[98] The local newspaper was of course enthusiastic in its claims for the new resort noting the upper classes were 'beginning to realise that when in search of health they can obtain what they need in Lincolnshire and need not journey to the land of saurkraut and Teutonic rapacity'.[99] The syndicate achieved some success; the number of visitors arriving by rail are reported to have risen from less than 16,000 before the development to 47,700 in 1889.[100] In the two decades following its launch in 1888 Woodhall prospered as a small health resort attracting members of the social elite. The spa attraced a number of German visitors with the local newspaper reporting that those from Kreuznach, 'speak of Woodhall Spa as a serious rival to their institution'.[101] A London architect, Richard Adolphus Came was employed on plans to extend the village with shops, guesthouses and a tall water tower in German medieval style. The Royal Hotel which opened in 1897 provided a glazed winter garden and became an alternative to the Victoria Hotel close to the spa baths. Woodhall later benefited from the patronage of Baroness Von Eckhardstein, the heiress to Sir Blundell Maple's fortune made through furniture stores, who visited the resort from the 1900s. Following her divorce and remarriage to Archibald Weigall, the couple settled at Petwood House which had grounds adjoining the spa complex. They entertained lavishly and had many society friends, including Princess Alexandra, who became patroness of the local hospital.[102] By 1912 the bath complex included facilities for what had by now become standard treatments at all the elite spa resorts; the Aix and Vichy systems of massage douche and a range of electric baths.[103] The approach taken by the syndicate at Woodhall demonstrates contemporary perceptions of what constituted an elite spa; at the heart of the enterprise lay medical endorsement of the mineral waters and specialist personnel to administer an increasing number of complex treatments. The relative remoteness of the small spa and the limited accommodation available served to maintain its exclusivity.

The resurgence of interest in spa treatments was sufficient to encourage investment at Leamington, Bath and Cheltenham in the final decades of the nineteenth century. At Leamington the Pump Rooms, which had been saved from closure in the 1860s by being taken into public control, had been remodelled to provide a range of facilities aimed at both residents and visitors. These included medical baths, slipper baths, a Turkish bath and swimming pool.[104] The importance of medical bathing to the enterprise and to the town was shown by the establishment of a Medical Advisory Committee composed of a number of local practitioners who advised the municipal authority on facilities and treatments. The building was extensively refurbished in 1887 to provide facilities for a full range of hydropathic treatments in 'warm, medicated, douche and shower baths all being provided with large and convenient dressing rooms, fitted up in a superior style'.[105] Medical practitioners played an important role in publicity and policy, for example Eardley-Wilmott, also a member of the municipal council, authored a new guide to the Leamington waters and presented a paper to the annual meeting of the BMA in July 1890.[106]

Enthusiasm for public investment to retain viable spa facilities in Cheltenham was much more muted. The majority of the private spa facilities had closed by the 1870s and although a new municipal authority was created in 1876 it was not until the early 1890s that it took the only remaining pump rooms, those at Pittville and Montpellier, into public ownership. While these provided grand assembly rooms suitable for drinking the water there was no provision for medical bathing in the town and the costs and potential benefits of investing in new facilities were hotly debated. A significant lobby emerged who argued that even if the spa ran at a loss the spin-off benefits to the town's economy outweighed these considerations. '… probably there is not a health resort in the world in which the attractions provided by the Municipality pay for themselves. They are not intended to pay as trading concerns; they are designed to bring visitors who will spend money in the town and so maintain it in prosperity.'[107] By 1901 the argument for the value of image and reputation was won. Over the next five years the Corporation developed facilities for drinking the mineral waters in the new Central Spa at the Town Hall to complement those at Pittville and upgraded the bathing complex at Montpellier.[108] The decision taken to invest was clearly influenced by the urgent need to upgrade infrastructure if the town was to maintain its association with the elite group of spas. Despite the composition of its mineral waters, which were closer to those at Carlsbad and Vichy than those at any other British spa, the facilities were manifestly insufficient to meet the growing consensus of what constituted a medical spa. The publication of *Climates and baths of Great Britain* in 1895 had also served to underscore Cheltenham's relative decline compared to other resorts. Archibald Garrod opened his remarks with the comment that 'the present is not by any means a favourable time for reporting upon Cheltenham as a mineral water resort' and was unable to call on any up-to-date comments on the therapeutic value of the mineral waters.[109] In contrast the first publication by the BSF in 1918 was able to commend the medical baths which provided brine baths and facilities for the Aix douche in addition to other hydropathic baths and to state that 'Cheltenham is once again restored to her former position as a British Spa.'[110]

Marketing the health resorts

In the second half of the nineteenth century the existence of natural mineral or thermal waters became fundamental to designation as a spa but a wider group of resorts were classified as health resorts on the basis of criteria including climate and facilities available for therapeutic bathing. The establishment of the BSF led to development of a strategy to delineate the elite spas from other resorts. The BSF had been formed soon after the outbreak of the First World War in order to promote home resorts to the British population as it was realised that the war offered a 'unique opportunity' when 'all things German are loathsome to British people' to put the 'legitimate claims' of the British resorts forward. Although the particular attributes of each resort were described, promotional material also stressed that together the British spas offered 'the health seeker all those advantages it was once fondly thought were obtainable only at a foreign Spa, together with others which no enemy Spa has ever possessed'.[111] Their common distinctive characteristic was Britain's maritime climate, so different from that on the Continent, being relatively cool in summer and mild in winter. In general this meant that the British spas were more tonic than the European ones although this could be modified as necessary by careful selection of resort and time of year for treatment. The guide made it clear that spas were the premier centres for treatment and that the BSF would work to raise standards through a process of validation of medical expertise and facilities. However there were many other inland and seaside towns that also fell within the category of health resort all of which were enthusiastically endorsed. 'The Home Spas may be looked upon as an inner circle of inland health resorts – varying in altitude, temperature, sedative or stimulant air, and so on. Around the circle of Spas is a much wider circle of moorland and marine health resorts, with every possible aspect and exposure, some in the fine rarified air of the north, some on the bracing easterly shores, some in the soothing west, some on the sunny southern coasts'.[112]

The increasing emphasis given to climate is illustrated by the rebranding of Malvern as a climatic resort as its reputation as a centre for hydropathy began to fade.[113] The association of local environmental conditions with the relative healthiness or unhealthiness of specific places dates to the classical foundations of the western medical tradition, notably Hippocrates' *Airs, waters and places*. From the late eighteenth century onwards the mapping of the global distribution of diseases was recorded on a more systematic basis under the aegis of the new discipline of medical geography.[114] From the mid-nineteenth century the collection of mortality data and public health reports presenting mortality and morbidity statistics facilitated comparison of the relative healthiness of places and these were soon incorporated into profiles for resorts along with information on geology and meteorology. By the 1880s specific emphasis was also given to commenting on local solutions to the contemporary problems of sanitation and air pollution.[115] Climate continued to be used to underpin discussion of the healthy attributes of resorts into the twentieth century; detailed discussion of statistics on rainfall, temperature, hours of sunshine and the direction of the prevailing wind became a standard part of the promotional literature used to classify particular climates and make the case for their suitability for specific groups of patients. The benefits of the warmer southern European and north African climates for invalids suffering from bronchial complaints was well established. Throughout the nineteenth century many patients suffering from tuberculosis travelled abroad seeking to alleviate their condition or mitigate the worst effects of the disease.[116] From the 1860s the potential to use climate in active treatment was also receiving more attention. Use of the high-altitude Alpine resorts such as Davos Platz to treat the early stages of tuberculosis was discussed among the British medical profession.[117] Ralph Grindrod engaged directly with this debate, making the case that Malvern, despite an altitude of between 750 to 900 feet above sea level, far lower than the high altitudes of the Alpine resorts, offered a suitable micro-climate for the treatment of many bronchial afflictions, asserting the main reason for this to be the dry, pure air. Effective treatment nevertheless necessitated a properly ordered hygienic regimen that included diet, exercise and suitable accommodation as well as medical expertise. Grindrod was also interested in the idea that therapeutic micro-environments could be helpful and his hydro, Townshend House, included a purpose-built room where patients could sit and breathe compressed air.[118]

From the last quarter of the nineteenth century climatology provided an analytical framework used to compare and measure distinctions between resorts using the principal factors identified as shaping the climate of a particular place – latitude, altitude, proximity to the sea, geology and the prevailing winds. Climate was believed to affect the whole metabolism and was described according to its relative stimulating effects on the body; tonic or bracing climates were contrasted with sedative or relaxing ones.[119] A tonic climate was one with 'plenty of sunshine, little humidity, and a temperature which is comparatively cool but with a fair daily range'. In contrast a sedative climate was more humid with a smaller temperature range, higher rainfall and less sun. The therapeutic effects of a tonic resort were to stimulate 'the vigour of the body, thus enabling it to combat or overcome the onslaught of disease' while sedative resorts were suited to more delicate individuals, including the very young and old.[120] In contrast to Britain, inland spas and mountain centres became the premier health resorts across Europe while the seaside remained relatively underdeveloped until the 1920s.[121]

Herman Weber noted that the chief feature distinguishing the climate of the British Isles was its equable nature. Extremes of heat or cold were rare with noticeably cooler summers and warmer winters than much of Europe due to the moderating influence of the Gulf Stream. The daily range of temperature was also less than at the European inland areas. Although the rainfall was not necessarily higher it was more equally spread across the year contributing to a reputation for fog and rainy days. In general, Weber considered the British climate to be 'tonic' and although 'somewhat dull and not exhilarating' nevertheless beneficial for those in generally good physical condition as it encouraged 'health and longevity'. The winds and the frequent changes in temperature kept the various organs in good working order and developed their 'power of adaptation and resistance'.[122] In 1939 Bonacina described the country's climate as characterised by the 'almost regular alternation of tonic and sedative types of weather, or what might be described as a happy blend of bracing and relaxing elements'.[123] The extensive comparative statistics detailing meteorological information demonstrated significant regional variations in climate with the eastern and south-eastern seaside resorts drier and colder, and therefore more bracing, than those in the south-west. Local factors also influenced tonicity especially the degree of exposure to the elements and the availability of shelter from wind and rain. As these concepts developed they were widely incorporated into the marketing literature for the British health resorts as a group as well as guides to individual towns.

Guide books to individual spas and resorts proliferated from the eighteenth century onwards. During the nineteenth century these were supplemented by a range of new media including newspapers, hydropathic manuals, accounts by patients, gazeteers to British and European resorts, specialist magazines and railway advertising. The rapid growth in the popularity of hydropathy was encouraged by extensive media coverage in the lay and medical periodical press and by a number of influential monographs produced by both patients and practitioners. Most authors sought to take advantage of the publicity potential of hydropathy's controversial reputation by clearly aligning themselves as either supporters or opponents of the new system. While hydropathic manuals written by practitioners were part of well-established genres of advice literature or medical treatises, the periodicals were a new medium that flourished from the early decades of the nineteenth century. The first edition of the satirical magazine *Punch* was published in 1841, the year before hydropathy was introduced to Britain and the system's novel techniques and accoutrements proved to be a rich source for amusing illustrations and satirical comment in that magazine and other publications. Figure 2.6, a cartoon from *The water cure* published in 1880, is typical of this genre. The image alludes to the early decades of hydropathy, showing a naked, shivering patient taking a bath in his simply furnished bedroom. The lack of plumbing is apparent with water applied from a watering can held aloft by a fit-looking bath attendant. The vulnerable patient, sitting alone and exposed in his sitz bath, is at the mercy of this practitioner, and dutifully endures the gush of cold water intended to invigorate his system. The 'rules' posted on the wall suggest that once the patient has entered the world of the hydropathic institution he forgoes the right to make his own decisions and instead is forced to submit to the regime laid out for him in the hope of improving his health and vigour. The piece assumes the reader has some familiarity

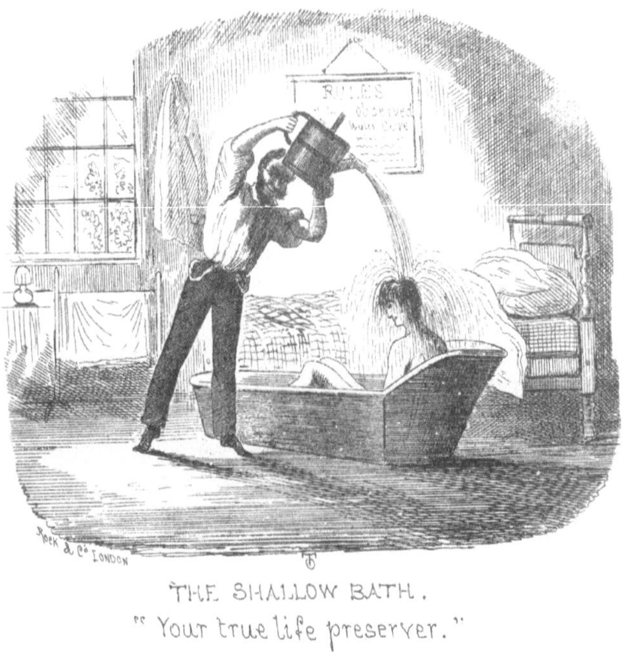

Figure 2.6: 'The shallow bath' from *The water cure* (Rock & Co., London, c. 1880).

with the routines and techniques of the hydropathic system in order to appreciate the joke.

The public dispute over hydropathy in the medical press, discussed in Chapter 1, encouraged patients to publish works describing their experiences and proclaiming the benefits and the safety of the system. These included several first-hand accounts authored by members of the London-based literary set. The earliest such account was *Confessions of a water patient* by the popular author Edward Bulwer Lytton, first published in the form of an extended letter in Henry Colburn's *New Monthly Magazine* in 1845 but later reprinted several times. Bulwer Lytton, who suffered from poor health and was a regular spa-goer, claimed that he achieved positive health as a result of Wilson's 'diligent, patient, care'. Commenting directly on the dispute between hydropathists and the orthodox profession he commented 'you cannot expect a doctor of drugs to say other than that doctors of water are but quacks', implying it was for patients to exercise their own judgement based on evidence available to them.[124] Richard Lane, a popular lithographer who published an illustrated diary of a month spent at Malvern with his son in 1845, noted his intention to 'establish a sort of peaceable agitation, a gentle movement against that hostility to the water'.[125] Further publications followed throughout the 1850s and 1860s, several of which were also by authors well connected to the London-based publishing world.[126] What readers made of these accounts remains conjectural but evidence of reprinting suggests they were popular. Whatever the protestations of the authors, they were written and published with an eye for profit, aimed at the middle-class readers of the competitive periodical market. Although they traded on the new and exotic elements of hydropathy, balancing fear and excitement, they were for the most part an endorsement of the new system, providing examples of personal experience and heartfelt recommendation. At the very least they made information about the new system available to a wider audience of potential patients. The popularity of such testimonials continued into the 1860s, well after the initial controversy over hydropathy had faded. In 1852 Macleod's methods were described anonymously in *Memorials from Ben Rhydding* while the Ilkley Wells Hydro was given positive publicity in works by Reverend Thomson and Captain Lukis.[127] Foster's journal describing life at Smedley's hydro published in 1864 is discussed in more detail in Chapter 4.[128] The Reverend Paxton Hood wrote an account of treatment at Townshend House in Malvern in the 1860s.[129]

These personal accounts tend to a similar pattern, comprising a narrative of breakdown in health followed by hard-won improvement through dedicated application by both therapist and patient, interspersed with vignettes of daily routine and social life at the hydros. The fact that they continued to be published over a period of some twenty years attests to ongoing interest in hydropathy and to the wider popularity of invalid narratives in the Victorian period.[130] Analysis of selected accounts is integrated into discussion of the cultures of the water cure in Chapter 4.

Another new source of information for the potential patient was the increasing number of published guides providing comparative information on resorts. Although these were sometimes directed at medical practitioners the mix of theoretical explanation, discussion of treatment options and general information on facilities and practical details for travellers meant these were of wider interest too. Granville's relatively comprehensive two volumes on British watering places aimed to be of interest and use to visitors in selecting a resort. A direct competitor to Granville was a shorter guide by Edwin Lee, also published in 1841 but revised and updated in 1854.[131] The next substantial compendium of British spas was John Macpherson's *Our baths and wells: the mineral waters of the British Islands*, published in 1871.[132] This was followed in 1875 by Hermann Weber's translation of Braun's work on European spas to which Weber added comments on British resorts.[133] In contrast to Granville these guides were primarily intended for medical practitioners although they may also have been of interest to a general reader with an eye for detail. The Ord and Garrod publication in 1895, prepared under the auspices of the Medical and Surgical Society, was again primarily intended for general medical practitioners as a guide to how to prescribe spa treatment for their patients.[134] The volume edited by Neville Wood in 1912 was prepared as an update to the 1895 work and was compiled with the help of an advisory committee of the B&CS section of the RSM.[135] In contrast T. D. Luke addressed his 1919 guide to a more general audience dedicating it 'To those who enjoy poor health, to those who are sick, to those who are well and wish to keep so'.[136] Weber and Parkes Weber's magisterial compendium on European spas was prepared for the medical profession; first published in 1889 it was substantially revised and enlarged in 1907.[137] Burney Yeo's publications on health resorts in 1882 and 1904 were targeted at both the profession and the general reader.[138] All these publications were essentially reference works, intended to be used as a guide to the conditions treated at the various spas, the main therapies used and the facilities available. As the number of resorts and research papers on balneology and climatology proliferated from the third quarter of the nineteenth century these compendium volumes tended to grow larger and larger. Despite this they quickly became outdated due to the frequent upgrading of facilities at resorts. A further limitation, from the publicity angle, was that professional protocol meant that works aimed at the medical profession could not include direct advertising for individual centres or businesses.

The recognition that resorts would benefit from more general publicity and advertising led to a variety of new publishing initiatives from the 1880s including commercial periodicals aimed at the public, the development of specialist medical journals and sustained efforts to publicise the use of resorts to the wider medical profession. The *Journal of British and Foreign Health Resorts* (*JBFHR*) published between 1890 and 1894 aimed at a readership that included consumers, medical practitioners and municipal authorities, all seen as essential to the development of a successful spa industry. The journal's subtitle '*A Monthly Record of Baths, Climate, Spa News and Spa Gossip*', reflected the broad scope covered in articles which were intended both to inform the reader and to publicise resorts. Each issue included a detailed article on a featured health resort along with anonymous reviews, details of royal visits to spas, the opening of new facilities as well as articles on baths, massage and other forms of treatment available. An article on Bath in February 1890 updated readers on the excavations of the Roman baths then under way which reinforced the longevity of the city's reputation as spa and provided a detailed description of the facilities at the New Massage Baths which had been extensively refurbished over a period of two years to provide facilities for the Aix douche and other hydrotherapeutic treatments. It continued with a call to the Corporation for further investment to maintain Bath's competitive edge against European rivals before providing a summary of conditions that could benefit from a course of the waters.[139] Although choosing to remain anonymous in the pages of the publication, the founding editor of *JBFHR* was Samuel Hyde, a qualified medical practitioner and hydropathist working in Buxton where he ran his own hydropathic business. An anonymous article in August 1890 praised both Hyde and his hydro as progressive and modern, illustrations emphasised the luxurious accommodation and facilities while the text credited him with 'an entirely original and most efficacious way' of applying the Buxton waters in his 'Thermal Cure'.[140] Examples of such blatant self-publicity ran alongside reprints of articles from the *Lancet* on climatology and the use of health resorts in orthodox medical practice as well as detailed explanations of the bathing and massage techniques commonly used.

The eclectic mix of advertisement and instruction contained within the *JBFHR* proved to be unstable and within five years it had disappeared to be replaced by periodicals aimed at either a lay audience or medical specialists. This trend highlights the difficulties of balancing professional etiquette that forbade the promotion of self-interest with the need for appropriate marketing within a competitive marketplace. The launch of the *JB&C* in 1897 as the official organ of the SB&C addressed this problem by creating a specialist forum for medical practitioners active in this area or interested in knowing more about the subject. This was one of a number of new specialist medical journals that proliferated by the end of the nineteenth century. Its role in developing a separate identity for balneologists and climatologists is discussed further in Chapter 1. Thus by the end of the nineteenth century there was a greater separation between publications intended for medical professionals and media addressed to a lay audience. Information about health resorts and promotional articles aimed at the general public continued to circulate in newspapers including the *Times* and general interest magazines including *Queen*.[141] These publications reviewed health resorts as part of the broader mix of tourist destinations. More specialist titles, such as *Health Resort: an illustrated journal of spas and sanatoria* and the *Invalid* targeted information at a smaller, more distinctive group of consumers interested in treatment. These titles published a wide variety of articles; some of those on baths, bathing and associated treatments were of a similar technical level to those addressed to general practitioners and suggest that patients wanted to be well-informed. Other copy emphasised the more general attractions of resorts as leisure destinations. Most importantly they were able to provide the consumer with up-to-date information as resorts vied with each other to upgrade facilities and introduce new treatments. The range of publications demonstrates the considerable knowledge and sophistication of discerning consumers as well as the complexity of the market for health and leisure resorts.

The Health Resorts and Watering Places Act, which came into effect in 1921 was the result of several decades of lobbying from resorts for legal powers to raise a local rate to fund publicity. The act allowed towns to use the profits from municipal enterprises of up to the equivalent of a penny rate on advertising in newspapers, handbooks, leaflets and railway placards. Further acts followed in the 1930s increasing the powers of local authorities to begin to develop comprehensive publicity. Unlike some European countries, including France and Belgium, the central British state did not take a lead role in tourism and instead developments were pushed through by a number of campaigns and associations of interested parties. For example, the 'Come to Britain' movement set up in 1926 has been described as using 'a well tried model of voluntary coalition of trade interests, led by the great and the good. Shipping lines, railways, London stores and the Association of Health and Pleasure Resorts were all represented'.[142] As recognition of the potential economic value of the tourism sector grew so too did support for state-funded promotional activities. In 1928 a temporary grant of £5,000 was awarded to a new organisation, the Travel Association, and in 1931 the Local Authorities Publicity Act allowed municipal funds to be used to promote Britain overseas. Many of these collaborative ventures pushed the attractions of Britain generally but this was also a period when images for particular towns were created, for example through the use of slogans and poster images. Some spas used associations with European spas as shorthand for their own attractions; Woodhall was described as 'The English Kreuznach' while Cheltenham's particular ambience was described as 'continental' and the tag the 'English Carlsbad' used in publicity. In contrast Buxton emphasised its natural surroundings and bracing English climate through the description the 'Mountain Spa'.[143]

The scope of promotional activity undertaken in the inter-war period is illustrated by measures put in place at Leamington coordinated by W. J. Leist, appointed as manager of the municipal Pump Rooms in 1924. A budget of £400 was set for the year of which £250 was allocated to initiatives with Great Western Railway, £45 to advertising in various publications, £77 paid to the BSF and £28 to the ISMH.[144] Publicity was directed at two separate audiences, the public and the medical profession, and comprised of a mix of individual and collaborative ventures, some of which promoted spa treatment in general and some of which publicised the town and its spa facilities. Two booklets were printed, one, aimed at the general public, was to be self-funding through charging businesses for advertising, while the other, with no advertisements, was distributed to doctors in the Leamington area.

Some 10,000 copies of the general booklet were produced of which 7,000 had been circulated by the following year, distributed via Great Western Railway, Cunard, Thomas Cook and several other large shipping lines and travel bureaux. A copy had also been sent to every librarian in the Library Association Year Book in Great Britain, Australia, America, India and Africa and to every doctor in Warwickshire.[145] In 1925 two thousand copies of the medical booklet were printed and distributed to doctors in Birmingham and surrounding towns as well as to a selection of practitioners in London and the provinces.[146] Advertisements were placed in a selection of national newspapers and periodicals including the *Times, Observer, Daily Telegraph, Morning Post, Daily Mail, Daily Chronicle, Observer, Sunday Times, Church Times, Queen, Lady* and the *Gentlewoman*. These had been carefully selected to target an appropriate market; as Leist remarked, 'I think it can be justly claimed that the needs of a resort such as ours are filled by the foregoing list, which I think is comprehensive, Of course, if Leamington catered wholesale for the tripper element, a very different list of media would have been used.'[147]

Advertising by railway companies became increasingly important with the production of illustrated tourist brochures and colour posters focused on resorts served by their networks.[148] The four railway companies that emerged from a reorganisation of the industry in 1921 each developed their own style of advertising. Leamington was served by Great Western Railway, a company renowned for its 'impressive range of handbooks and guides' although its posters have been described as having 'an old-fashioned feel' which 'lacked both imagination and style'.[149] In 1923 the company published an illustrated booklet targeted at the general public which provided a brief description of resorts on the network together with details of tourist and weekend railway tickets. The entry for 'Leafy Leamington' emphasised the genteel urban pleasures of the town, including the excellent shops, the beauties of the Jephson Gardens and range of all-year entertainments available in addition to the up-to-date treatment facilities.[150] A poster advertising the town featured a middle-class clientele enjoying the waters, gardens and sports facilities in the Pump Rooms and Jephson gardens.

As noted already, publicity policy at spas was influenced by the conventions of professional behaviour which deprecated advertising of the services of individual practitioners.[151] An important vehicle for reaching other medical practitioners who might recommend patients to visit a spa was the BSF's annual handbook prepared for the medical profession. The BSF also represented the interests of spas within organisations with a wider remit such as the BHRA which aimed to use 'all legitimate ways in which publicity may be given to British Health Resorts' and to develop the understanding of the medical profession and the laity of their potential therapeutic uses.[152] The directors of the company included several influential members of the medical elite, including Lord Horder, Sir Humphrey Rolleston and three current or past Medical Officers of Health.[153] Reiterating the long-held belief in the detrimental effects of modernity on health, the association's literature suggested that the sedentary life of town-dwellers, compounded by the 'nervous stresses inseparable from civilisation' could result in the 'fatigue-factor' that contributed to increased pathology.[154] A well-directed course of treatment at a health resort would improve overall health and mitigate these deleterious effects. The Association funded an annual guide, *British Health Resorts,* also compiled by Fortescue Fox, which provided brief details of member resorts and organised the contribution of promotional articles to the lay and medical press. It also maintained an information bureau in London for the dissemination of publicity material to potential visitors and held regional conferences on topical issues of both general and medical interest. For example the 1937 conference included sessions on 'The spa as a national asset in the maintenance of physical fitness', opened by Lord Horder and a technical forum on 'Hydrological methods in the treatment of injuries and diseases of the joints' opened by Dr F. C. Thomson, physician at the Royal United Hospital Bath and a former chairman of the BMA.[155] The Association was also interested in improving standards at resorts and set up a system of visits and inspections of spas in 1935. In addition emphasis was given to promoting the use of resorts outside of the summer months with several entries for towns providing tabular details of sunshine and rainfall in the winter period. It was argued that the facilities available, the range of treatments offered and the quality of accommodation provided meant that many resorts could be comfortably used throughout the year.

Conclusion

This chapter has explored the development and marketing of specialist spa and hydropathic resorts. The nineteenth century saw growing demand for resort towns stimulated by rising incomes, a separation of work and leisure time and the commercialistion of leisure activities. The evidence presented here makes the case that health has been underplayed as a factor in consumer demand and argues that centres providing spa and hydropathic treatments flourished partly because they were recognised as a distinctive type of resort. For these resorts it became more rather than less important to secure medical endorsement of their natural assets and man-made facilities and to become associated with health rather than leisure pursuits. At Buxton and Harrogate, the water cure remained the cornerstone of the resort's economic life while Cheltenham and Leamington grew into larger residential towns with more diverse economies, becoming, to paraphrase Granville, towns with spas rather than spa towns.[156] In an age characterised by industrialisation, small rural spas offered a vision of respite from dirty urban environments, particularly in the middle of the century before widespread sanitary improvements. The new hydropathic resorts at Matlock, Malvern and Ilkley traded on their natural assets and simple pleasures. By the 1880s a small group of elite English spas, presented as comparing favourably with European spas, was clearly delineated within the broader category of health resorts. This trend was further consolidated by measures taken by the BSF to restrict entry to the Federation to a small minority of resorts which were actively promoted on the basis of their natural mineral waters, facilities and expertise.

Although private investors were the driving force behind expansion and development in the early part of the nineteenth century, a variety of other medical and non-medical actors also contributed to the creation of these resorts, including local government, railway companies and charitable and mutual societies. It has been argued that the role of medical practitioners has been underplayed and emphasis has been given here to illustrating their important contribution. Medical expertise had long been used to justify the clinical efficacy of mineral waters, typified by the medical treatises of authors such as Jameson at Cheltenham or the clinical reputation of Jephson at Leamington, but practitioners also undertook a range of other roles. Charles Hastings was instrumental in the early development of Droitwich, investing in new enterprises while the example of A. B. Granville highlights the important role of medical authors in the transfer of knowledge and the development of consumer awareness in the developing market for health resorts. The advent of hydropathy demonstrates the entrepreneurial drive of practitioners in establishing individual businesses in an emerging marketplace and their crucial roles in both publicity and wider resort development. The market for water cures continued to develop in size and scope throughout the century, demonstrated by real growth in the number and size of specialist resorts and the emphasis given to bathing suites and hydrotherapeutic establishments. Although the discussion in this chapter has focused on drawing out the increased emphasis given to medical validation it is recognised that the overall success of resorts relied on attracting a broad range of consumers from the industrial and commercial middle classes. As Bernard Jennings comments of Harrogate, 'Connoisseurs of mineral waters, invalids seeking the latest scientific treatment, people coming to atone for a year's overeating, dabblers in the cults of hydropathy and electrotherapy, and holiday makers could all find what they wanted in Harrogate.'[157] Economic viability depended on both individual business initiative and the development of a public infrastructure to attract a broad public. This included baths, pump rooms, assembly halls, parks and gardens. The changing provision of facilities for recreation and the intersection between therapeutics and leisure activities are discussed in Chapter 5 after further exploration of evidence of the specialist treatment functions that developed at water cure resorts.

Notes

1 Hembry, *British spas from 1815*; Borsay, 'Health and leisure resorts'; Patmore, 'Spa towns.'

2 P. J. Corfield, *The impact of English towns 1700–1800* (Oxford: Oxford University Press, 1982); Borsay, *English urban renaissance*.

3 Walton, *English seaside resort*, pp. 7–9; J. A. R. Pimlott, *The Englishman's holiday: a social history* (London: Faber and Faber, 1947), p. 46.

4 Pimlott, *Englishman's holiday*, p. 185.

5 Blackbourn, 'Taking the waters,' pp. 453–4 and 441.

6 Jon Stobart, 'In search of a leisure hierarchy: English spa towns and their place in the eighteenth-century urban system,' in Borsay, Hirschfelder and Mohrmann (eds), *New directions in urban history*, 19–40.

7 Walton, *English seaside*, pp. 3–4.

8 S. V. Ward, *Selling places: the marketing and promotion of towns and cities 1850–2000* (New York, Routledge, 1998).

9 'What is a spa?,' *AMH*, 17 (1939), p. 124.

10 'The work of the British Health Resorts Association, 1931–1938,' BHRA, *British health resorts* (1939), p. 9.

11 Granville, *Northern spas*, p. xxxv.

12 Granville, *Midland and southern spas*, p. 403.

13 Granville, *Northern spas*, p. xxxvi.
14 Granville, *Midland and southern spas*, p. 375.
15 Granville, *Midland and southern spas*, p. 629.
16 Hembry, *English spa 1560–1815*, pp. 197–201.
17 Hembry, *English spa 1560–1815*, pp. 289–94 and 300.
18 Jameson, *Cheltenham waters* (1814).
19 Hembry, *British spas from 1815*, pp. 36–7.
20 Hembry, *British spas from 1815*, pp. 33 and 39.
21 Granville, *Midland and southern spas*, pp. 285 and 228.
22 Hembry, *British spas from 1815*, p. 45.
23 'The sayings and doings of Cheltenham', *Cheltenham Looker-on* (4 October 1851), 632–3; (26 June 1852), 434–5; (6 December 1856), 1173.
24 'The sayings and doings of Cheltenham', *Cheltenham Looker-on* (3 July 1852), 450; Hart, *Cheltenham*, p. 317.
25 Hart, *Cheltenham*, p. 317.
26 H. G. Clarke, *Royal Leamington Spa: a century's growth and development* (Leamington: Courier Press, 1947), p. 93.
27 Pimlott, *Englishman's Holiday*, pp. 96–7; Walton, *English seaside*, pp. 51–9.
28 Granville, *Northern spas*, p. xxix.
29 Hembry, *British spas from 1815*, Appendix 1, p. 249.
30 Charles Hastings, *Illustrations of the natural history of Worcestershire* (London: Sherwood, Gilbert & Piper, 1834).
31 Charles Hastings, *On the salt springs of Worcestershire: a lecture delivered before the members of the Worcestershire Natural History Society* (Worcester: Chalk and Holl, 1835). These were to be found at Evesham, Dudley, Droitwich, Hasler, Defford, Barn Bank, Upton, Churchill, Spetchley, Stonebow Turnpike, Cauldwell, Abberton, Pinvin,Tewkesbury, Walton and Redmarley.
32 Hastings, *Salt springs*, pp. 25–6.
33 John Wall, *Experiments and observations on the Malvern waters* (London: W. Sandby, 1756); Wall, *Medical tracts of the late John Wall.*
34 Mary Southall, *A description of Malvern* (London: Longman, Hurst & Co., 1822), pp. 11–19 and 53–6.
35 Hastings, *Natural history of Worcestershire*, p. 119.
36 *M. Billing's Directory and Gazetteer of the county of Worcestershire* (Birmingham: M. Billing, 1855), pp. 206–7.
37 *Birmingham Gazette* (30 August 1832), quoted in Weaver, *Droitwich Spa*, p. 1; Percy A. Roden, *Droitwich and its brine baths* (Worcester: Worcester Herald Office, n.d. but c. 1887), p. 6.
38 *Berrow's Worcestershire Journal* (24 September 1835) (1 October 1835); Weaver, *Droitwich Spa*, p. 10.
39 Weaver, *Droitwich Spa*, pp. 13–14.
40 Hembry, *British spas from 1815*, pp. 87–9; Ken Hillier, *A history of Ashby de La Zouche* (Leicester: Jones & Co, 1998). Hillier draws on notes taken from records held at the Bute archive.

41 David Cannadine, *Lords and landlords: the aristocracy and the towns, 1774–1967* (Leicester: Leicester University Press, 1980), part 3, 'The Devonshires and Eastbourne'.
42 Granville, *Midland and southern spas*, pp. 111–12.
43 Granville, *Midland and southern spas*, pp. 154–68.
44 Langham and Wells, *Baths at Buxton Spa*, p. 46.
45 Granville, *Northern spas*, p. 37.
46 *Visitor's vade mecum, being an historical and descriptive sketch of Harrogate* (Harrogate: P. Palliser, 1838).
47 Granville, *Northern spas*, pp. 61–2.
48 Hembry, *English spa 1560–1815*, pp. 219–22.
49 Langham and Wells, *Baths at Buxton Spa*, pp. 73–4.
50 Langham, *Buxton*, pp. 17–22.
51 Charles Scudamore, *A chemical and medical report of the properties of the mineral waters of Buxton, Matlock, Cheltenham [et al]* (London, printed for the author, 1820); Charles Scudamore, *The analysis and medical account of the tepid springs of Buxton* (London, printed for the author, 1833).
52 Langham, *Buxton*, p. 25.
53 W. H. Robertson, *A handbook to the peak of Derbyshire or Buxton in 1854* (London: Bradbury and Evans, 1854). The book was reprinted into the 1880s.
54 Blackbourn, 'Taking the waters', p. 441.
55 Richard Metcalfe, *The rise and progress of hydropathy in England and Scotland* (London: Simpkin, Marshall, Hamilton, Kent, 1906), p. 98.
56 Joseph Buckley, *Matlock Bank as it was, and is* (London: Job Caudwell, 1867), pp. 6–8.
57 Claridge, *Hydropathy*, James Wilson, *The water cure: a practical treatise on the cure of diseases by water, air, exercise and diet* (London: J. Churchill, 1842).
58 Browne, 'Spas and sensibilities', pp. 102–3.
59 James Nott, *The story of the water cure* (Malvern: Stevens and Co., 1900), pp. 2–3.
60 Browne, 'Spas and sensibilities', p. 103.
61 *Shuttleworth's guide book to Ilkley and vicinity*, 2nd edn (Ilkley: J. Shuttleworth, n.d., c. 1867), p. 42.
62 *Shuttleworth's Ilkley* (1867), pp. 55–7.
63 *Shuttleworth's guide book to lIkley*, 3rd edn (Ilkley: J Shuttleworth, 1882), pp. 42–3.
64 *Shuttleworth's Ilkley* (1882), pp. 50–1 and 54–7, 'Register of apartments' before p. 1.
65 Derbyshire Record Office (DRO), D1397 B/B 20, 'Matlock Bank hydropathic establishment, copy of rules and regulations with short prospectus' (1858).
66 Smedley, *Practical hydropathy*, 13th edn (London: W. Kent & Co., 1870), p. 11.
67 DRO D1397 B/B 20, 'Matlock Bank rules' (1858).
68 Smedley, *Practical hydropathy*, 13th edn, p. 12b.

69 Buckley, *Matlock Bank*, pp. 7, 37–41 and advertisements in the back of the book. These show that the smaller hydros were charging about a guinea a week with better rooms costing up to 25 shillings a week, compared to two guineas at Matlock Bank. Children were charged at a lower rate, 15 shillings in the smaller hydros compared to one guinea a week at Smedley's.

70 *Derbyshire Post Office Directory* (London: Kelly, 1864), pp. 46–7.

71 DRO, D1397 B/B 29, Smedley's Hydropathic Establishment prospectus, p. 4.

72 This is discussed further in Chapter 4.

73 Harcup, *Malvern water cure*, pp. 46–7; J. Morris, *Dr Gully and Malvern* (Malvern: Malvern News, 1872), p. 15.

74 Nott, *Story of the water cure*, pp. 60–2.

75 Metcalfe, *Rise and progress*, p. 284.

76 Metcalfe, *Rise and progress*, pp. 209, 106–9 and 117–19.

77 Durie, *Water is best*, p. 89.

78 DRO, D1397 B/B 14, Bill for a seven-day stay at Smedley's Hydro by Mr and Mrs Haworth in September 1878.

79 T. D. Luke, *Spas and health resorts of the British Isles* (London: A. & C. Black, 1919), pp. 98 and 300.

80 Langham, *Buxton*, pp. 107–9.

81 W. H. Robertson, *Guide to the Buxton waters*, 19th edn (Buxton: John Cumming Bates, 1876), pp. 12–13

82 Langham, *Buxton*, pp. 58–9; Robertson, *Buxton waters*, 19th edn, pp. 19–22.

83 Devonshire Collections, Chatsworth, Buxton Estate Records, 1860–1890.

84 Adams, 'Accommodating the poor', pp. 183–8. These developments are discussed further in Chapter 3.

85 Robertson, *Buxton waters*, 19th edn, pp. 20–2.

86 Grayson Carter, 'The case of the Reverend James Shore', *Journal of Ecclesiastical History*, 47 (1996), 478–504, pp. 494–5.

87 Langham, *Buxton*, p. 122.

88 Jennings, *Harrogate*, pp. 408–9.

89 Jennings, *Harrogate*, pp. 300, 311 and 315.

90 Metcalfe, *Rise and progress*, pp. 213–14; Jennings, *Harrogate*, p. 415.

91 Jennings, *Harrogate*, p. 423.

92 Jennings, *Harrogate*, p. 429.

93 Hembry, *British spas from 1815*, pp. 152–4.

94 W. H. Bainbrigge, *Remarks on the Droitwich saline springs* (Worcester: Worcester Journal office, 1871).

95 Weaver, *Droitwich Spa*, pp. 54–61.

96 Lionel Calthrop, *A guide to the bromo-iodine mineral water and spa baths, Woodhall Spa* (Woodhall Spa: no publisher, n.d. but c. 1912), pp. 4–7 and 27–8.

97 Anon., *Woodhall Spa: the English Kreuznach* (1886), pp. 5–6 and 17.

98 'The inaugural day at Woodhall Spa', *Horncastle News and South Lindsey Advertiser* (26 May 1888), quoted in Marjorie Sargeant, *Woodhall Spa and the*

world 1885–1890 (Woodhall Spa: Woodhall Spa Cottage Museum, 2006), pp. 79–81.

99 *Horncastle News and South Lindsey Advertiser* (21 August 1888), cited in Sargeant, *Woodhall Spa*, p. 124.

100 *Horncastle News and South Lindsey Advertiser* (22 February 1890), cited in Sargeant, *Woodhall Spa*, p. 122.

101 *Horncastle News and South Lindsey Advertiser* (9 August 1890), cited in Sargeant, *Woodhall Spa*, p. 130.

102 Helen Mary Webb, 'Woodhall Spa: functional aspects of an inland resort town', BA dissertation, University of Durham, 1978, pp. 25–37.

103 Calthrop, *Bromo-iodine water, Woodhall Spa*, pp. 24–5.

104 The varied uses of this building are discussed in Chapter 4.

105 *Leamington Spa: a history of the Royal Pump Room bathing establishment, a description of the renovated pump room and new baths, illustrations of the baths – past and present; a report of the opening ceremony on Wednesday, June 1st 1887, Leamington Spa Chronicle* (4 June 1887). Reprinted separately, p. 2.

106 R. Eardley-Wilmot, *On the natural mineral waters and spa of Leamington* (Leamington: W. H. Smith, 1890).

107 'The Spa question', *Cheltenham Examiner* (23 January, 1895).

108 'New spa opened', *Cheltenham Looker-on* (23 June, 1906).

109 Ord and Garrod, *Climates and baths*, Vol. 1, pp. 589 and 591.

110 BSF, *British spas and health resorts* (London: E. J. Burrow, 1918), p. 28.

111 F. C. Broome, 'The British Spa Federation', *British spas and health resorts* (1918), pp. 11–12.

112 R. Fortescue Fox, 'The spas of Britain', *British spas and health resorts* (1918), pp. 3–10, p. 6.

113 R. B. Grindrod, *Malvern; its claims as a health resort; with notes on climate … also an exposition of the physiological and therapeutic influence of compressed air* (London: Robert Harwicke, n.d. but c. 1871).

114 A useful introduction is N. A. Rupke (ed.), *Medical geography in historical perspective, Medical History*, Supp. No. 20 (London: Wellcome Institute for the History of Medicine, 2000).

115 For example, Walter Tyrrell, *Notes of the climate of Malvern, with reference to its effect on disease*, 2nd edn (Malvern: Advertiser, 1894).

116 James Clark, *The sanative influence of climate with an account of the best places of resort for invalids in England, the south of Europe, etc.* (London: John Murray, 1841); Vladimir Jancović, *Confronting the climate: British airs and the making of environmental medicine* (Basingstoke: Palgrave Macmillan, 2010).

117 For example, Hermann Weber, 'On the influence of the Alpine climates on pulmonary consumption', *BMJ* (20 July 1867), 41–2.

118 R. B. Grindrod, *The compressed air bath: a therapeutic agent in various affections of the respiratory organs, and other diseases* (London: Simpkin, Marshall & Co, 1860); Grindrod, *Malvern: claims as health resort.*

119 Hermann Weber, *Climatotherapy* (London: Smith, Elder and Co., 1896).

120 E. Hawkins, *Medical climatology of England and Wales* (London: H. K. Lewis, 1923), pp. 257–9.
121 John K. Walton, 'Spas and seaside cultures in the age of the railway: Britain and France compared', in Cossic and Galliou, *Spas in Britain and France*, 475–98.
122 Weber and Weber, *Climatotherapy and balneotherapy*, pp. 234–5.
123 L. C. W. Bonacina, 'Climate, health and the British resorts', in BHRA, *British health resorts: spa, seaside, inland, including the British dominions and colonies* (London: BHRA, 1939), 50–2, p. 52.
124 Bulwer Lytton, 'Confessions of a water patient', pp. 14–15.
125 Lane, *Life at the water cure* (1851), p. xxiv.
126 John Leech, *Three weeks in wet sheets: being the diary and doings of a moist visitor to Malvern*, 4th edn (London: Hamilton Adams, 1858); Timothy Pounce, *Malvern as I found it* (London: published for the author, 1858) and Oddfish, *Health and pleasure or Malvern punch* (Malvern: J. Burns, 1863).
127 Anon., *Memorials from Ben Rhydding: concerning the place, its people, its cures* (London: Charles Gilpin, 1852); R. Woodrow Thomson, *Ben Rhydding: the asceplion of England* (London: Nelson & Sons, 1862); J. H. Lukis, *The common-sense of the water cure* (London: Robert Hardwicke, 1862).
128 Foster, *Journal*.
129 Paxton Hood, *The metropolis of the water cure or records of a water patient at Malvern* (London: Simpkin, Marshall and Co., 1858).
130 Frawley, *Invalidism*.
131 Lee, *The mineral springs of England*.
132 John Macpherson, *Our baths and wells: the mineral waters of the British Islands* (London: Macmillan, 1871).
133 Braun, *Spas of Europe*.
134 Ord and Garrod, *Climates and baths* Vol. 1.
135 Wood, *Health resorts of the British Islands*.
136 Luke, *Spas and health resorts*, dedication before p. vii.
137 Weber and Weber, *Climatotherapy and balneotherapy*.
138 I. Burney Yeo, *Health resorts and their uses* (London: Chapman and Hall, 1882); Burney Yeo, *Therapeutics of mineral springs*.
139 'The baths of Bath', *JBFHR*, new series 1.2 (February 1890), pp. 9–14.
140 'A modern hydro', *JBFHR*, new series 1.8 (August 1890), pp. 87–9.
141 Steward, 'Representations of spa culture'.
142 J. Beckerson, 'Marketing British tourism: government approaches to the stimulation of a service sector, 1880–1950', in H. Berghoff, B. Korte, R. Schneider and C. Harvie (eds), *The making of modern tourism: the cultural history of the British experience* (Basingstoke: Palgrave Macmillan, 2002), 133–57, pp. 140–1.
143 Luke, *Spas and health resorts*, BSF advertisement p. 1, after p. 318; *Woodhall Spa: the English Kreuznach; The Carlsbad of England: the official handbook of the Cheltenham corporation* (Cheltenham: Cheltenham Corporation, c. 1925).
144 Leamington Spa Art Gallery and Museum (LSAGM), Pump Room and baths' manager's report book, 1916–1927, M 4348.1995, 4 June, 1924.

145 LSAGM, Pump Room and baths' manager's report book, 1916–1927, M 4348.1995, 23 April 1925.
146 LSAGM, Pump Room and baths' manager's report book, 1916–1927, M 4348.1995, 23 April 1925 and 26 June 1925.
147 LSAGM, Pump Room and baths' manager's report book, 1916–1927, M 4348.1995, 23 April 1925.
148 Ward, *Selling places*, p. 35.
149 B. Cole and R. Durack, *Railway posters from the collection of the National Railway Museum, York* (London: Lawrence King, 1992), p. 9.
150 Anon., *Spas and inland resorts: health giving centres in the midlands, the west of England and central Wales* (London: Great Western Railway, 1923). This included Bath, Cheltenham, Church Stretton, Droitwich, Leamington Spa, Malvern, Torquay, Weymouth and the Welsh spas.
151 Anon., 'Medical ethics for spa practitioners', *AMH*, 13 (1935), p. 51.
152 TNA BT 31/35556/267466, *Annual Report of the BHRA 1937/8*, p. 2. Twenty-four of the forty directors were medical practitioners.
153 TNA BT 31/35556/267466. Annual Return of the BHRA, 19 October 1932.
154 'British Health Resorts Association: first spa conference', *BMJ* (28 May 1932), p. 1001.
155 'Health Resorts conference at Bath: the spa as a national asset', *BMJ* (11 December 1937), pp. 1184–6.
156 Granville, *Northern spas*, p. xxxix.
157 Jennings, *Harrogate*, p. 430.

3

Specialisation at the water cure: institutions and skilled workers

It has been argued that from the mid-nineteenth century the English spas and water cure centres were presented as places providing specialist facilities and treatment and that the therapeutic possibilities they offered continued to be a draw to patients suffering from a variety of complaints. This chapter assesses the extent to which this can be substantiated by examining detailed evidence from institutional records, census returns and local authority sources. Despite the fragmentary evidence available it is clear that the growth and operation of large institutions including hospitals, bathing establishments and hydropathics along with growing numbers of skilled workers support the claims made in promotional literature that these resorts did offer increasing levels of specialist expertise. The analysis begins by tracing trends in the development of therapies and facilities; in the 1840s most hydropathic treatments were provided in patients' bedrooms delivered by skilled bathmen and women using basins, jugs and sheets, but by the 1860s more extensive bathing facilities were widely provided in private rooms equipped to deliver bathing and douche treatments. Developments in plumbing and heating technologies added further potential for bathing contrivances using water at a variety of temperatures in diverse applications. By the 1880s the premier hydros and spa bathing establishments offered broadly similar facilities which included a variety of hydropathic baths as well massage-douches. In the early twentieth century innovation continued, for example more extensive use was made of applications using mud and commercially produced electrical treatments became popular. Facilities made provision for separation of male and female clients either through the provision of discrete suites or by allocating them separate treatment sessions within the working day. Increasing emphasis was also given to the separation of social classes and it was not uncommon to have two sets of baths for paying clients in addition to those for charity patients. The voluntary hospitals were the main mechanism through which access to spa treatment for the working class was introduced. The origins of these institutions lay in bathing charities developed to channel and control access to the spa waters for the vagrant poor, thus fulfilling both social and medical functions.

The rigorous regimes developed from the 1840s required skilled personnel to provide the wide range of physical treatments offered. Although the medical profession sought to control access to treatment through enforcing the necessity for a medical assessment, treatments were delivered by other practitioners who were able to influence and shape therapeutic practice. Towards the end of the nineteenth century their skills and knowledge gained more formal recognition through the development of professional associations for practitioners of medical gymnastics and massage.[1] Patients were able to tailor their regimes, choosing to visit an inpatient hydropathic institution or to create a more individual package of accommodation and treatment by selecting from the medical practitioners, bathmen and women and masseuses working in a resort. The discussion considers the extent to which the medical profession achieved professional dominance over the water cure. As argued in Chapter 1, by the 1870s the attacks on hydropathy's radical therapeutic approach had declined and its practices were broadly adopted within mainstream medicine. In the 1890s this endorsement by the medical establishment was demonstrated by efforts to establish the new specialty of balneology and climatology. Despite these trends and an expansion in medical influence at resorts achieved through employment in new institutions or serving on medical advisory committees, the orthodox medical profession found it difficult to establish dominance in this specialised marketplace. Watering-places remained sites of competition for the custom of patients with a variety of practitioners providing a choice of treatments and models of care, depending upon the size of the patient's purse.

Hydropathics, bath houses and therapeutic innovation

Vincent Preissnitz's hydropathic system, popularised from the 1840s, sparked decades of innovation in therapeutic techniques that continued into the 1930s. Hydropathy introduced a myriad of external applications, including baths, showers and a variety of wraps and packs as well as encouraging patients to drink copiously. Figure 1.1, reproduced from the frontispiece from Claridge's work on hydropathy published in 1842, shows the standard methods of early hydropathic practice; the wet pack, the sitz bath, the douche, the full immersion bath and a variety of partial baths.[2] In comparison to earlier spa practices they are innovative in two ways; the increased privacy of treatment and the number of specialist applications. Each image shows a single patient undertaking treatment sometimes supported by one or two specialist attendants. Most treatments represented are delivered in a simply furnished bedroom and even though the douche and the plunge bath required larger, more specialist bathing facilities the patient is still shown being treated alone. These methods continued to be used into the twentieth century although many successful hydropathists were innovators, willing to adapt the techniques developed by Preissnitz in their own practice to meet the requirements of their patients.

The versatility and invention so characteristic of hydropathy is illustrated by the practice of John and Caroline Smedley who developed a signature 'mild cure' which used tepid and warm water in addition to the cold water originally endorsed by Preissnitz. Among the treatments they developed were baths using mustard and chilli and the running sitz which incorporated a flow of water over the abdomen. Several of these, such as the ladies sitz or baths for the immersion for an arm or leg, could be taken partially clothed. Baths were carefully adjusted to the needs of each patient and detailed attention paid to the temperature of the water applied. By 1873 the 'bath book' for their hydro listed some 242 different treatment options.[3] On admission, each patient was assessed by one of the Smedleys, Caroline dealing with the female patients and children and John with the men. An individual bathing regime, tailored to each patient's particular complaint, was marked up in the patient's personal copy of the institution's bath book using numbers to refer to the specific treatments to be given. Prescriptions for diet and exercise were also included. To supplement the information in the bath book, patients were encouraged to purchase a copy of either John Smedley's *Practical hydropathy* or Caroline Smedley's *Ladies' manual of practical hydropathy* which gave full explanations of the principles of the system used at Matlock as well as an up-to-date list of the bathing treatments used.[4] In general patients had a hydropathic treatment before breakfast, one later in the morning and another in the afternoon.

After John Smedley's death in 1872 the institution was re-launched with the new owners determined to maintain its reputation for excellent treatment. Up-to-date facilities were integral to this and a pattern of sustained investment can be traced through the Hydro's publicity material. The 1882 prospectus advertised a Turkish bath and facilities for electro-therapeutics in addition to hydropathic baths.[5] The bathing facilities were once again substantially upgraded in 1894 at a cost of over £20,000 to create sixteen bathrooms, each with four private packing or dressing rooms administering an extensive range of baths.[6] Additionally, there was a new suite of Electric Baths, separate Turkish Baths for male and female patients, Russian Baths and facilities for the provision of medicated baths. Massage or medical rubbing was also available, based on the Weir Mitchell method. This American system which used bed rest, aggressive feeding, massage and electrotherapy in an intensive treatment cycle, was developed in the 1870s based on Weir Mitchell's experiences of treating wasted, nervous Civil War veterans. In England the method was adapted by W. S. Playfair for use with female patients and became popular at many health resorts, particularly for patients suffering from neurasthenia.[7]

A rare surviving case book for a patient treated at Smedley's demonstrates the longevity of the treatment approach. Isaac Bradburn, assessed as having a disordered liver, was treated in September 1896.[8] His booklet set out his treatment regime by listing the numbers of the baths to be given. By referring to the bath list the following routine is revealed. Bradburn's day started with a glass of hot water at 7 a.m. followed by a bath before breakfast and another mid-morning. After lunch he was to take a walk and have a foot bath including treading in cold water. In the evening he would be given a brief rub until the skin glowed following which a wet bandage would be wound around his waist and worn overnight. In case of sluggish bowel action, a warm water enema was to be given. In addition he was to drink a glass of cold water shortly before each meal and a glass of hot water afterwards, leaving at least an hour after eating. He was also to fit in three or four more short walks of twenty minutes each day. Due to his liver problems his diet was to avoid fat as far as possible – which meant no sauces, stuffings, sweet puddings, meat or bacon fat. Yorkshire pudding was also banned. The baths given in the mornings were varied according to the day. The one taken before breakfast used hot and cold alternating water either in a sponge bath taken standing in a sitz, or under a spray or rain bath. Mid-morning on Monday, Wednesday and Friday he was to be given a twenty-minute liver pack comprising of a hot wet pad applied around the trunk secured by a blanket. On top of this a hot stomach tin was applied with a hot water bottle to his feet. On Tuesday and Saturday the pack was replaced with a brief Turkish bath followed by soaping and a warm spray bath. On Thursdays he was to have his back sponged with a hot mustard concoction for four minutes, rinsed off with cold water. The daily routine has much in common with that followed by Claridge in Gräfenburg in the 1840s although with less emphasis on walking and drinking large quantities of water. Despite the new treatments introduced since John Smedley's death over twenty years earlier, the sitz bath, pack and his signature mustard bath were still at the heart of Bradburn's treatment plan. Despite this, investment in new techniques was publicised. An article in *Health Resort* in January 1905 emphasised the wide range of electrical treatments recently made available at the hydro including heat and light baths, D'Arsonval High Frequency Current, Röntgen Rays Apparatus and the Finsen lamp.[9]

Spas were also investing in similarly elaborate bathing facilities. The Presidential address to the Harrogate Medical Society in 1893 noted a rapid increase in the number of patients treated from the late 1880s with the numbers of baths delivered increasing from 20,822 in 1882 to 33,688 in 1893. Receipts had risen from £1,979 to £3,750 over the same period.[10] The main bathing provision was at the Victoria Baths which had been purchased by the town's Improvement Commissioners in 1870 and expanded to provide two wings, one for male and one for female patients, each with eighteen bathrooms, four showers, vapour baths and a swimming pool.[11] Table 3.1 shows the bathing treatments given in 1893.

Far and away the most popular treatment was an immersion bath in the naturally occurring sulphur water although considerable numbers of more complex treatments were also being delivered. The number of Aix douches delivered had doubled from 2,000 the previous year and it was 'bidding for first place in the public favour' despite the higher price charged.[12] The period from the late 1880s was one of extensive investment in medical bathing facilities at every premier English spa although all were overshadowed by the Royal Baths in Harrogate which were constructed at a cost of over £120,000 in 1897. In addition to immersion, sitz, showers and douches there were special facilities for the Harrogate massage douche, advertised as an improvement on the Aix system, rooms kitted out for Vichy massage and a luxurious suite of

Table 3.1: Breakdown of baths given at the Victoria Baths, Harrogate, 1893.

Type	*Number*
Ordinary sulphur baths	20,874
Needle showers	5,707
Aix douches	4,062
Rain water baths	957
Liver packs	921
Thermal sulphur baths	709
Dry rubbing	184
Vapour baths	173
Shower baths	101
Total	33,688

Source: *Extracts relating to baths, wells, etc. from the presidential address delivered before the members of the Harrogate Medical Society*, 16 November 1893 (Harrogate: R. Ackrill, 1893).

Turkish baths.[13] Also advertised was the Harrogate special combination bath that delivered a mix of 'shower, wave ascending, descending and spinal douches' and incorporated a hydraulic floor. This apparatus was first developed by William Burkinshaw, one of the technicians needed to keep the baths running smoothly and was first described in 1891 as the 'wonderfully ingenious' Harrogate universal bath capable of delivering a tailor-made combination of showers able to reach any or every part of the body from head to heels. Both comfort and safety had been considered with an electric bell provided to warn if 'the water is rising toward a temperature which might be dangerous'.[14] A photograph of the universal bath (see Figure 3.1) was included in the Corporation's publicity brochure from 1898 onwards. The Harrogate baths were intended to place the resort in the first rank of European spas, to rival Baden-Baden and Aix-les-Bains and set the standard for other English spas to emulate. The tiled room with decorative ceramics on the walls denotes an upmarket bathing establishment while the impressive tangle of pipes and valves on the right of the image demonstrates the technical expertise needed to deliver extensive hot and cold water sufficient to feed

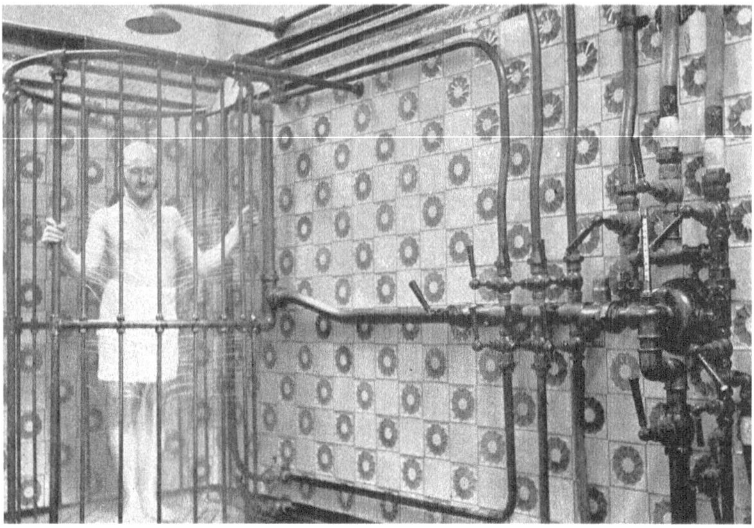

Figure 3.1: The Harrogate combination bath, 1898.

the numerous jets and sprays of the complicated apparatus. Although not depicted, a bath attendant would have been on hand to set up the apparatus for each patient and to wrap them in towels at the end of their treatment session. The controls are out of reach of the bather who is portrayed holding onto the bars of the shower, perhaps helping to withstand the assault of water from every angle. A slight smile suggests the experience is not only exceptional but also enjoyable.

In 1905 Harrogate introduced facilities for the Plombières douche, a treatment first developed at the French spa, Plombières-les-Bains to treat diseases of the intestinal tract. The potential benefits of the method had been aired in an article in the *Lancet* the previous year.[15] The specially designed suite of rooms provided facilities for 'an internal douche for washing out the bowel' followed by 'an immersion bath with an external or "Tivoli", or "submassive" douche to the abdomen, given under water'. Despite an outlay of £3,000 the investment proved profitable with over 2,000 treatments given in the first three months.[16] In 1912 the treatment rooms were moved to a purpose-built suite and in 1928 the Medical Advisory Committee recommended the accommodation should be doubled to provide twelve baths for women and eight for men. This report also noted the increase in provision for electrical treatments since

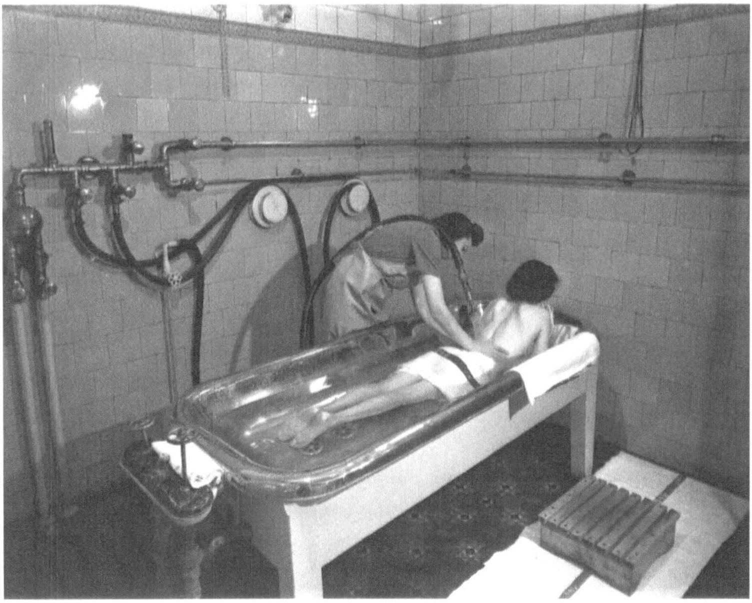

Figure 3.2: Buxton douche massage, 1947.

the opening of the Royal Baths some thirty years earlier.[17] These trends in provision are also apparent at other major spas.

At Buxton the Devonshire estate sold the baths complex to the Urban District Council in 1904. By 1907 provision had been made for the provision of the Plombières douche, the Buxton moor bath using local peat and the Dowsing Radiant Heat and Light bath.[18] The Buxton douche massage (see Figure 3.2) was also popular. This was a local variant of the Vichy massage in which the patient lay on a slab to be massaged by a skilled practitioner with the additional application of water. Vichy apparatus commonly had a spray over the slab but at Buxton a hose able to provide a more vigorous application of water was used. This image, dated 1947, attests to the enduring popularity of these methods over several decades. The photographic images of bathers printed in promotional brochures from the end of the nineteenth century included both men and women, always presented in private rooms being treated by attendants of the same sex. Early images show female workers and patients modestly dressed in loose garments perhaps with bare legs and arms if required for the treatment depicted. This image, from the mid-twentieth century, is striking for the degree of nudity presented, but the angle of the shot preserves the anonymity of both patient and practitioner. The tiled walls, shining metal ware, plumbing apparatus and freshly laundered towels create an impression of cleanliness, while the masseuse's air of concentration and careful attention to her patient emphasise expertise and quiet competence.

Plans for further modernisation of the natural baths were in preparation by 1912 although not started until 1922 when funds were secured through a loan of £19,500 from the Ministry of Health (MoH). As well as upgrading facilities in the bathing areas additional electrical treatments were also provided.[19] Despite these newer treatments the communal pools continued to be used, offering the opportunity for immersion baths with the patient able to move about freely or take more structured exercises in water. Figure 3.3 shows one of the men's baths at Buxton in 1947 with a patient being lowered into the water in a specially designed chair. A therapist in the water offers support to the patient. Photographs of male and female attendants actively treating patients in bath and douche rooms featured extensively in promotional material for bathing suites from the end of the nineteenth century. Representations of treatments such as the Aix douche (Figure 1.2) or the Buxton douche (figure 3.2) show skilled men and women attending to patients in private settings. Despite some emphasis given to cleanliness and plumbing, it is the intimacy and physicality of the treatments that is the central focus of these images. Hydrotherapeutic treatment remained labour-intensive with the patient's experience dependent on the expertise and approach of attendants. While hoists and special chairs offered facilities for frail clients, their safety and comfort ultimately depended on the staff employed in the bathing enterprises (see Figure 3.3).

The Leamington Corporation also continued to improve facilities with the support of the local Medical Advisory Committee. Delegations visited Bath, Cheltenham and Harrogate to inform the redevelopment plans for the Royal Pump Rooms. Among the new treatments introduced in the 1920s were the Dowsing Radiant Heat equipment, Bergonie apparatus, Diathermy, a Plombières Suite, Berthollet Steam treatment and Paraffin Wax baths.[20] The Dowsing and Greville apparatus were commercially produced pieces of equipment designed for the application of heat and light and hot air respectively. Their growing popularity at the elite spas is evidence of continued pressure for standardisation in the treatments provided, a trend towards the application of heat through

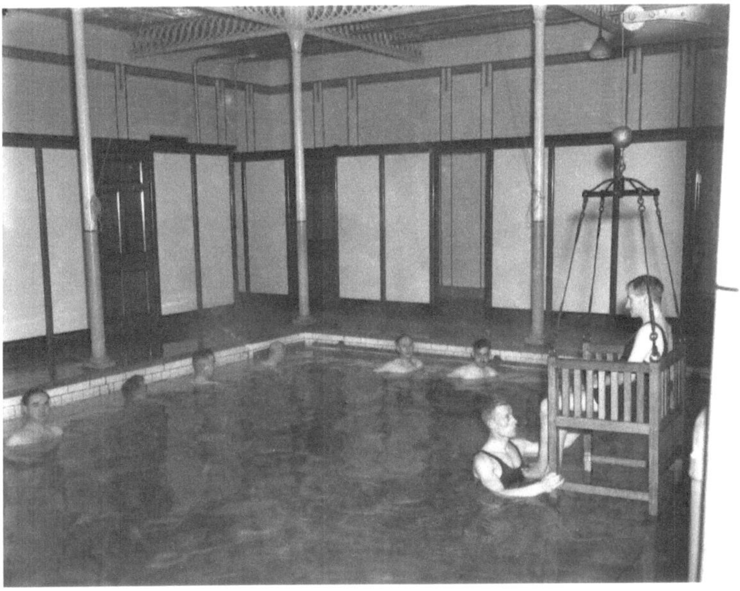

Figure 3.3: Natural baths, Buxton, 1947.

media other than water and a developing market in the commercial manufacture of electrical baths. As discussed in Chapter 1 increased emphasis given to hydrotherapeutic techniques rather than the action of minerals or heat in natural waters undermined the unique appeal of individual resorts. By investing in technical equipment, facilities and trained personnel institutions or resorts hoped to build a reputation for specialist expertise.

The Nauheim cure for heart disease is an example of this. The Schott brothers working at Bad Nauheim developed a treatment comprised of a series of baths taken in the naturally effervescent brine waters heated to different temperatures combined with a graduated exercise programme. The therapeutic potential of the treatment was introduced to British doctors through articles written by Theodor Schott published in the *Lancet*.[21] These posited that the treatment could be successfully provided anywhere using plain water with the addition of salt in specified quantities. The treatment generated strong debate among the medical profession in Britain with a number of articles published from 1891 either supporting or denigrating the approach. Disagreement was such that the *Lancet* established a committee to review the evidence which concluded that it had much to recommend it. [22] The Nauheim treatment became available at several centres in England; for example W. Bezley Thorne, one of the earliest promoters of the treatment, recommended Malvern to his London-based patients. Alternatively they could arrange for home treatment under the supervision of a competent nurse.[23] Samuel Hyde was another early advocate of the treatment and incorporated the terraced walks laid out on the Slopes to provide the graduated exercise regime for patients taking his Buxton 'terrain cure'. [24] These examples show the drive for innovation in therapeutic applications from the 1840s into the inter-war period which meant that these resorts came to offer an extensive variety of baths and auxiliary treatments delivered by skilled workers using specialist equipment.

Work at the water cure

The 1861 census records for Malvern record thirty-three people working in occupations directly associated with the water cure, seventeen men and sixteen women. Fourteen men were listed as bath man or bath attendant, one was listed as a bath chairman, and two as medical rubbers. The occupations of all the women were recorded as bath woman or bath attendant.[25] It is significant that the number of male and female employees was roughly equal, indicating that both male and female patients were treated at the resort and confirming the convention that patients were treated by members of their own sex. In a number of instances, several family members are recorded with similar occupations, for example, George and Hannah Grant at Link Common, Elizabeth and Ivory Nott at the Well House in Malvern Wells and Louise, Elizabeth and Richard Page from the Wytch. The model of the family firm, in which both male and female family members worked in the same occupation, was well suited to the water cure, as it meant that the business could treat all patients.

As Malvern expanded specialist practitioners were attracted from other parts of the country. Mr Kent, who had practised under Dr Carstairs in Buxton, moved to Malvern in the 1850s where he advertised his services as shampooer and medical manipulator, offering to provide treatment within a radius of one mile of the hydros.[26] J. Steele, medical rubber, advertised consultations and treatment either at his premises in Lansdowne Crescent or in the patient's private rooms.[27] Medical rubbers Angus Cameron and Thomas Milne, in Malvern in 1861, were born in Edinburgh while Andrew and Betsy Hamilton, recorded in the 1881 census, were from Fife.[28] Census information indicates increasing numbers of medical rubbers or masseurs in the town, six by 1881, of which four were women, again demonstrating their participation in this expanding area. Both men and women are also recorded as managing bath houses in the vicinity, suggesting that managerial roles were filled by both sexes.[29] These practitioners worked with patients both with and without medical recommendation and supervision. Thus patients attending the West Villa baths at Malvern had the option of attending there to consult with Dr Grindrod at designated times or to arrange baths directly with the superintendent either at the bath house, in their lodgings or at Grindrod's hydro.[30]

Records kept by Smedley's manager, Jonas Brown, show that the hydro employed 136 people in April 1871, evidence of the complexity of the organisation and its focus on cure and care. There were forty-four employees in the bathing department, fifty-nine domestic staff, twenty-two working in the dining room and eleven in the maintenance department.[31] Roughly equal numbers of men and women were employed as bathing attendants; thirteen men and eleven women. They would have each had to deal with eight to ten patients, wrapping and unwrapping them, preparing baths, bathing, rubbing and drying and cleaning up. Many treatments were provided in patient's bedrooms, requiring the transport of water, baths, sheets and blankets around the premises. The twenty special nurses provided additional assistance and support to those who needed it. After Smedley's death, the bathing department continued to expand. In 1893 the hydro had a bathing staff of thirty-five to forty 'skilled attendants', men and women, classified as bath attendants, special nurses, masseurs or electricians. Bathing was segregated by sex, each under the control of a head bath man or woman responsible for all treatments in the bathrooms.[32]

Jonas Brown's account book records the weekly wage rates for 1871 of 18 shillings for bath men, 9 shillings for bath women, and 7 shillings for special nurses.[33] These rates work out to £23 per annum for bath women and £18 for the special nurses, putting them in the range of salaries offered to trained staff nurses in the last quarter of the nineteenth century, estimated at between £15 to £30 in poor law hospitals and £20 to £30 in general hospitals.[34] The rates paid confirm that bathing attendants were considered to have specialist skills which exceeded those of special nurses, who provided personal care and support to individuals. The rates paid to both male and female bath attendants exceed those paid to the keepers at the Wolverhampton asylum in 1859, for example, which were £25 for the head male attendant and £15 for the head female attendant.[35] The inequality between male and female workers at Matlock was addressed to some extent the following year when Caroline Smedley approved increases to 10s 6d a week for bath maids and 8s 6d for special nurses over twenty years of age.[36] However, the pay differential continued to be marked, and in 1877 male bath attendants attending patients on an out-patient basis were charged at £2 2 shillings a week, double that of female workers.[37] In addition to working with patients in the hydro, bath men and women also provided hydropathic care to patients in their own homes with charges levied to cover wages, board and lodging, and travel expenses.[38] One of the Smedleys' stated aims was to provide their patrons with the opportunity to gain 'a thorough knowledge ... of the domestic application of Hydropathy, and general personal management as regards bath, diet, clothing etc.'[39] This facility was available to those living locally and to patients returning home from the hydro and clearly required competent staff to undertake treatment and training away from the home institution.

Salaries paid at the Buxton Baths complex, managed by the town council from 1904, also indicate the need to pay for highly specialist skills, especially for those in managerial roles. The council employed separate male and female superintendents at the hot baths complex, paying the male supervisor £83 and the female supervisor £60 a year. Each headed their own team of staff comprising a masseur or masseuse and bath attendants. Despite attempting to tap into the market for experienced spa managers by advertising in the Buxton, Bath and Harrogate newspapers, they failed to recruit to the female superintendent post until the salary was raised to £80, when they appointed Miss Kemp, previously staff masseuse at the hospital in Bath.[40] After further difficulties the committee decided to restructure and appoint a single overall spa manager, advertising in the *Manchester Guardian, London Daily Telegraph* and '2 or 3 continental newspapers'.[41] Despite offering a salary of up to £200, this failed to attract a suitable candidate and a local man, John Hatton, was eventually appointed on the strength of his managerial capacity, despite having no previous relevant experience or specialist skills.[42] Hatton's appointment proved to be a success and in 1909 he moved to take up an appointment at the spa facilities at

Bath, working there until his retirement in 1948.[43] The Baths and Wells Committee then advertised the post as Bath Manager and Head of Publicity, appointing Fred Broome who stayed some five years before moving to take up a role as manager of the Harrogate baths.[44] Broome became the first honorary secretary to the BSF and took a leading role in negotiations with the MoH over financial support for spa treatment in the inter-war period. This is discussed in more detail in Chapter 6. William Leist, who worked as Broome's assistant at Harrogate, was later appointed as General Manager at Leamington. The duties of spa managers were extensive and included publicity and advertising as well as management responsibility.

Access to scientific and technical skills became increasingly important. In 1912 the Harrogate Corporation commissioned a new analysis of the waters by Professor Smithells of Leeds University to focus particularly on the radioactive attributes of the water. On the basis of his recommendation they employed Arnold Woodmansey as Borough Analyst to undertake the 'scientific supervision' of the waters.[45] In 1928 Woodmansey worked closely with Broome in the production of publicity material for a new 'fango' treatment to be used in full baths or as local packs applied, for example, to the ankle. Interest in the use of pelloids, the mineral-rich mud found close to springs, increased in the inter-war period prompting a search for suitable deposits at Harrogate. Broome wrote a pamphlet aimed at patients outlining the new treatment for joints affected by rheumatism, neuritis and certain diseases of the liver.[46] Woodmansey co-authored a paper directed at the medical profession which described the treatment's use of electricity to maintain heat as 'diathermy-fango' and explained its therapeutic action as being due to ions, mechanical and thermal effects. Brief case studies were included to demonstrate its effects in reducing pain and improving mobility in patients suffering from osteo- and rheumatoid-arthritis and fibrositis.[47]

The construction of elaborate baths also required skilled technical staff to keep equipment in good running order. Need for high standards of maintenance and the ability to innovate meant that a competent team of technicians and mechanics were an integral part of the spa workforce. At Harrogate these technical duties were the responsibility of the Borough Surveyor and his team of skilled plumbers and engineers. The creative and technical contribution of one mechanic, William Bintiff Burckinshaw, was celebrated in an article in the *Harrogate Advertiser.*

In 1887 Burckinshaw built a working model of a new bath designed by Councillor Hargreaves for the Victoria Baths for which he was rewarded by the Corporation with the gift of £10 plus a salary increase from 28s to 35s a week. Some years later, in the planning phase for the new Royal Baths, Burckinshaw was asked to 'try and get something new for the bathing scheme' and given a budget of £2 to build a prototype. The result was the Harrogate universal bath later known as the Harrogate combination bath discussed earlier in this chapter and shown in Figure 3.1.

The approach to remuneration and employment conditions for more junior staff was often less generous than for senior employees. At Buxton strategies adopted to reduce staff costs included both seasonal employment contracts and attempts to restrict private practice.[48] The terms of employment for Miss Davenport, appointed in 1905 as superintendent for the ladies' section at both the natural and hot baths, stipulated that she was not permitted to treat private patients in the town.[49] Even working under these restrictive terms, she was told that she would be suspended between the end of October 1910 and the beginning of April 1911 along with other staff who were also to have their wages reduced or be laid off over the winter months.[50] Staff objections resulted in further negotiations. Davenport was eventually offered the choice of £2 a week for six summer months or 25s a week in the summer season and £1 for the remainder of the year. She chose the option of reduced pay in winter.[51] Policies implemented at the Buxton Baths had an impact on the health economy of the whole town. When a dry massage department was opened in 1907 private practitioners complained that prices at the baths were too low and undercut the informal local agreement on rates for private treatments. Practitioners also requested that a list of private masseuses be displayed at the baths in the same way that a list of medical practitioners was made available to visitors.[52]

For many hydropathists training was undertaken on the job, based on learning by doing. Practical experience, often through working as an assistant to an established practitioner, provided a path to later independent practice. John and Caroline Smedley are good examples of the self-taught hydropathists of the mid-nineteenth century who developed their techniques and knowledge through empirical methods, in their case through treating patients at their free hospital in Lea Mills. Henry Steer, in his laudatory account of the Smedleys' careers, describes how Caroline's expertise was developed over twenty years but that her lack of formal instruction in physiology and pathology was not seen as a drawback or omission by those attending for treatment. 'It was not, therefore, regarded as either strange or dangerous that Mrs. Smedley should direct the application of simple remedies according to the prescribed formulae of the water-cure system'.[53] Despite recognising her courage and individual qualities, Steer indicated that the Smedleys were not unique but representative of 'the hydropathic practitioners, who began to spring up rapidly at this time, [who] did not wait until they were qualified by having passed medical and surgical examinations prior to opening their respective establishments, and prescribing hydropathic treatment. They began as boldly as if they were entitled to put M.D. after their names.'[54]

This emphasis on practical skills and personal reputation is similar to the situation described for nurses prior to the introduction of formal training schools in the 1880s.[55] For employees, training was provided by the employer and was directed towards their specific needs and requirements, as was the case at Matlock. Smedley notes he 'repeatedly tried medical assistants and failed', and instead came to rely on a staff of bath men and bath women trained in his own bathing techniques.[56] Well-trained and compliant bath attendants, who attended patients in their bedrooms and in the special bathrooms, were crucial to the provision of an effective and safe treatment regime for patients. The 1858 prospectus for Matlock Bank Hydro set out bathroom rules addressed to both 'bath-attendants and patients' encouraging compliance with the detailed and sometimes tedious methods on the part of both parties as 'the success of the treatment mainly depends upon attention to all these subsidiary appliances, and it is sometimes owing to practitioners not having patience and perseverance in these minutiae, that the treatment fails'. Emphasis was placed upon the safety and comfort of patients; thermometers were to be used to check water temperatures and bath attendants were instructed not to leave patients alone when taking baths using hot water, vapour or the spirit-lamp.[57] Publicity for Harrogate also emphasised the skills of trained staff; the brochure for 1929 noted that the Royal Baths employed over 200 people, declaring that the 'Staff is Medically Trained, Medically Examined and Medically Certificated as being competent in both the Theory and Practice of Spa work'. This was achieved through bi-weekly lectures to staff from members of the Harrogate Medical Society along with at least eighteen months of practical work. Successful candidates were awarded either a primary or final certificate.[58] In practice many of the staff were far more experienced than this having been employed for many years.

While opportunities for more formal training began to be introduced by the end of the century their impact on the water cure remained limited. The most marked shift in training in the auxiliary methods of the water cure was associated with massage tuition which was available from the 1880s mainly at private schools in the London area. Two of the earliest were Dr John Fletcher Little's London School of Massage and Dr H. Tibbits' West End School of Massage which offered four to six months training for both male and female practitioners. Massage tuition was popular with some trained nurses who took courses to enhance their nursing certificates, some encouraged by medical practitioners such as Playfair at King's College Hospital.[59] Massage continued to increase in popularity, sometimes provided in massage houses with little or no medical involvement. An article in the *BMJ* in July 1894 drew attention to a situation it described as a scandal, asserting that several London 'massage shops' were little more than 'houses of accommodation'. This assertion was followed up by a special report published in booklet form later that year outlining 'astounding revelations'.[60] One consequence of this adverse publicity was the development of a formal association for female practitioners. In 1895, Rosalind Paget, a trained nurse, and others founded the Society of Trained Masseuses to establish a clearer distinction between those working in the medical and leisure markets, organising exams and setting up a register of trained masseuses. Candidates for the exam were required to take a training course of a minimum of three months duration at either a private massage school or in one of the increasing number of hospitals providing training in massage. In 1905 some thirty schools entered candidates for the Society's exams.[61] The founder members, mindful of the implications of the massage scandal, adopted a rule that members were to give massage only on medical direction and also banned advertising in all but medical publications.[62]

The expansion of bath houses and hydros clearly increased opportunities for employment by specialist workers although some of this was on a seasonal or part-time basis. Other practitioners worked outside these institutions in their own businesses. For example in the preface to the second edition of *Life and electricity in health and disease*, William Hardy reflected on a career of twenty-two years as an electrician, many of which he had spent practising from Volta House in Harrogate.[63] Treatments available there included a 'Hydro-Electric Vapour Douche' first developed by Dr Bennett of Harrogate which he claimed had been endorsed by the BMA in 1869. Case studies included in the booklet suggested he treated a wide range of complaints with galvanism including 'change of life' and nervous depression. Another staple treatment in his repertoire was the use of electric belts whose efficacy was supported by testimonials which attested to their usefulness in treating swollen and painful joints and extremities due to rheumatism and poor circulation.[64] Although electrical treatments became popular at spas from the mid-nineteenth century the first formal association was not established until 1902 when the British Electro-therapeutic Society was set up. The first examination in medical electricity was held in 1915.[65] The evidence presented here, drawn from fragmentary records of various specialist institutions, census returns and local authority records, supports the claims made in promotional literature that visitors could access a variety of treatments delivered by skilled personnel.

The growth and impact of charitable and mutual institutions

Specialist hospitals also influenced the character of the nineteenth-century medical spa. Bathing charities and institutional provision were integrally linked to social attitudes towards the poor and the focus on spas as elite resorts has underplayed this aspect of their history. Charitable organisations have been associated with the English spas from at least the end of the sixteenth century with customary rights of free access to mineral waters accepted in principle even if practical difficulties mitigated against the poorer classes exercising this right. The expense of travel and treatment at a spa was considerable with costs to be covered including not only medical advice and access to wells and bath houses but also accommodation and living expenses. With most patients staying for at least three weeks, the cost of visiting a spa was beyond the means of the majority of the population. Although John Jones suggested in 1572 that wealthy visitors to Buxton should give a donation, according to their means, to fund treatment for the poor there is no evidence that this idea was put into practice until the eighteenth century.[66] In 1609 Thomas Bellott endowed a small hospital at Bath with twelve beds providing free treatment for men but this remained the only formal institution offering access for the poor to English mineral waters.[67] This restricted access was in line with the spirit of legislation passed in 1597 which sought to limit the number of those travelling to spas. While the right of genuine patients to have access to the water was accepted, beggars and vagabonds were viewed less favourably. Large numbers of poor people close to the baths and pump rooms were a potential source of unruly or intimidating behaviour that might well deter paying visitors. The legislation of 1597 restricted the right to travel to Bath and Buxton to those sponsored by their local parish who were also certified as being genuine patients able to benefit from taking the waters. Potential patients unable to fund their own treatment required a licence signed by two justices of the peace along with confirmation that their travel and other costs would be paid by their local poor law union. The expiry of this legislation in 1714 has been cited as one of the factors that contributed to the campaign to set up a mineral water hospital at Bath to act as an alternative mechanism for controlling access by the poor to the town and baths.[68] Patients unable to afford their own treatment were entitled to free care if sponsored by a subscriber to the infirmary charity. The hospital provided medical assessment and accommodation with patients taking baths at the public facilities. Patients were obliged to follow the rules of the institution which included restrictions on leaving the premises to wander around the town.

The Bath General Infirmary (BGI), which opened in 1738, was based on the administrative model developed at other early English voluntary hospitals. Payment of an annual subscription or a donation sufficient to be recognised as a life governor gave subscribers the right to recommend patients for treatment. The rules were explicit about the admission process to ensure that potential beneficiaries were both medically and socially worthy of charitable help.

> The Person proposed shall first have his Case drawn up by some Physician or skillful Person in his Neighbourhood, which, being duly attested by the Minister and Church-Wardens of the Parish he resided in, and transmitted to the Physicians of the said *Hospital,* [at Bath] together with the age of such Person, shall by them be carefully considered and examined; and if they find that the Person is a proper Object of this Charity, they shall signify such their Judgement to the Minister of the said Parish; and so soon as there is a Vacancy in the said *Hospital,* shall notify it to him by Letter, for the Person to come within a limited Time, who is to bring back these Letters of the Physicians to the Minister; by which he or she is to be admitted

> into the said *Hospital;* and if any Person shall come to *Bath*, under pretence of proposing himself to the *Hospital*, contrary to this Order, he shall not only be refused Admittance, but be treated as a Vagrant, with the utmost severity of the Law.[69]

The hospital was a success and soon developed a waiting list to cope with excess demand. Despite this, the model of institutional management was not taken up at other spas until almost a century later. Table 3.2 provides a summary of the foundation dates of hospitals at spas together with the number of beds provided when they opened and in 1926. The next to be established was a small institution for twenty-five patients opened at Harrogate in 1826, almost a century after the Bath institution. This was followed by the Warneford Hospital at Leamington in 1833 which provided access to bathing treatments as well as general medical services. Neither of these competed with the BGI in terms of size or national prestige. The first real rival was the Devonshire Royal Hospital (DRH) opened in Buxton in 1859 with 150 beds. After expansion to 300 beds in 1881 this became the largest of the British mineral water hospitals. The Bath Hospital at Harrogate was substantially expanded in the 1880s, a decade which also saw the foundation of purpose-built hospitals at Droitwich and Woodhall Spa. Thus within fifty years specialist hospitals to provide treatment with mineral waters had been established all the larger English spas, and three of these, at Bath, Buxton and Harrogate were large organisations with over 100 beds.

Table 3.2: Dates of foundation and bed numbers at English mineral water hospitals.

		Date	*Beds on foundation*	*Beds in 1926*
Bath	Bath General Infirmary	1738	100	136
Harrogate	Royal Bath Hospital	1826	25	150
Buxton	Devonshire Royal Hospital	1859	110	300
Droitwich	St John's Hospital	1881	15	40
Woodhall	Alexandra Hospital	1890	12	30

Source: Annual reports of named institutions.

These bathing institutions were part of a broader trend in hospital development in England that gathered pace from the early eighteenth century onwards. The extensive historiography of hospitals has emphasised the complex social, cultural and medical functions of these institutions, shaped by both national and local factors.[70] The voluntary subscription infirmary was the dominant model of English hospital organisation providing treatment for the deserving poor. The quotation from the rules of the BGI given above illustrates how prospective patients were required to pass through social and medical filters in order to direct charity towards those capable of benefiting from but also deserving of treatment. The BGI was unusual in providing treatment for patients from anywhere in the country and in specialising in treatment with mineral waters. Most general infirmaries in the eighteenth and nineteenth centuries provided services for their local population. By 1900 a wider range of institutions had developed including specialist hospitals focusing on specific diseases and dispensaries which provided outpatient care. Over the course of the nineteenth century hospitals came to provide a greater range of medical treatments including the expansion in surgery from the 1840s onwards. They also played a greater role in medical education and research. Close examination of the organisation and administration of the hospitals at English spas demonstrates their influential role in shaping the development of the medical spa of the nineteenth century.

As Table 3.2 shows, the model of institutional provision adopted at Bath was not followed at other spas until the nineteenth century. Despite Jones's call for a charitable fund in Buxton in 1572 his suggestion was not followed up for a further two centuries. However in 1779 a proposal to fund treatment for the poor led to the establishment of the Buxton Bath Charity. The cost of accommodation and subsistence was to be funded from money collected from wealthy visitors by the hoteliers and innkeepers in the town. Access was open to anyone living over three miles from Buxton and was controlled through a system of written recommendations similar to those in place in Bath. A patient was required to secure sponsorship from a responsible citizen such as a poor law overseer or churchwarden along with a certificate from a medical practitioner confirming their condition was suitable for treatment with the Buxton waters. Services funded by the charity included assessment by a medical practitioner who prescribed the use of waters as appropriate.[71] In 1795 the small allowance given to patients for accommodation and board was 6 shillings a week.[72] It is significant that the launch of the charity coincided with the redevelopment of the bathing complex in the 1780s to provide facilities offering greater segregation of the sexes and classes. The new facilities included a separate bath for the poor fed by the overflow from the principal bath for gentlemen.[73] By the end of the eighteenth century investors and owners of spa buildings were giving consideration to the needs and preferences of various social classes with expansion plans based on an assumption that the poor should be able to access treatment. Robertson, writing in 1854, cited a printed document dated 1785 which noted that the Buxton Bath Charity treated sixteen patients at any time and only operated during the summer season. These numbers increased in the early decades of the nineteenth century. Using statistics from the annual reports of the charity Robertson calculated that 33,709 patients had been treated between 1820 and 1853, an average of around a 1,000 a year.[74] In the 1830s Charles Scudamore described many of those seeking relief as working-class factory hands and mill workers from the developing industrial areas in the North and Midlands.[75]

A small bathing charity was also started in Harrogate in the early nineteenth century, founded with a capital sum of £200 collected from visitors. As at Buxton, the fund was used to provide an allowance for accommodation, set at 7 shillings a week and by 1821 was treating around 140 patients a year.[76] Soon after this steps were taken to establish a hospital funded by subscription and a twenty-five bed institution opened in Low Harrogate close to the Bog's Field. The hospital closed for two months each year from early July as the demand from paying guests in the high season was such that water at all wells was reserved for their use. Granville commented that the closure, whatever the justification, ensured that elite visitors did not have to mix too closely with the poorer classes.[77] Although the hospital was expanded to thirty-five beds in 1838, it remained a small institution, providing access to the poor who lived more than three miles from Harrogate and continuing to close in the summer months until 1867.[78] The size and organisation of these bathing charities indicates that they were arranged as much for the benefit of elites as for the poor who might benefit from them. Numbers treated were low and the rules required each individual patient to be screened, arrangements designed to minimise inconvenience to paying visitors.

Another important role of these charities, properly administered, was to create publicity for the local mineral waters and thus enhance the reputation of a spa with the wider public and, in particular, the upper and middle classes targeted for donations. The committee of the Leamington Charitable Bathing Institution set up in 1831 argued that in addition to benefiting poor invalids the charity was a powerful mechanism to advertise the town 'diffusing as widely as possible the usefulness and celebrity of the LEAMINGTON WATERS and BATHS ... and thereby increase the welfare and general interests of the place'.[79] Promotional events included charitable balls, fundraising bazaars and church sermons that all served to integrate medical charity into the social and cultural life of the spa.[80] The 1831 venture was an effort to re-launch an earlier organisation that had fallen into disuse. The Leamington Spa Charity is reputed to have been set up in 1806 by the town's acknowledged founder, Benjamin Satchwell, and was recorded as having provided 'upwards of 2,000 baths' by 1816.[81] Publicity for the Bathing Institution stated that the charity would cover costs of medical assessment with free baths and drinking water provided at the Pump Rooms for poor people from outside the town. Accommodation costs would not be covered and instead patients would be directed to cheap lodgings costing between 5 shillings and 15 shillings a week.[82] The re-launch of a separate bathing charity was part of more widespread efforts to deal with the perceived social problems of an expanding town, including vagrancy and begging. Another venture launched in 1831 was the Benevolent Society which sought to dissuade general alms-giving by visitors by directing their generous impulses towards organised charities which would target who was helped and how.[83] A charitable appeal to fund the building of a general hospital to supplement provision of medical services at the town's dispensary was also launched in the same year.[84] The aims of the two medical charities were distinct as the hospital would provide general medical services for the local population while the bathing charity was intended to improve access to the Leamington waters. Hospital development was also being promoted at Cheltenham and a report in the *Leamington Spa Courier* cited the move to expand the Cheltenham Dispensary and Casualty Hospital with a planned 100 beds as evidence that Leamington now needed its own hospital.[85] The Leamington infirmary appeal did not attract the support its promoters had hoped for and although the charity began to treat patients in 1833 the new premises opened with only twenty-four beds in use despite greater capacity. Even this limited success owed much to the large donations from Samuel Warneford and his daughter who donated more than £2,500 between them. The bathing charity had also failed to attract sufficient support to get off the ground and Samuel Warneford, the principal donor to both organisations, proposed their merger into the Warneford General Bathing Institution and Leamington Hospital.[86] Some potential supporters were fearful the charity would attract poor vagrants to the town, something many wished to discourage. At the end of the first year the committee took the opportunity to emphasise 'that the proportion of patients from Leamington, for the last year, is nearly 3 to 1; viz. Leamington 117 – other places 44 – which they trust will be sufficient evidence of the actual benefit which this Town derives from the Hospital, in its present and incomplete state'.[87] The promise of a substantial annual subscription of 100 guineas from Henry Jephson, the town's most celebrated spa physician, finally enabled the Committee to open a further ten beds 'for the suffering poor'. Jephson's total subscriptions to the hospital were £1,270 and he showed further support for the organisation by serving as Vice-President and as a governor from 1839.[88] Unlike the hospitals at Bath, Buxton and Harrogate, the Leamington hospital was a hybrid acting as both general hospital and specialist mineral water facility. While Warneford was attracted to support the institution at least partly due to a desire to expand access to the town's saline waters, members of the local population and medical fraternity had a vision of a general hospital providing services for the local population.

A review of the activities of the first forty years of the hospital, published in 1873 referred to this ongoing tension, presenting statistics to show that the use of baths at the hospital were in decline by the 1850s (see Table 3.3). In 1832 an average of three baths per patient were given which if continued would have meant 10,000 bathing treatments in 1872 rather than the 191 recorded. During his lifetime Warneford had sufficient influence to ensure that bathing treatments continued to be offered and his dedication to this cause was reflected in the terms of his will. After his death in 1855, support to the hospital continued via the Warneford Trustees but only on condition that access to the baths was provided. The Committee were obliged to continue to report on the 'number and character of the diseases treated by the Leamington Waters'. In 1872 provision was made to pipe saline water directly into the hospital in a scheme intended to ensure that the hospital continued

Table 3.3: Patients and mineral-water baths, Warneford Hospital, 1832–72.

Year	*Inpatients*	*Outpatients*	*Total patients*	*No. of baths*
1832	76	195	271	813
1842	188	278	466	2,153
1852	208	610	818	1,456
1862	273	1,349	1,622	1,170
1872	486	2,402	2,888	191

Source: Warneford Hospital Annual Report, 1873, p. 9.

to meet the requirements of Warneford's legacy despite the decline in the use of baths.[89] The management committee at Leamington favoured the development of general medical facilities over specialisation. The prime function of the hospital was to serve the local community and developments included increasing the overall numbers of beds and making provision for children and fever cases. The hospital at Cheltenham which grew out of a dispensary charity was also intended as a general hospital to serve the local population, with no special access to spa waters for patients. Medical charities at other spas tended to diverge, with the mineral water charities developing as specialist institutions while the medical needs of the resident population were met by a range of dispensaries, infirmaries and other institutions. For example in Bath, the United Hospital was formed in 1826 from the merger of two earlier organisations, the Casualty Hospital founded in 1788 and the City Infirmary and Dispensary. By 1820 there was also an Eye Infirmary, a Lock Hospital treating women for venereal diseases, a Lying-in hospital and a Childbed Charity.[90] At Harrogate a small six-bed hospital and dispensary opened in 1870 to provide general medical services. The institution, later extended and renamed the Harrogate Infirmary, remained separate from the Bath Hospital.[91]

The first of the specialist mineral water hospitals to rival Bath in size and reputation was the DRH at Buxton, founded as part of the major redevelopment of the spa by the Devonshire estate in the 1850s. The scheme included provision of new charity baths with hot bathing facilities for the growing numbers of patients treated by the Buxton Bath

Charity.[92] The popularity of this scheme led the committee to press for a mineral water hospital for the town. The local medical profession were in favour and the project secured the support of the Duke of Devonshire. His donation of £100 launched the appeal for the new institution and a search began for a site sufficient for a sizeable purpose-built institution of some 80 beds. Publicity for a fundraising bazaar for the project described the benefits of an inpatient institution for patients as being due to 'the distance from the Baths at which so many of the Charity Patients are at present compelled to lodge, render it both difficult and in many cases when crippled or infirm, very distressing to them to reach the baths with that regularity which is so essential to ensure them the greatest possible amount of good to be derived from the Waters.'[93] The limited allowance provided for lodging costs meant that most patients stayed in poorer districts away from the bathing complex. A hospital would ensure that patients had access to good quality accommodation close to the baths. The site finally selected was the great stables, owned by the Devonshire estate and originally built to accommodate the horses and carriages of wealthy visitors. This impressive building based on a classical circus design was constructed in the 1780s at the same time as the Crescent was developed to provide hotel accommodation and public facilities. By the 1850s demand for stabling had decreased as although there was as yet no railway station in the town the development of a national network meant that many visitors travelled at least part way by train, continuing by coaching services.[94] The building was in an ideal situation allowing easy access by patients to the charity baths situated at the back of the Crescent without crossing the resort areas reserved for the use of wealthier visitors. An agreement was reached to convert half of the building to provide accommodation for 100 patients, 65 men and 35 women. The new hospital opened in 1859.

In the first year of the hospital's operation 622 patients are recorded. By 1872 this had increased to 1,403 inpatients with a waiting list in the summer months.[95] The committee, among whom was Henry Robertson, the leading medical practitioner in the town, pressed the Devonshire estate for the release of the remainder of the building for conversion to additional ward space, arguing that this was justified on the grounds of both Christian charity and the general economic interests of the town which would only benefit from 'increasing celebrity'. However costs of conversion were prohibitive and it was not until 1876 when the trustees identified an external source of funding that the ambitious scheme became viable.

The source identified was the Cotton Districts Convalescent Fund (CDCF). This organisation was formed in 1875 to disburse funds remaining in a number of charities set up to provide support to cotton workers during a sustained period of unemployment in the early 1860s when supplies of American cotton to the English factories were disrupted by the Civil War. Once cotton production recommenced these surplus funds were directed to projects for the benefit of residents of named Poor Law Unions in Lancashire, Yorkshire and Chester. One of the sectors the CDCF invested in was the provision of convalescent homes and hospitals and the organisation made large capital donations to the DRH and the Southport New Convalescent Home to provide 150 additional beds in each institution.[96] The DRH had already been associated with efforts to relieve the effects of the famine in the area by launching a special fund to treat 100 young women in the hospital over the winter of 1862–63.[97] Discussions with the CDCF for capital funding continued over several years, with estimates of the cost of the project rising substantially. The eventual grant of £24,000 was sufficient to fund the conversion of the remainder of the stables into hospital accommodation.[98] The scheme attracted considerable national attention, not least because the conversion included the construction of a domed roof to cover the original open circus reputed to be among the largest domes in the world. The project was featured in the *Builder* of July 1880 and the grand opening in October 1881 reported in the medical press and London papers, including the *Illustrated London News*.[99] The resulting building was very prestigious, an undoubted architectural asset to the townscape. It provided a large specialist facility of 300 beds ably used by the Buxton doctors to develop their reputation in the emerging specialism of balneology and hydrotherapy.

Under the terms of the arrangement the CDCF had first rights to arrange for the referral of patients into the 150 beds created as part of the extension. Patients came from one of seventeen named infirmaries in the surrounding industrial towns and cities including Manchester, Salford, Ashton-under-Lyne, Blackburn, Preston, Stockport, Wigan, Oldham, Macclesfield and Lancaster. Regular statistical reports produced by the CDCF provide details of the age, gender and occupation of patients funded at all their homes (Table 3.4). Male and female patients were

Table 3.4: Age and gender of patients sponsored by the CDCF in 1890.

Age	*Male*	*Female*	*Total*
<20	85	121	206
21–30	128	171	299
31–40	152	90	242
41–50	127	74	201
51–60	78	54	132
61–70	43	28	71
Total	613	538	1,151
	53%	47%	

Source: CDCF Annual Report, 1890

fairly evenly balanced; of the 1,151 patients sponsored in 1890, just over half were men (53 per cent). The majority of those treated were of working age with 742 (65 per cent) between 21 and 50 years old.

The occupation with the highest recorded numbers for both men and women was weaving, reflecting the origins of the fund and the age and sex structure of the workforce in cotton and woollen mills (Table 3.5).These 375 workers accounted for 33 per cent of the total number of patients funded and was the largest occupational group for both men and women. Other categories of skilled male workers were mechanics (12 per cent), colliers (5 per cent), clerks, commercial travelers and apprentices (19 per cent) and those working in clothing trades (3 per cent). Together these categories of skilled worker made up 68 per cent of the male patients funded. Unskilled porters, labourers and stablemen accounted for a further 18 per cent while 4 per cent of men were recorded as having no occupation. A smaller proportion of the female patients were skilled workers; weavers accounted for 36 per cent of the total number of female patients while a further 9 per cent worked in the clothing industries. After weaving the most commonly recorded occupational groups were servants and charwomen (22 per cent) and housewives (22 per cent), with 9 per cent recorded as having no occupation.

Table 3.5: Recorded occupations of patients sponsored by the CDCF in 1890.

Occupation	*Male*	*Female*	*Total*	*Male*	*Female*	*Total*
Weavers	179	196	375	29%	36%	33%
Servants, charwomen		119	119		22%	10%
Housewives		118	118		22%	10%
Clerks, commercial travellers, apprentices	114		114	19%		10%
Porters, labourers, stablemen	109		109	18%		9%
No occupation	27	47	74	4%	9%	6%
Mechanics	72		72	12%		6%
Clothing trades	22	46	68	3%	9%	6%
Colliers	29		29	5%		3%
Painters, plumbers, shopkeepers	29		29	6%		3%
Joiners	21		21	3%		2%
At school	11	12	23	1%	2%	2%
Total	613	538	1,151	100%	100%	100%

Source: CDCF Annual Report 1890.

The CDCF was charged around 15s a week to cover the subsistence costs for each patient at the DRH and these ongoing charges may explain why the average number of beds used remained as low as thirty in many years. The annual report for the hospital in 1883 recorded that of the 2,230 patients treated only 303 had been referred by the CDCF scheme. However, demand from other users of the hospital was sufficient to ensure that much of this spare capacity was used. Other patients were referred from smaller welfare organisations, in particular from Friendly Societies. A review of hospital records has shown that over the course of the nineteenth century the proportion of hospital subscription income given by institutions rather than private individuals increased.[100] This pattern is clear at the DRH where, as shown in Table 3.6, subscriptions from Friendly Societies and Poor Law Unions rose substantially from 1858 to 1892. In 1892 they totalled £505, some 17 per cent of the £2,936 annual subscriptions due for the year. Other workers' funds, companies and infirmaries also contributed to the hospital. For example the 1872 Annual Report lists subscriptions from the following; infirmaries at Leeds, Huddersfield and Nottingham; the Oaks Colliery Accident Fund, Staunton Iron Works Company, Kingston Mill Working People; Sheffield and Rotherham Banking Company and the London and North Western District Rail Company.[101] This range of donors suggests that the treatment available at Buxton was valued by workers, employers and welfare organisations.

Table 3.6: Friendly society and poor law union subscribers to the DRH, 1858–92.

	1858	*1872*	*1882*	*1892*
Friendly Societies				
No. of subscribers	17	82	111	149
Subscriptions (Guineas)	20	134	245	354
Poor Law Unions				
No. of subscribers	18	36	40	38
Subscriptions (Guineas)	54	142	140	151

Source: DRH Annual Reports for selected years.

The occupational analysis of patients treated in the hospital in 1892 shows a broader mix than those groups targeted for support by the CDCF (see Table 3.7). Of those helped by the CDCF, 33 per cent were classified as weavers (see Table 3.5) while cotton operatives, weavers and knitters together only accounted for 10 per cent of the total numbers treated at the DRH. The annual report listed 221 different occupational groups of which the largest was domestic duties. These accounted for 24 per cent of the total number with a further 9 per cent recorded as working as servants or in domestic jobs. Some 12 per cent were labourers and a further 12 per cent worked in a variety of retail trades and commercial occupations, and another 28 per cent worked in a wide variety of industries, of which the largest single categories were mining and textiles. The building trade accounted for 7 per cent. The numbers

Table 3.7: Occupations of inpatients at the DRH, 1892.

Occupation	*Number*	*Percentage*
Domestic duties	431	24%
Labourers	224	12%
Retail and commerce	220	12%
Other industrial trades	172	10%
Servants and domestics	160	9%
Building trades	126	7%
Colliers and miners	106	6%
Cotton operatives	101	6%
Weavers and knitters	76	4%
Children	39	2%
Clerical	31	2%
Mechanics	31	2%
Nurses and teachers	30	2%
Agricultural	27	1%
Other	33	1%
Total	1,807	100%

Source: DRH Annual Report 1892.

listed from agricultural occupations was very low – just 1 per cent and other occupations listed included white-collar clerical jobs and nurses and teachers. The DRH annual reports also provided statistics of the diseases treated. The medical report for 1892 classified the 2,359 patients treated according to the major disease category they were suffering from. The figures for 1892 set out in Table 3.8, show the institution had become a specialist centre for rheumatic disorders. Some 82 per cent of all patients treated were classified as suffering from diseases of the locomotary system and 12 per cent from nervous diseases. Further breakdown of rheumatic diseases provided showed 53 per cent of these cases were male and 47 per cent female (Table 3.9).

Table 3.8: Analysis of cases treated at the DRH, 1892.

Treatment	*Number*	
Locomotary system	1,924	82%
Nervous system	278	12%
Anaemia/old injuries	84	4%
Respiratory system	37	2%
Surgical cases	16	0%
Alimentary system	15	0%
Urinary system	5	0%
Total	2,359	100%

Source: DRH Annual Report, 1892.

Table 3.9: Cases of rheumatism, rheumatoid arthritis and sciatica treated at the DRH, 1892.

	Male	*Female*	*Total*
Chronic articular rheumatism	359	374	733
Chronic non articular	185	109	294
Convalescent from rheumatism	219	146	365
Sciatica	133	31	164
Rheumatoid arthritis – hip	51	10	61
Rheumatoid arthritis – other	77	230	307
Total	1,024	900	1,924
	53%	47%	

Source: DRH Annual Report, 1892.

The DRH developed into a premier mineral water hospital to rival the institution at Bath. In the early decades of the twentieth century it took steps to develop its own specialist facilities. New mineral water baths constructed within the hospital were completed in 1914 providing separate facilities for men and women comprising immersion, douche and steam baths as well as facilities for Plombières and massage baths.[102] In 1939 plans to further update these facilities were delayed due to the outbreak of war. In 1945 the bathing department comprised ten douche immersion baths, two douche massage baths, two aerated baths, one whirlpool bath, two Plombières douche rooms, two vapour cabinets and two needle sprays. These facilities had delivered 23,448 baths to male patients and 20,592 to female patients (Table 3.10).[103]

Table 3.10: Treatments provided at the DRH in 1945.

	Male	*Female*
Hydrotherapy		
Immersion baths	12,312	12,067
Buxton massage	6,553	4,020
Vapour baths	3,208	2,088
Aerated bath	1,240	2,229
Plombières douche	109	70
Whirlpool bath	26	118
Total	23,448	20,592
Physiotherapy		
Massage	8,344	8,162
Electrical	6,736	6,068
Exercises	6,236	6,009
Heat (infra red, radiant heat, wax)	5,948	5,042
Sunlight	708	831
Cautery	610	690
Total	28,582	26,802

Source: DRO, D4508/7/3/4. Buxton co-ordinating committee, information requested by Professor Cohen, MoH, 1945.

The massage department opened in 1902 and was at first staffed by honorary personnel working on a voluntary basis.[104] Costs were kept to a minimum by using qualified staff to supervise students, a model which saved some £536 a year on employing additional trained staff. In 1930 the staff complement comprised one full-time masseuse, one staff assistant and nine students providing about 700 treatments each week. A proposal to employ an additional staff assistant to allow student numbers to increase to twenty was approved.[105] By 1945 the school had 84 students. By the 1940s the DRH provided a mix of physical therapies to its patients. Hydrotherapy treatments accounted for almost half the treatments given and despite the development of combination therapies the immersion bath in Buxton's natural water accounted for 24,379 (24.5 per cent) of a total of 99,424 treatments.[106]

The prestige and national publicity of these institutions encouraged the view that all spas of the first rank should have their own specialist hospital. The Bath Hospital at Harrogate was substantially expanded in the 1880s with the help of a generous donation from the Rawson family. At Woodhall publicity for the new spa promoted from the late 1880s included reference to a charitable hospital 'national in its character, open to all comers on the presentation of a Subscriber's order', clearly a strategy to assert the medical credentials of the spa and attract the support of wealthy patrons.[107] The Alexandra Hospital opened in 1890 with twelve beds but despite its small size the Princess of Wales, who had friends at Woodhall, consented to become President.[108] A hospital was also proposed as part of the expansion of Droitwich spa from the late 1870s and St John's Brine Bath Hospital opened in 1881 moving to new premises in 1892 with accommodation for forty patients.[109] Patients were treated at the second-class Royal Baths.

The increase in voluntary hospital provision provided the main vehicle through which access to spa treatment was extended beyond the middle classes. By the early twentieth century some mutual societies also became interested in investing in homes at spas and health resorts to provide convalescence or treatment for members. For example, in 1916 the Birmingham Hospital Saturday Fund (BHSF) opened Highfields hospital in Droitwich to provide accommodation for men and women with treatment for rheumatism arranged at the brine baths. Between 1919 and 1923 between seven to eight hundred patients a year were being treated.[110] In 1927 bed numbers were increased to seventy-eight and in 1938 more than 1,000 patients received treatment for rheumatism at a cost of over £7,000.[111] In 1936 Highfields was adapted to provide on-site facilities for auxiliary treatment including a gymnasium, light and heat therapy and massage.[112] The BHSF opened St Ann's convalescent home for women in Malvern in 1916 accommodating twenty-nine patients and treating 400–700 patients a year between 1917 and 1923. In addition to homes at these inland resorts the fund also provided convalescent homes on the North Wales coast and in 1933 opened a new home for women close to Weston-super-Mare. St Ann's was then converted to a convalescent home for girls with accommodation, later transferring to larger premises built at Hugh Sumner House in Malvern.[113] This detailed evidence from Buxton and Droitwich shows that by the twentieth century spa treatment was attracting support from a number of institutional supporters including Hospital Saturday fund schemes, friendly societies and the CDCF. This demonstrates that the specialist role of mineral water hospitals within the broader pattern of institutional provision of medical care was recognised and that treatment available at spas was valued by organisations providing health care for the working class. The introduction of National Health Insurance (NHI) in 1911 offered the opportunity for spas to gain more comprehensive support from the central state. The extent to which this was achieved is considered in Chapter 6.

Medical authority and the growth of paramedical groups

By focusing on the detailed practices of the water cure, and directing attention to those who provided treatments as well as those who prescribed them, this chapter has highlighted that numbers of skilled practitioners working in spas and hydros rose from the mid-nineteenth century. Practices at the water cure were notable for innovation, building on traditional spa treatment by incorporating hydropathic methods, electrical treatments and massage to deliver intensive personalised regimes. These rigorous approaches required skilled personnel to provide the wide range of physical treatments. Opportunities for both male and female workers grew in a number of roles including giving baths, nursing, massage and management positions. The history of auxiliary health workers in the nineteenth century has been largely neglected with the development of formal training and professional associations receiving particular attention in the historiography.[114] In contrast this study has focused on charting the expansion in skilled roles that occurred and understanding the organisation of therapeutic practice.[115]

The medical profession had always claimed a monopoly on the prescription of spa regimens and by the 1870s sought to extend this principle to hydropathic treatments. Gerald Larkin has argued that medical practitioners, although perhaps sceptical about the therapeutic value of some physical therapies, were nevertheless concerned about competition for private patients from specialists in massage and electricity. They therefore supported the Board of Trade regulations for the incorporation of the Society of Trained Masseuses which stipulated that no massage was to be undertaken without medical prescription as they wished to see a register of trained practitioners that recognised their own superiority in the medical hierarchy.[116] Even if medical practitioners at spas were convinced of the value of hydrotherapy and other physical approaches some tension remained. Although medical practitioners remained responsible for prescribing treatments they lacked the expertise of the therapists who delivered them and whose training and skills exceeded their own. This included the ability to give an extensive range of baths, wraps and packs, to provide massage or to operate and supervise equipment for exercises or electrical treatments. Larkin concedes that medical influence was far greater over those masseuses who worked in hospitals than those employed in private practice and argues that the main area of dispute with the medical profession was over 'private practice in areas of treatment neglected by the modern medical profession'.[117] In practice it was difficult to assert medical authority on many practitioners or on patients. Men were excluded from membership of the Society of Trained Masseuses in its early years and some female therapists chose not to join it. Many therapists at watering places worked in organisations where medical influence was tempered by other interests, principally by investors in bathing institutions, while others took advantage of opportunities to work independently as self-employed practitioners. Patients were frequently charged separately for medical advice and the treatments provided by the therapist and opportunities existed to bypass medical advice and involvement.

Despite this, medical practitioners were able to exert influence over the water cure through a number of other strategies. Although appointments at the mineral water hospitals were honorary, they nevertheless played an important part in enhancing the professional reputation of the individual medical practitioners associated with them. Leading spa doctors at the resorts supported these new institutions. For example Henry Jephson was a founder member of the Warneford Hospital at Leamington in the 1830s and continued to work actively on the committee into the 1850s. William Henry Robertson (1810–97) worked tirelessly first for the Buxton Bath Charity and later for the DRH. He was one of several medical authors who wrote popular guides to resorts and the use of waters in addition to texts aimed at the medical profession.[118] By the end of the nineteenth century spa practitioners were also seeking to establish a more corporate identity, differentiating themselves as specialists within the medical profession. This was in line with broader trends with groups establishing clubs and setting up journals targeted first at general practitioners and later at members of their own community.[119] An honorary appointment brought access to patients and opened up the opportunity for research, an activity that became increasingly important in the inter-war period as discussed in Chapter 6.

Opportunities for paid work were also available at hydros. For example, at Rockside Hydro in Matlock, owned and managed by the Goodwin family from the 1890s, treatment was provided under the supervision of Marie Goodwin-Orme and her husband, both qualified doctors, supported by a team of specialist staff, including masseurs and hospital-trained nurses.[120] This model was similar to that at Smedley's where William Hunter was appointed after Smedley's death. The medical department continued to be supervised by qualified practitioners until the hydro's closure. By the end of the nineteenth century the most prestigious hydros reckoned that an association with a qualified doctor was likely to appeal to patients despite the fact that within these institutions patients might be able to use the baths and treatment facilities without first seeking medical advice. Smedley's charged an additional fee for a medical consultation and offered the option to deal directly with the employees providing the treatments and thereby avoid this optional charge. The smaller Matlock hydros did not employ qualified medical practitioners at all, but nevertheless continued to attract patients and to apply the simple hydropathic methods first promoted by the Smedleys.

Local authorities, which became increasingly important in running bathing establishments from the 1860s onwards, continued to value medical endorsement of the waters and by the end of the nineteenth century all were setting up more formal links with the profession. When the municipal authorities at Buxton took over management of the baths from the Devonshire estate in 1904 they set up an advisory committee to formalise communications with representatives of the local medical community. The advisory committee was asked to comment on equipment, treatments and staffing levels with some becoming involved in staff training and recruitment. However investment decisions and management responsibility remained with the local authority. Some issues, including the need for medical prescriptions, remained contested. In 1910 the Buxton spa committee agreed to display notices in the baths stating that a medical prescription was recommended and that management was empowered to refuse treatment to bathers without one. However the policy shied away from making a medical prescription compulsory.[121]

Conclusion

This chapter has presented evidence to show how the development of medical institutions and the presence of growing numbers of skilled workers shaped the character of English spas from the mid-nineteenth century. The methods of the water cure were transformed from the 1840s onwards prompted by the popularity of new hydropathic methods and auxiliary physical treatments and the need for individual businesses to maintain a competitive edge. There was a notable expansion in both the diversity of therapies employed and an increase in the intensity of therapeutic regimes. Innovation arose from personal experimentation by practitioners such as John Smedley and through a review of treatments and techniques available elsewhere. Some innovations at English spas were prompted by new bathing techniques imported from abroad, for example the development of massage douche at Aix-les-Bains and Vichy. The extent of this proliferation in techniques and therapies is neatly summed up by the advertisement for the Buxton Baths in 1906 which advertised that '100 medical treatments' were available.[122] Sixteen categories of treatment practices were in regular use, including ordinary baths at different temperatures, vapour and steam baths, sea water, natural mineral water and artificially prepared mineral, medicated, nutrient and aromatic baths and showers, douches, wet packs and sponging. In addition, there were sun baths, hot air baths – such as the Greville or Dowsing methods – mud and peat baths, mustard, bran and sand baths. Associated physical methods included massage, gymnastics and Swedish exercises. Various complex treatments, incorporating several of these methods, were widely available, including the Vichy Douche and the Nauheim method for cardiac cases. Some of these required one or two specialists per patient to prepare baths and give massages while further workers were needed to maintain facilities, including electrical and mechanical equipment.

The sector offered a variety of employment opportunities for practitioners in hydros, specialist bathing establishments and in hospitals, but also the option to work on a self-employed basis either alone or in small family-run businesses. The water cure was labour intensive, requiring the skills of large numbers of specialist bath men and women, medical rubbers and electricians to provide treatments. Despite the desire of the medical profession to assess and prescribe for patients, their ability to dominate therapeutic provision at the water cure was tempered by competition with other specialists and interests. In practice, patients were able to exercise choice in selecting an advisor and accessing the treatments offered by a number of independent businesses including hydros, bath houses and independent practitioners. At mid-century these skills were developed through hands-on experience but towards the end of the period under consideration more formal methods of training developed as part of the increasingly complex market for medical workers. Bathing facilities were segregated by sex, and this convention ensured that women were fully integrated as practitioners, working as bath women, masseuses and electricians. In institutional settings, there was scope for women to take up supervisory and managerial roles, although at all levels they were paid less than their male counterparts. A popular model for many women was the family business, which allowed them to participate as therapists and, as shown by Caroline Smedley and a cluster of family partnerships in Matlock, gave them the opportunity to shape and influence the practice of the water cure. In contrast to the image of women as subordinate workers in the medical hierarchy, specialising in caring rather than curing, the evidence presented shows that many women were recognised as skilled practitioners and worked in positions of considerable independence and autonomy.[123] Thus the water cure remained an area in which medical professionals faced difficulties in asserting dominance over therapeutic practice.

The discussion has also highlighted the important role of voluntary hospitals in shaping the medical spa. Originating in bathing charities which provided accommodation for poor patients, these institutions had a key role in expanding access for the working class to spa treatment. They attracted support from mutual societies and worker's funds and demonstrate that hydrotherapy treatment was perceived as offering real benefits to workers by those interested in their welfare. From the 1890s these institutions provided a platform for spa practitioners to promote the development of the new medical specialty of balneology. Chapter 6 will consider how further schemes to improve access for the working class were pursued in the inter-war period.

Notes

1 Jean Barclay, *In good hands: the history of the Chartered Society of Physiotherapy 1894–1994* (Oxford: Butterworth Heinemann, 1994); Gerald Larkin, *Occupational monopoly and modern medicine* (London: Tavistock, 1983), pp. 92–124.
2 Claridge, *Hydropathy*, opposite title page.
3 Smedley, *Practical hydropathy*, 17th edn (London: James Blackwood & Co., 1877), bath list dated January 1873, pp. 479–88. Descriptions of some baths were supplemented with images. See for example Smedley, *Practical hydropathy*, 13th edn, pp. 69a–69b.
4 Smedley, *Practical hydropathy*, 11th edn (London, W. Kent and Co., 1869), p. 12a. Sales figures quoted were 40,000 for *Practical hydropathy* and 30,000 for the *Ladies' manual*.
5 DRO, D1397 B/B 29, Smedley's Hydropathic Establishment, prospectus, p. 13.
6 DRO, D1397 B/B 35, W. B. Hunter, 'Smedley's as a winter resort for invalids'.
7 Silas Weir Mitchell, *Fat and blood; and how to make them* (Philadelphia, J. B. Lippincott, 1882); Hilary Marland, '"Uterine mischief": W. S. Playfair and his neurasthenic patients', in M. Gijswijt-Hofstra and R. Porter (eds), *Cultures of neurasthenia from Beard to the First World War* (Amsterdam and New York: Rodopi, 2001), 117–39.
8 DRO D3219/1/1–2, Smedley's Hydro case book for Isaac Bradburn.
9 'Hydropathic news', *Health Resort*, 6 (January 1905), 360–2.
10 Anon., *Extracts relating to baths, wells, etc. from the Presidential address delivered before the members of the Harrogate Medical Society*, 16 November 1893 (Harrogate: R. Ackrill, 1893).
11 Harrogate library, local studies, PH 615.49; Francis Barber, *The passing of the Victoria Baths: its significance, cost and consequence* reprinted from the *Harrogate Herald*, 16 September 1931 (Harrogate: R. Ackrill, 1931), p. 1.
12 Anon., *Extracts relating to baths and wells*, p. 5.

13 *Harrogate as a health resort* (Harrogate: Harrogate Corporation, 1898), p. 21. This was the first of a series of lavishly illustrated annual guides to the spa produced by the corporation.
14 'Improved bathing appliances at the Victoria Baths designed by William Bintiff Burkinshaw, Corporation mechanic', *Harrogate Advertiser* (11 April 1891), transcript in Harrogate Library, local studies, PH 615.49.
15 De Langenhagen, 'The treatment of muco-membranous colitis', *Lancet*, 4209 (30 April 1904), 1186–96. This article was cited in *Harrogate as a health resort* (Harrogate: Harrogate Corporation, 1908), p. 41.
16 *Harrogate as a health resort* (1908), p. 41.
17 Memorandum from the Harrogate Medical Society to the Baths and Wells Committee of the Harrogate Corporation, 'Better accommodation for, and more efficient treatment of patients at the Royal Baths', 4 December 1928. Harrogate Library, local studies, PH 615.49.
18 DRO, D1323/2/9/1, Buxton baths and wells committee minutes 1904–09, January 1907.
19 Langham and Wells, *Baths at Buxton Spa*, pp. 101–3.
20 LSAGM, M 4151 1994, Medical advisory committee minutes, 21 January 1920 'Report on a visit to Bath', 15 November 1923, 1 May 1924.
21 'Theodor Schott, 'The treatment of chronic diseases of the heart by means of baths and gymnastics', part 1, *Lancet*, 3534 (23 May 1891), 1143–4; part 2, *Lancet*, 3535 (30 May 1891), 1199–200.
22 Report of the *Lancet* commission on the balneological and gymnastic treatment of heart disease at Nauheim', *Lancet*, 3809 (29 August 1896), 619–21; 'Report of the *Lancet* commission on the balneological and gymnastic treatment of heart disease at Nauheim', *BMJ* (16 October 1897), 423–4.
23 W. Bezley Thorne, 'Chronic diseases of the heart by baths and exercises according to the method of Drs Schott', *Lancet*, 3688 (5 May 1894), 1117–20.
24 Samuel Hyde, 'The treatment of cardiac disease by baths, exercises and climate', *JB&C*, 2 (1898), 119–35.
25 Census enumerators' books, Great Malvern, 1861.
26 *Malvern Advertiser* (20 June 1857).
27 *Malvern Advertiser* (18 May 1861).
28 Census enumerators' books, Great Malvern, 1861 and 1881.
29 Census enumerators' books, Great Malvern, 1881.
30 *Malvern Advertiser* (1 June 1861).
31 DRO, D1397 B/B 1, Account and memorandum book J. J. (Jonas) Brown, April 1871.
32 DRO, D1397 B/B 35, Hunter, 'Smedley's as a winter resort', p. 15.
33 DRO, D1397 B/B 1, Account book, J. J Brown, p. 58.
34 Christopher Maggs, *The origins of general nursing* (London: Croom Helm, 1983), pp. 126–7.
35 Leonard D. Smith, 'Behind closed doors: lunatic asylum keepers, 1800–1860', *Social History Medicine*, 1(1988), 301–27, p. 310.

36 DRO, D1397 B/B 1, Account book, J. J. Brown, p. 71.
37 Smedley, *Practical hydropathy*, 17th edn, p. 4.
38 DRO, D1397 B/B.1, Account book, J. J. Brown, pp. 3–5.
39 Smedley, *Practical hydropathy*, 13th edn, Publicity insert for Matlock Bank Hydropathic Establishment, p. 446.
40 DRO, D1323/2/9/1, Buxton baths and wells committee minutes, 9 May 1905.
41 DRO, D1323/2/9/1, Buxton baths and wells committee minutes, 14 April 1905.
42 DRO, D1323/2/9/1, Buxton baths and wells committee minutes, 15 December 1905.
43 DRO, D1323/2/9/1, Buxton baths and wells committee minutes, 17 January 1909.
44 DRO, D1323/2/9/2, Buxton baths and wells committee minutes, 4 December 1914.
45 Arthur Smithells, *Report of a scientific survey of Harrogate spa waters (made in 1912–1919) for the Corporation of Harrogate* (Leeds: Chorley and Pickergill, n.d. but c. 1919), pp. 3–4, Harrogate Library, local studies, PH 615.9.
46 F. J. C. Broome, *The Harrogate fango treatment* (Harrogate: Harrogate Corporation, n.d. but c. 1928), Harrogate Library, local studies, PH 615.9.
47 D. Durward Brown and A. Woodmansey, 'The "fango" method of treatment in rheumatism', reprint of article published in *British Journal of Physical Medicine* (July 1935), Harrogate Library, local studies, PH 615.9.
48 DRO, D1323/2/9/1, Buxton baths and wells committee minutes, 23 March 1905.
49 DRO, D1323/2/9/1, Buxton baths and wells committee minutes, 6 September 1905.
50 DRO, D1323/2/9/2, Buxton baths and wells committee minutes, 20 September 1910, 29 November 1910.
51 DRO, D1323/2/9/2, Buxton baths and wells committee minutes, 7 January 1911, 10 April 1911.
52 DRO, D1323/2/9/1, Buxton baths and wells committee minutes, 21 October 1907.
53 Henry Steer, *The Smedleys of Matlock Bank: being a review of the religious and philanthropic labours of Mr. and Mrs. John Smedley* (London: Elliot Stock, 1897), pp. 93–4.
54 Steer, *Smedleys of Matlock Bank*, pp. 93–4.
55 Maggs, *General nursing*, p. 11.
56 Smedley, *Practical hydropathy*, 11th edn, p. 12b.
57 DRO, D1397 B/B 20, Matlock Bank Prospectus with rules and regulations, 1858.
58 *Harrogate cure* (Harrogate: Harrogate Corporation, 1929), p. 25.
59 Barclay, *In good hands*, p. 15.
60 'Immoral 'Massage' Establishments', *BMJ* (14 July 1894), p. 89; BMA, *Astounding revelations concerning supposed massage houses or pandemoniums of vice, frequented by both sexes, being a complete exposé of the ways of professed*

masseurs and masseuses (London: Skeats, 1894). For a discussion of the massage scandal in the context of contemporary concerns about sexuality and immorality, see Sheryl Root, 'The healing touch: spiritual healing in England, c.1870–1955', PhD thesis, University of Warwick, 2005, pp. 146–62.

61 Barclay, *In good hands*, pp. 38–9.

62 Root, 'Healing touch', pp. 153–4.

63 William Hardy, *Life and electricity in health and disease*, 2nd edn (Harrogate: T. Hollins Advertiser Office, 1870), p. iiii.

64 Hardy, *Life and electricity*, pp. 121–2.

65 Barclay, *In good hands*, p. 50.

66 John Jones, *The Benefit of the Auncient Bathes of Buckstones* (London: William Jones, 1572), cited in Langham and Wells, *DRH*, p. 9.

67 Robert Pierce, *Memoirs of Bath* (Bath: for the author, 1713), pp. 135 and 104–6, cited in Rolls, *Hospital of the nation*, pp. 3–4.

68 Anne Borsay, *Medicine and charity in Georgian Bath: a social history of the General Infirmary c. 1739–1830* (Aldershot: Ashgate, 1999), p. 232.

69 Broadside advertising the proposed hospital at Bath (1737), reproduced in Rolls, *Hospital of the nation*, p. 16.

70 See for example, John Woodward, *To do the sick no harm: a study of the British voluntary hospital system to 1875* (London: Routledge and Kegan Paul, 1974); John V. Pickstone, *Medicine and industrial society: a history of hospital development in Manchester and its region, 1752–1946* (Manchester: Manchester University Press, 1985); Hilary Marland, *Medicine and society in Wakefield and Huddersfield, 1780–1870* (Cambridge: Cambridge University Press, 1987); Borsay, *Medicine and charity*; Jane Adams, 'The mixed economy for medical services in Herefordshire, c. 1770–1850' (PhD dissertation, University of Warwick, 2004).

71 A. Jewitt, *The history of Buxton; and the visitor's guide to the curiosities of the Peak* (London: published by the author, 1811), pp. 65–7; Robertson, *Handbook to the Peak*, pp. 197–201; Buxton library local studies collection, Ernest Axon, 'Buxton Doctors since 1700, 8th paper, reprinted from the *Buxton Advertiser* (2, 9, 23 December 1939), pp. 7–11.

72 W. Bott, *A description of Buxton and the Adjacent Country or the New Guide etc* (Manchester: J. Harrop, 1796), cited in Langham and Wells, *DRH*, pp. 11–13.

73 Langham and Wells, *Baths at Buxton spa*, p. 36.

74 Robertson, *Handbook to the Peak*, p. 200.

75 Scudamore, *Tepid springs at Buxton*, pp. 3–6 cited in Langham and Wells, *DRH*, p. 13.

76 E. P. L. Dixon, 'Harrogate Royal Bath Hospital and Rawson Convalescent Home', typescript (1956), Harrogate Library, p. 1.

77 Granville, *Northern spas*, pp. 72–3.

78 Dixon, 'Harrogate Royal Bath Hospital', pp. 2–5; Jennings, *Harrogate*, pp. 297–9.

79 'Leamington Charitable Bathing Institution', *Leamington Spa Courier* (30 April 1831).
80 Adams, 'Accommodating the poor', p. 163.
81 J. Bissett, *A descriptive guide to Leamington Priors*, 2nd edn (Coventry: J. Bisset, 1816), pp. 37–8; *Warneford Hospital Annual Report* 1873, pp. 5–7.
82 'Leamington Charitable Bathing Institution', *Leamington Spa Courier* (30 April 1831).
83 'Leamington Benevolent Society', *Leamington Spa Courier* (8 January 1831).
84 'Leamington General Hospital and Dispensary', *Leamington Spa Courier* (22 January 1831).
85 'Leamington General Hospital and Dispensary', *Leamington Spa Courier* (15 March 1834).
86 'The Warneford General Bathing Institution and Leamington Hospital', *Leamington Spa Courier* (10 May 1834).
87 'The Warneford General Bathing Institution and Leamington Hospital', *Leamington Spa Courier* (31 January 1835).
88 Eric Baxter, *Dr Jephson of Leamington Spa*, Joan Lane and Robert Bearman (eds) (Warwick: Warwickshire Local History Society, 1980), p. 38.
89 *Warneford Hospital Annual Report* 1873, pp. 9–13.
90 Rolls, *Hospital of the nation*, p. 42.
91 *Harrogate Cottage Hospital, its history and developments* (Harrogate: R. Ackrill, 1896) reprinted from *Harrogate Advertiser* (11 January 1896).
92 Robertson, *Handbook to the Peak*, p. 203.
93 'Advertisement for a bazaar and fancy fair', reprinted in Langham and Wells, *DRH*, p. 22.
94 Langham and Wells, *DRH*, pp. 21–8.
95 DRO, D4508/10/1, *Devonshire Hospital Annual Report*, 1872.
96 Manchester local studies library, M558/1/1/1, CDCF, Governors committee minutes, 24 July 1875.
97 *Devonshire Hospital Annual Report*, 1862, p. 6.
98 CDCF, Governors committee minutes, 20 January 1879.
99 'Devonshire Hospital Buxton', *Builder* (10 July 1880), p. 4; and 'Devonshire Hospital Buxton', *Illustrated London News* (12 October 1881), p. 7.
100 Martin Gorsky, Martin Powell and John Mohan, 'British voluntary hospitals and the public sphere: contribution and participation before the NHS', in Steve Sturdy (ed.), *Medicine, health and the public sphere in Britain, 1600–2000* (London: Routledge, 2002), 123–44, pp. 126–9.
101 DRO, D4508/10/1, *Devonshire Hospital and Buxton Bath Charity Annual Report*, 1872, pp. 37–47.
102 DRO, D4508/31/2, DRH, Plan of proposed new baths, 1913.
103 DRO, D4508/7/3/4. Buxton co-ordinating committee, DRH, Information requested by Professor Cohen, MoH, 1945.
104 *Devonshire Hospital Annual Report*, 1904, cited in Langham and Wells, *DRH*, p. 106.

105 DRO, D4508/4/3/2, Minutes of honorary medical staff; Mercia M. Heyworth handwritten report 'Suggestions for re-organisation of the Massage department,' dated May 1930; DRO, D4508/4/3/3: Typed statement of review of Massage department and school 1925–31.

106 DRO, D4508/13/4, 'A plan for the Buxton centre for the treatment of rheumatism in a national scheme'.

107 Anon., *Woodhall Spa: English Kreuznach*, pp. 16–17.

108 Anon., *Woodhall Spa* (London: Ward, Lock and Co., 1902), p. 17.

109 Weaver, *Droitwich Spa*, pp. 80–2.

110 Birmingham Hospital Saturday Fund (BHSF), *Report and Annual Statement of Accounts*, 1918–23, 'Services provided for convalescent and brine bath treatment and surgical aid'.

111 Anon., *Birmingham' s triumph: The Hospital Saturday Fund* (Birmingham: BHSF, 1938); p. 13; BHSF, *Report and Annual Statement of Accounts*, 1938, p. 229.

112 BHSF, *Report and Annual Statement of Accounts*, 1936, p. 10.

113 Anon., *Birmingham's triumph*, p. 17; BHSF, *Report and Annual Statement of Accounts*, 1918–23, 'Services provided for convalescent and brine bath treatment and surgical aid'.

114 Jane H. Wicksteed, *The growth of a profession, being the history of the Chartered Society of Physiotherapy 1894–1948* (London: Edward Arnold, 1948); Barclay, *In good hands*.

115 A rare example of a detailed study of auxiliary workers other than nurses is Len Smith's work on asylum keepers in Smith, 'Behind closed doors'.

116 Larkin, *Occupational monopoly*, pp. 93–5.

117 Larkin, *Occupational monopoly*, pp. 92–3.

118 Obituary, William Henry Robertson', *JB&C* 1 (1897), 374–5. His two most popular works were *A guide to the use of the Buxton waters* (London: John Churchill, 1847) and *Handbook to the peak*, first published in 1854.

119 Lindsay Granshaw, '"Fame and fortune by means of bricks and mortar": the medical profession and specialist hospitals in Britain 1800–1948', in Lindsay Granshaw and Roy Porter (eds), *Hospitals in history* (London: Routledge, 1989), 199–220, p. 214.

120 DRO D3932/2. Promotional brochure for Rockside Hydropathic after opening of new wing, 1904.

121 DRO, D1323/2/9/2, Buxton baths and wells committee, 18 October 1910.

122 Frederick Roberts, 'Some general comments on balneology and associated methods: and on spas', *JB&C*, 10 (1906), 165–94.

123 For the relationship between the emerging nursing profession and medical practitioners in the nineteenth century see Robert Dingwall, Anne Marie Rafferty and Charles Webster, *An introduction to the social history of nursing* (London: Routledge, 1988), pp. 48–61; Brian Abel-Smith, *A history of the nursing profession* (London: Heinemann, 1960).

4

Water cure, regimen and healthy living

A conviction that regimen was an important influence on health was fundamental to the Greek concept of hygiene which recommended close attention be paid to air, exercise, sleep, diet, evacuations and the passions. [1] These ideas continued to influence both orthodox medicine and lay and popular healing traditions into the nineteenth century.[2] This chapter examines the appeal of the water cure for patients and practitioners in the context of ideas and concerns about health and healthy living. The close attention paid to the rituals of daily life at spas and hydropathic resorts contributed to their wider relevance and influence. Although spa medicine and hydropathy made use of many of the same water treatments and both gave advice on diet and exercise there were marked differences in the way the two systems were perceived depending on the broader beliefs and attitudes of individuals.[3] Accounts by patients and practitioners are used to explore the scope of interests that shaped individual experience and local practice and to trace the ways in which the principles of water cure were influential in both radical and mainstream health movements. Regimen was integral to the agenda of various health and social reform groups including those interested in temperance. While some of these ideas were associated with radical agendas including anti-vaccination, others were integrated with more broadly based movements such as physical fitness. The twentieth century brought renewed interest in regimen from both orthodox and unorthodox practitioners, reflected in increased emphasis given to health promotion by public health professionals and the rise of naturopathy as a healing approach distinct from orthodox medicine.

For some health reformers one aspect of regimen became the focus for action – for example diet was central to the developing vegetarian movement. Others within the diverse group of nineteenth-century medical irregulars were concerned with the full development of the individual and promoted the principles of self-management and lay expertise.[4] For many, an interest in health reform was integral to involvement in other campaigns, for example the promotion of dress reform or early feminism.[5] Hydropathy's association with fringe medicine around the 1840s was due in part to its links with the radical political and social reform movements of the period including Unitarianism and religious reform.[6] The system's emphasis on improving personal habits also tapped into a shift towards the domestic sphere as an important site for a broad reform agenda around mid-century.[7]

The appeal of water cures to a generation facing the social upheavals of the early industrial period is explored through the records of both patients and practitioners. Worry about how to counter the deleterious effects of more sedentary lifestyles and manage the stresses of contemporary urban life were real concerns for many.[8] Published accounts by patients detailing their experiences made a substantial contribution to the dissemination of both practical and theoretical information about hydropathy and helped to ensure its commercial success. These works were part of a wider genre of patient narratives dealing with illness and responses to it that were peculiar to the mid-Victorian period.[9] They provide a rich seam through which to explore the context of conviviality and community that underpinned the enduring popularity of water cures by satisfying 'a deep desire that the healing enterprise should proceed within frameworks essentially sociable in their nature, and suffused with symbolic cultural meanings'.[10] Health topics, including hydropathy, also provided popular subject matter for several of the new periodicals including *Punch* and *The Illustrated London News*. Many hydropathists produced works aimed at a general audience and urged active engagement in managing their health. For example the works of John and Caroline Smedley promoted hydropathy's potential to transform physical and spiritual health as well as fostering a spirit of self-reliance.[11]

The growing convergence in methods used at spas and hydropathic resorts from the 1870s has been seen as marking a decline in the practice of hydropathy as a distinctive form of unorthodox healing in Britain.[12] However the system's underlying principles of natural healing approaches and opposition to the use of drugs continued to influence health reform movements. Thomas Low and Mary Gove Nichols who came to England after the outbreak of the American Civil War were among those who propagated American ideas of health reform in Britain.[13] Hydropathy in America was influenced by the ideas of Sylvester Graham who propounded the benefits of the 'Science of Health' in the 1830s and by the 1850s the water cure movement had become integrated with a newer manifestation of health reform – hygeiotherapy – which promoted rules for healthy living.[14] The Nichols's periodical, *The Herald of Health*, was an example of an expanding range of specialist titles dealing with health and health-related matters which developed to cater for specific interest groups within a segmented market, including those attracted to the water cure. Edited by Thomas Low Nichols from its launch in 1875 to at least 1890, the paper continued to run into the twentieth century under the same title. The Nichols were active in the English food reform movement from the 1870s and promoted a wide range of causes in the pages of the *Herald of Health*.

American and European ideas were important to the re-emergence of natural healing practitioners in Britain in the early twentieth century.[15] American nature cure pioneers, including Benedict Lust and Henry Lindlahr, were influenced by developments in German approaches in the last quarter of the nineteenth century promoted by Sebastian Kniepp, Adolf Just and others who had adapted Preissnitz's methods. Lust is credited with coining the term naturopathy in 1901 and this term came into use in Britain around the same time. By the 1930s the number of practitioners calling themselves naturopaths exceeded a hundred and the system was being actively promoted as part of a healing tradition quite separate from orthodox medicine.[16] The basis of the naturopathic approach was that health was the natural state of the body and that disease arose from a failure to follow nature's laws through incorrect regimen. The task of the practitioner was to use natural methods, principally fasting and adjustments to diet, but also hydropathic baths, physical manipulation and other 'drugless' methods to encourage the body's natural propensity to heal itself.

The last decades of the nineteenth century brought a transformation in the concept of the ideal body for both men and women with increased emphasis given to exercise and fresh air to counter the effects of modern life.[17] It is argued that ideas expressed by hydropathists and embodied in water cure regimes as early as mid-century were forerunners to these trends and that practices developed at water resorts not only reflected changing health cultures but also influenced their formation. Hydropathic patients such as Bulwer Lytton celebrated a renewed feeling of positive health and vitality. At Malvern and Ilkley both male and female patients were encouraged to exercise and spend time in the fresh air and by the 1850s institutions at both resorts were promoting the new methods of physical training developed in Sweden. Spas were among the first places to make provision for a growing number of sports for both sexes including archery, croquet, swimming, tennis and golf. The specialist watering place offered not only a literal change of air but also the opportunity to dedicate the whole day, or the greater part of it, to staying or getting well. These principles appealed both to naturopathic practitioners who openly claimed to offer an alternative to orthodox medicine and the physical culture movement which was associated with a more mainstream interest in health, fitness and the outdoors.

Regimen and early nineteenth-century spa culture

The principle that a healthy regimen was fundamental to gaining and maintaining good health lay at the heart of both spa therapy and hydropathic practice. These principles can be traced back to classical notions of health and disease expressed in the work of authors including Hippocrates and Galen which emphasised the importance of six influences on the health of an individual; air, motion and rest, sleep and waking, substances taken, substances voided or retained and what happens to the soul. These factors were later termed the non-naturals, meaning factors external to the body, and were described as surroundings, exercise, sleep and rest, ingested substances (including food, drink and medicine) excretions and secretions (including sweat, urine and faeces) and the emotional state. In the early modern period these factors were used to maintain health (prophylaxis) as well as relieve symptoms and cure illnesses.[18] By 1800 disease was increasingly considered to be manifested locally, situated in individual organs and later cells, but despite this the overall physiological system continued to be recognised as important. A holistic model in which disease was understood to affect the whole being – or what was termed as the physical and the psychical – remained influential and regimen was used to influence both bodily and mental states. Water could be incorporated in a number of ways, for example advice to maintain a smoothly functioning digestive system might recommend the use of mineral waters as purgatives or laxatives to encourage the body to cleanse itself through emptying the stomach or bowels. Iron-rich chalybeate waters were commonly used as natural tonics to boost health. Attention to regimen was believed to be as important for healthy people as for those who were unwell, and was used to manage a variety of complaints. An underlying principle was the belief that therapies should be adjusted to the individual, taking account of their physical condition and mental state as well as their constitution.

One of the most celebrated English spa practitioners was Henry Jephson who worked in Leamington from the mid-1820s until his retirement in 1848. Jephson's practice attracted both upper- and middle-class visitors including the nobility and military. His reputation rested on his belief that 'most of our ailments sprang from bad habits of eating and drinking, so that in almost all cases he insisted upon a rigidly plain diet and abstinence from stimulants'.[19] The day started early with patients required to take a glass or two of mineral water, walk for twenty minutes, drink more water and take a further twenty-minute walk before breakfast. Baths or showers, if prescribed, were taken later in the day. Despite his reputation Jephson left no written account or case notes to explain his therapeutic approach. However, evidence drawn from scattered correspondence and diaries show that a plain diet was the norm, principally meat and bread with no soups, sauces, pies, fruit or cheese. Important principles underlying his treatment methods were minimal interference and recognition of the body's capacity to do much to heal itself if lifestyle was adjusted appropriately.

Directions given to Margaret Moss were for a very restricted dietary plan:

> Luncheon at one o'clock – a slice of lean meat or a mutton chop with stale bread, or dry toast, no liquid must be taken during the meal, but in half an hour after it one glass of sherry without water.[20]

The advice given to individual patients could be detailed as shown in this letter to Colonel Newdigate in August 1837.

> I recommend you use a tepid shower bath every morning with your head covered and your feet placed in water; and to take the mixture and pills now prescribed for four or five weeks.
> You must vary the dose of the pills according to the effects they produce upon your bowels.
> Walk for an hour before each meal.
> Live upon plain meat, poultry, game, mealy potatoes, stale bread, plain puddings, eggs lightly boiled, sherry, toast and water, black tea and butter only.[21]

John Ruskin received similar advice, with dinner and supper to consist of meat and bread only. He was also advised to walk morning and afternoon and to go to bed early. The importance of keeping quiet and ensuring sufficient rest was particularly emphasised.[22] Another patient, Dr Thomas Guthrie, was advised to abstain from 'all stimulants to the *body* and the *mind*' and told that 'he must talk less' to avoid over-stimulating the brain – advice he found hard to stick to.[23]

Jephson's insistence on the importance of walking was well known; even celebrated in comic verse as 'the main business of life' as shown in this extract from the anonymous poem *Leamington Peripatetics;*

> They WALK if they're Commoners, WALK if they're Peers;
> They WALK whether young, middle ag'd, or in years
> EPILEPTIC, DYSPOEPTIC [*sic*], NEURALGIC, what not,
> No matter what ails them, they SET OFF FULL TROT!
> ... In short, he makes those WALK who have ne'er walked before;
> And those who have always WALKED, here WALK still more ...[24]

Jephson expected his advice to be followed but was aware that some patients found difficulty in sticking to the restrictive regimes. He is reputed to have regularly attended the Pump Rooms or joined patients in their walks to provide gentle but firm supervision and support and even visited their hotels to ensure they were complying with his strictures. One report records him upbraiding an offending patient caught with an unsuitable hot buttered roll that was not on the list of recommended foods with the words 'Your Lordship may trifle with your stomach, but certainly not with my reputation'.[25]

Jephson does not appear to have participated in the public debate about hydropathy that raged during the 1840s. Although he did not, as far as we know, incorporate hydropathic baths into his practice, his advice to Colonel Newdigate, quoted above, included directions on showers and baths within the context of broader guidance. Although hydropathic treatment regimes gave greater emphasis to the internal and external application of water they too incorporated recommendations on other aspects of lifestyle including diet and exercise. Despite, or perhaps because of, his celebrity Jephson attracted allegations of quackery from some in the medical fraternity due to the emphasis he gave to the importance of the digestive system. Writing in 1861, J. C. Jeaffreson, another Leamington physician, noted that 'Most physicians would now disdain to give dietetic instruction to a patient beyond the most general directions.'[26] Still at the height of his powers when the uproar over hydropathy broke out, Jephson apparently preferred to quietly continue with his own successful practice and to eschew any publicity generated either through support of or opposition to the new system. Evidence from his practice illustrates his continued belief in the therapeutic potential of the non-naturals to address the health problems of his patients. His advice to John Ruskin in the 1840s shows that regimen remained at the heart of his approach, encouraging him to believe that 'there *is* nothing whatever the matter with me that I cannot conquer by quiet, regularity and exercise.'[27]

Hydropathy, healing and the pressures of modernity

Patient testimonials were key to the rapid growth in popularity of hydropathy in the early 1840s with works by Richard Claridge and others spreading knowledge about the system. Claridge described his personal experience of the strange, potentially dangerous and then little-known methods of hydropathy with the avowed intention to make better known a therapeutic system with a growing reputation on the continent. He promoted the system through a series of lectures throughout Britain and Ireland in 1842 and 1843 with his book going into a fifth edition within a year.[28] Claridge's work was a testimonial to the healing potential of hydropathy and its rigorous therapeutic regimes. He and his family stayed at Gräfenburg for three months, following a daily routine set out by Preissnitz. They not only gained health but also learned how to preserve it, ' ... we had been at Graffenburg 3 months, during which time ... health ... was perfectly established; we acquired the habit of living more moderately, of taking more exercise, of drinking more water, and of using it more freely in external ablutions than we were accustomed to; and I may add, that we have learned how to allay pain, how to ward off disease, and I hope, how to preserve health.'[29] Claridge's testimonial emphasised both hydropathy's potential to treat chronic conditions and its uses as a system of health maintenance to reduce troublesome symptoms from recurring.

The earliest published account by a patient describing their experience of hydropathy in England was authored by Edward Bulwer Lytton in 1845.[30] His public support for hydropathy tapped interest in the system from the literate middle classes among whom information was already circulating through informal networks.[31] The members of the literati who took the Malvern cure included Charles Darwin, Alfred Tennyson, Thomas Carlyle, John Ruskin and Harriet Martineau. Several individuals associated with the London-based publishing world authored articles and books recounting their experiences. The anonymous 'Life at the cold water and brandy cure', published in *Punch* in 1846 has been attributed to Douglas Jerrold, playwright and journalist.[32] John Leech, a caricaturist who described his stay in Malvern in *Three weeks in wet sheets*, worked for Jerrold's *Shilling Magazine*.[33] Richard Lane, who published an illustrated diary of a month spent at Malvern in 1845, which proved popular enough to be republished in 1851, was an established lithographer.[34] The contemporary interest in hydropathy was deemed to be of sufficient interest to some of those who made their living from these magazines for them to dedicate time to try it, spend time writing about it and to believe that it was of sufficient appeal to their readers to be featured in commercial periodicals.

Despite an enviable list of successful publications and an established reputation as an author, Bulwer Lytton considered himself an invalid, his health impaired by the rigours of life. Commenting on his frequent use of metaphors of 'wear and tear' and 'depletion' Maria Frawley argues that his work reveals deep-seated insecurities about the nature of mid-Victorian masculinity. He was an example of a seemingly increasing number of middle-class, often middle-aged men who suffered from 'overwork' or collapse due to an excess of 'brain work'.[35] Bulwer Lytton used his piece to call upon the brotherhood of those suffering nervous collapse due to hard mental work to dedicate themselves to a new way of living. The avoidance of artificial stimulants including alcohol and medical preparations or 'physic', adoption of the 'wonderful excitement' of hydropathic practice that acted on 'the passions and the mind' should be embraced by those wishing to journey 'towards recovery'.[36] As he declared 'at the water-cure the whole life is one remedy; the hours, the habits, the discipline – not incompatible with gaiety and cheerfulness tend perforce to train the body to the highest state of health of which it is capable'.[37] The vision of health Bulwer Lytton promotes is one of bodily vigour unimpeded by mental stress. He encourages others to try hydropathy and open themselves to experience 'the impatient rush into the open air … the sense of unwonted strength … the lush landscape far and wide below … exhilarating the blood, and lifting the spirits into religious joy … a hope that the very present was but a step … into a new and delightful region of health and vigour'.[38] Although the tone of much of the piece suggests the potential for hydropathy to effect a deep-seated transformation, there is recognition that the new state of grace may be hard won. After leaving Malvern Bulwer Lytton continued his treatment elsewhere and quotes 'a water doctor of repute at Brussels' as saying 'I do not expect you will be well while here – it is only on leaving me that you will know if I have cured you'.[39] Despite this, the overall message is one of optimism, a characteristic shared by other authors writing about Malvern. Richard Lane ended a schematic summary of his health problems endured over twenty-five years with the words 'advised to go to Malvern – went and took my boy to comfort me. Got well and wrote a book about it'.[40]

The appeal of the water cure was grounded in the fundamental economic and social changes of the early nineteenth century rooted in the industrial revolution. The generation reaching adulthood in the 1820s and 1830s was one in which significant numbers of educated men experienced work as alienating, often carried out in polluted urban environments and associated with dehumanising personal relationships.[41] Thomas Carlyle, treated by Gully at Malvern, compared his own life of speculation, writing and physical idleness, together with his failure to achieve an independent and productive career, with the more strenuous and active life of his father, James, who had worked as a stone mason and farmer.[42] In contrast to the healthy James who had spent his days in active and useful occupation, Thomas was an anxious, self-tormenting hypochondriac beset by chronic health problems put down to the pressures of modern life.[43] The link between mind and body had been undermined with deleterious effect on both. 'Men do less and speculate more. Thought without action has occasioned morbidity' so that 'modern thinking, self-conscious, logical, speculative, has become a stranger to itself'.[44] Carlyle understood his own poor health as intimately related to the wider unhealthy spirit of the age. In *Past and Present* published in 1843 he urged the need for both individual action to improve health and social measures including improved sanitary reform and the amelioration of degraded urban environments.[45] A potential solution for the individual was to harness nature's ability to cure in order to re-establish physical and mental equilibrium. Carlyle's decision to try the Malvern cure under the supervision of Gully was driven by a desire to relieve the physical and nervous symptoms brought on by the stresses of modern life through the natural processes of hydropathy.

For middle-class women this culture of invalidism was influenced by expectations of appropriate gendered roles regarding work inside and outside the home and concerns about the potentially harmful effects of intellectual activity. Adopting the role of a bed-ridden invalid was one option by which to navigate social pressures and expectations and thus gain a measure of control over one's life and offer a legitimate way to modify or avoid domestic duties. For Florence Nightingale time spent as an invalid offered respite from domestic responsibilities she was able to use to further her own interests outside the home.[46] Harriet Martineau perceived the collapse of her health in 1838 to be due to a combination of pressure to make a living as a writer and the stress of caring for her mother.[47] After some five years as an invalid, during which she had a prolonged stay at the seaside resort of Teignmouth, Martineau recovered her health through mesmerism. Nightingale undertook several stays at Malvern over the years as part of strategies to maintain her health and strength.

Nervous diseases had an importance in Victorian culture that went far beyond the medical profession and the individual patient. As Janet Oppenheim has noted, '[t]he nerves and their disorders were inextricably interwoven with nineteenth-century British assumptions about more than health and illness, or normalcy and deviance; they were interlaced with attitudes towards success and failure, civilisation and barbarism, order and chaos, masculinity and femininity'.[48] Nervous distress manifested itself in a variety of ways, through 'breakdown, depression, collapse, exhaustion, prostration, agitation and irritability', with symptoms including 'fatigue, insomnia, emptiness, weeping, impotence, obsessive fears, headache, backache, neuralgia, dyspepsia'.[49] These disorders were recognised as widespread from at least the eighteenth century onwards, called, among other labels, vapours, hysteria and hypochondria. In 1733 George Cheyne estimated a third of all disorders were some sort of nervous complaint, dubbing these the 'English Malady'.[50] There was a shift in ideas about the root cause of these disorders over the course of the nineteenth century. Whereas in the eighteenth century they were associated with politeness, affluence and excess, by the 1870s they were believed to be the result of stresses associated with labour in industrial society.[51] In the 1880s George Miller Beard, a neurologist and electrotherapist practising in New York, popularised a new term, neurasthenia, which he argued arose from the unique stresses of modern-day American life.[52] Although neurasthenia did not achieve the same popularity as a diagnosis in Britain as in America, the concept gained currency from the 1880s into the inter-war period, influenced by the experience of shellshock in the First World War. Neurasthenia became a convenient umbrella diagnosis for both men and women presenting with a wide range of symptoms which had no obvious origin and was particularly commonly used for middle-class private patients.[53] In line with contemporary understanding that the health of both the mind and the body had a physical basis, neurasthenia identified the nerves as the source of these disorders.

Spa treatment had an established pedigree in treating nervous complaints, used for example by George Cheyne who practised at Bath for a period each year, and hydropathy also became a popular treatment option for patients. The ability to adapt the system to either stimulate or pacify a patient meant it was well-suited to deal with the complex and often contradictory symptoms presented by patients.[54] Neurasthenia joined the already long list of disorders treated at spas and hydros. One popular treatment model was the 'rest cure' developed by Silas Weir Mitchell which used an intensive therapeutic package incorporating enforced bed rest along with food and massage. Several institutions, including Rockside hydro at Matlock headed up by the female doctor Maria Goodwin, gave their expertise in the 'Weir Mitchell treatment' considerable prominence in their publicity.[55]

Transformation, community and self-management

A wonderfully detailed account of the routines and vicissitudes of extended hydropathic treatment is provided in F. C. Foster's account of treatment at Matlock from August to October 1860. Published some ten years after his treatment, the journal was drawn from letters to his wife and family and describes the small steps towards recovery – often followed by reversals – experienced during his stay. Intended for a private rather than a public, commercial audience, it complements the more widely circulated accounts of treatment at Malvern. Foster believed he suffered from a nervous complaint brought on by 'study and exertion in my business' and made the long trip to Derbyshire from his home in Bridgewater, Somerset, seeking 'renewed health and vigour'.[56] His early days are marked by optimism; he records 'cases *precisely similar* to my own almost cured in a month'.[57] Despite a general feeling that the treatment is doing him good, Foster acknowledges that it could be tiring and tiresome. After a month of treatment he noted, 'My chest is become very sore with the continual mustard rubbings and this afternoon is unbearable. To-morrow is a day for rest and I am very glad of it'.[58] By early October, Smedley deemed Foster sufficiently recovered to alter his treatment with the intention of bringing on the crisis, designed to get the body to throw off morbid matter through encouraging eruptions on the skin. Foster's resigned comment that 'It will certainly torment me a little but I shall be very well compensated by the good results', is a testimony to the confidence he had built up in Smedley and his staff.[59] Foster found the treatment unpleasant, bringing him to a low ebb, causing him to 'feel languid and weak', reducing 'the buoyancy of my spirits', and resulting in considerable pain and discomfort through 'intolerable itching'.[60] Encouragement and support from the bath attendants and daily consultations with Smedley himself were important in maintaining his resolve to continue with the treatment and maintain a positive mental attitude. Smedley reassured him that he would feel better but only once he had had an opportunity to rest and recover as

> the system having become in great measure exhausted by the continual treatment, and from the exertions made by it to throw off the impurities contained therein, nature requires undisturbed rest and quiet in order that the body may gain its healthy functions and vitality which cannot be done while the system is being harassed by treatment.[61]

Although convinced that the system had done him good, Foster was only too ready to leave hydropathic treatment behind him when he returned home the following week at the end of his three-month stay.

Foster's account attests to the focus on healing at Matlock Bank under the guidance and management of the Smedleys. It highlights the individual care packages they developed for each patient and the importance of confidence in the hydropathic practitioner in ensuring a good outcome. Bulwer Lytton also emphasises the value of personal attention, noting 'the anxious, unaffected interest, which Doctor Wilson manifests to every patient'.[62] Confidence in the hydropathist and his system was central to the cure. One reason for Wilson's success, Bulwer Lytton suggests, was that 'he has that earnest faith in his own system, which begets an earnest faith in those to whom he administers'.[63] Hydropathy certainly required compliance from individual patients in attending to their own regime but also encouraged participation in the communal life of the institution. While the daily routine at hydropathic institutions was similar, the culture of each hydro reflected the personality and interests of the proprietor. The descriptions of life at Matlock and Malvern indicate that the shape of the patient's day at the English hydros closely followed the routine established by Preissnitz, organised around rising early, morning and afternoon treatments, three communal meals and an early bedtime. The limited time not dedicated to treatment was taken up with exercise or excursions with patients having some discretion in what they chose to do. Although Foster mentions that trips were organised to a variety of places of interest including Chatsworth, Lea Mills (Smedley's woollen factory) and Darby [*sic*] Dale during his stay, he refused some of these invitations, preferring to spend time walking with 'poor Brown', a friend from Bridgewater who was also in Matlock for treatment. Foster entered into a correspondence that secured funding to enable Brown, who had exhausted his own financial resources, to stay on at Matlock another month despite the likelihood that any further treatment was only likely to be of limited use.[64] Brown was not staying at the main hydro but nearby, perhaps in one of the cheaper establishments run by one of the Smedleys' employees. The two men met frequently to walk in the surrounding area and Brown also attended chapel at the main hydro. In addition to cultivating this link with home, Foster corresponded with family and friends and also had an unexpected visit from an acquaintance, William Haslam, who dropped in on his way from Bridgewater to Sheffield.[65] Thus despite being a considerable distance from his family for a period of some weeks Foster was supported throughout his extended treatment by a network of friends and acquaintances.

These personal accounts of life at hydros catering for the better off, such as those run by Wilson and Smedley, stress their domestic culture, which replicated that of the Victorian bourgeois home. John Tosh has described the period between 1830 and 1860 as the heyday of domesticity, arguing that it 'denotes not just a pattern of residence or a web of obligations, but a profound attachment: a state of mind as well as a physical orientation'.[66] Communal meals, parlour games, prayers, a piano and library all endorsed the ideals of middle-class family life. A few hours after dinner and before bed were set aside as a time for patients to socialise together in a variety of activities. For the hydropathic patient removed from the bosom of their family a hydro could provide a stable, safe and convivial environment in which to recover sufficiently to be able to return to their own home. One reason why the family business was so suitable for hydropathy was that there was a natural female figurehead to set an appropriate tone for female patients.[67]

For Foster, a practising Christian, one of the particular attractions and 'important and distinguishing' features of Smedley's establishment was 'its spiritual character', based on Christian values.[68] Foster was profoundly impressed by Smedley, describing him as a 'Christian Philanthropist of no common order'.[69] Prayers and bible readings were held each morning and evening with further services on Sundays. Although Smedley was deeply religious he was not associated with either the Anglican or organised free churches, and dedicated Sundays to preaching the gospel in a marquee, events that sometimes attracted up to fifteen hundred people.[70] In line with his principles, all patients were encouraged to attend the services at the hydro, whatever their spiritual preference. There was 'nothing sectarian, nothing biasing, nothing bigoted or narrow minded in the whole of the matter, but the services are left free and untrammelled, so as to be participated in by all'.[71] Patients were encouraged to actively contribute, for example Mr Binney, an established preacher from an 'independent persuasion of Christians', occasionally led prayers as well as officiating at several Sunday services.[72] Smedley publicly acknowledged his hydropathic practice was an integral part of a new life course based on Christian values chosen after recovering from a nervous collapse. Following successful treatment at Ben Rhydding and having 'found peace in believing', Smedley and his wife determined to dedicate themselves to 'a life of usefulness' for others, based around hydropathic practice and other philanthropic work.[73] Caroline Smedley also saw her practice as a hydropathist as fulfilling her Christian duty to be useful and charitable, despite personal sacrifice, recording that 'when we see the certain effects of our treatment, we cannot for a moment think of leaving such a glorious work, so long as God enables us to go on'.[74]

The Smedleys' influence among patients extended well beyond those treated at Matlock. Sales figures for their books given in 1878 were 85,000 for *Practical hydropathy* and 48,000 for the *Ladies' manual*.[75] In addition to promoting the hydro at Matlock, these books also aimed to educate the reader, 'to teach Hydropathic remedies for self-application', so that the working classes would be able both to maintain health and treat the early symptoms of diseases including fever, consumption, and inflammation from really taking hold of their system.[76] Patients who attended the hydro developed some expertise in self-management while the manual contained illustrations demonstrating the simple equipment needed and provided guidance on how to improvise kit at home. The basic equipment required for home treatment was available for purchase and details of recommended suppliers were provided. Railway transport and the improved postal service meant all these appliances could be easily obtained by readers. The popularity of *Practical hydropathy* was not limited to Britain. Metcalfe notes that Smedley's influence spread throughout the British empire; noting that he 'had men traveling the Colonies for years introducing the handbook, and making the Water Cure method known wherever there was a centre of population'.[77] In line with their view of themselves as health missionaries, the Smedleys gave advice by letter where patients could not travel to Matlock. Later editions of the books include some of this correspondence along with patient testimonials, recording the voice of patients in a limited manner through the recorded discussions of their experience of using the manual and knowledge acquired at the hydro. The works proclaimed the lifestyle changes needed to support good health such as 'the temperate use of plain and wholesome food, cleanliness, and taking proper open air exercise, with that proper denial in abstaining from intoxicating drink, smoking, and other pernicious habits, and a strict governance of the passions'.[78] Thus, although the Smedley's practice was rooted in Matlock, the extensive circulation of their manuals enabled their health message to reach a far wider audience, inviting engagement in a common journey from ignorance towards knowledge, mirroring the journey from disease towards health.

Hydropathic manuals such as those by the Smedleys continued a long-established tradition of self-care which aimed to promote the skills needed for effective self-management and the use of home remedies.[79] For some consumers the economics of capitalist medicine in which the doctor's financial interests were served by keeping patients ill, further encouraged the ideal of self-help and keeping healthy.[80] As opposition to hydropathy from orthodox practitioners declined, bathing and hydropathic applications for home use were increasingly included in a broad spectrum of advice literature written by both health reformers and more mainstream authors. Regular bathing was increasingly accepted as a part of a healthy regimen and its use in hygienic and beauty routines increased, promoted in articles in mainstream advice literature such as *The Domestic Magazine* and *Journal for the Household* and *Good Health:*

a Journal for Everybody.[81] Many manuals for domestic use included advertisements for products for home use including foodstuffs, domestic appliances, baths and clothing. By the 1880s the rising purchasing power of the late Victorian consumer as well as improved domestic water supplies further stimulated the creative use of hydropathy at home. [82]

Life reform and the radical tradition

Radical conceptions of lifestyle reform and a belief in the ability of education to promote good habits were central to the work of Mary Gove and Thomas Low Nichols who left America for England in 1861 at the outset of the Civil War. Both Mary and Thomas had been involved with water cure In North America for over twenty years. Mary had lectured on physiology and together they had edited health journals, run a hydropathic centre, a vegetarian community and the American Hydropathic Institute. Among the radical issues they embraced were dress and marriage reform, birth control, natural childbirth and anti-vaccination.[83] They arrived in England penniless, at first earning their living as journalists, contributing both fiction and non-fiction pieces to a variety of publications including Charles Dickens' *Household Words*. Their first years in England were fraught with financial and personal difficulties, compounded by the early death of their daughter, aged 14, in 1864. In 1867 they moved to Aldwyn Towers in Malvern and opened a water cure centre and by the 1870s were involved in a series of ventures promoting health.[84] Mary, now in her mid-fifties, losing her sight and in general poor health, took the lead at Malvern while Thomas concentrated on re-launching their work as health reformers in London. In 1868 *A woman's work in water cure*, a revised version of Mary's earlier *My experience in water cure*, was published, setting out the manifesto for their future work.[85] They were devoted to both 'teaching and healing', complementing a small hydropathic practice with 'teaching persons to cure themselves so they will neither require to come to me nor to go to any other physician'.[86]

The vehicle for their reform agenda was *The Herald of Health*, a fortnightly publication launched in 1875 which aimed to provide its readers with both information and inspiration. At first priced at 1d, by 1878 an expanded format was sold for 6d. Regular editions were later supplemented by an annual Almanac, priced at 1s. The publication reflected the Nichols's wide interests which included hydropathy, temperance and dietary reform. Each edition included one substantive article, frequently closely based on material from one of their publications such as *How to live on sixpence a day* as well as reprinted material from selected periodicals such as *Dietetic Reformer*, *Vaccination Inquirer* or the temperance journal *The Crusade*.[87] Their aim was to promote improved lifestyles and the magazine aimed to provide the wherewithal for readers to adopt reformed habits. A sizeable section was taken up with advertisements; all the Nichols own works were listed as well as numerous water cure appliances, several of which were their own invention. These included the Portable Fountain Bath 'for the home treatment of constipation, piles, fistula, protrusion of the lower bowel, falling and displacement of the womb, vaginal weakness. 63 shillings – carriage free' and the Turco-Russian Hot-Air or Vapour Bath that 'enables anyone to take the Turkish Bath or Steam Bath in his bedroom'. Vegetarian foodstuffs, including Nichols own make of bran were also advertised along with the associated Alpha restaurant, the first vegetarian restaurant in London which opened in 1879.[88]

The Herald of Health, through its continued promotion of a broad reform agenda was a vehicle for self-help, reaching out to a wider community of those attracted by its promise of health. The title was one of an extensive wave of new publications developed during the Victorian period that helped to shape new ways of living, providing both philosophical and practical guidance.[89] For the Nichols, hydropathy was part of a wider agenda aimed at producing a healthy individual in harmony with others. Considerable emphasis was given to instruction on the 'rules of health'. 'Health, in those who have the blessing of a good constitution, is maintained by a simple nourishing diet, pure air, exercise, cleanliness and the regulation of the passions'.[90] Their vision of health was grounded in holistic principles in which body and mind were united in useful purpose; health 'is the perfection of bodily organisation, intellectual energy, and moral power'.[91] Mary in particular was held up as an example; she had been a vegetarian for forty years, and was presented as devoted to unselfishly helping others despite the strains on her own physical and mental resources. In 'To my friends', written in 1880, she wrote 'My life is nearly lived and I want to make what remains of the greatest possible use'. To this end she intended to cease her hydropathic practice and instead dedicate her time to writing as a 'book may do for thousands, and for coming generations, what I may do by individual effort for very few'.[92]

The Nichols had developed their approach to water cure in the American context where hydropathy built on earlier established health reform movements. During the 1830s Sylvester Graham promoted the 'Science of human life', asserting the importance of adopting good habits and renouncing bad ones in order to maintain good health. James Whorton argues that it was the association of behaviour with personal morality that set Graham's system of healthy living apart from the regimen of classical times; whereas orthodox medicine asserted the benefits of moderation in all things, Graham's system banned various habits associated with immorality or excessive stimulation as well as prohibiting the use of medical drugs.[93] In addition to asserting the need for a vegetarian diet and the avoidance of alcohol and tobacco the Grahamite system also required avoidance of tea, coffee and spices and promoted the value of brown bread. In addition to these dietary rules prohibitions were set on other habits including sex which was to be limited to within wedlock. Masturbation, the solitary vice, was abhorred. Costume was to be adapted to promote health and allow free movement with particular criticism directed at the fashion of tight-laced corsets for women. Many of these Grahamite principles were endorsed by the next generation of American health reformers including Russell Trall and Joel Shew who also adopted the hydropathic system. By the 1850s the term hygeiotherapy was used to describe a broad approach that incorporated water cure along with diet and exercise in treatment regimes applied in a context of broader lifestyle reform. Graham was also a pioneer in the popularisation of his ideas through lectures, books and magazine articles and these became the standard methods used by later generations of health reformers.[94]

Mary Gove was introduced to the Grahamite movement in 1837 and became an active proponent of the system, introducing its principles into schools in Boston. She was one of the first cohort of female physiology lecturers dedicated to improving women's knowledge about their bodies and health and later graduated as a water cure doctor.[95] In North America, hydropathy was associated with the early women's movement and causes such as the training of independent women practitioners and the articulation of the need for dress and marriage reform.[96] Whorton argues that interest in hygeiotherapy was at its peak between the 1840s and 1870s, a period characterised by earnest optimism in the potential for individual and social improvement which later declined in the face of growing pessimism stimulated by the horrors of the Civil War and the increased consumerism that developed from the 1880s.[97] Although hygeiotherapy was not widely promoted under that term in Britain, the launch of the London Vegetarian Society in 1872 and Nichols's *Herald of Health* in 1875 demonstrates growing interest in a broad health reform agenda. P. S. Brown notes the influence of other Americans, including Lorenzo Niles and Lydia Folger Fowler and Emmet and Helen Densmore, in disseminating hygienic principles and the importance of natural healing in Britain in the late nineteenth century.[98]

The appeal of social and lifestyle reform movements for many of those espousing the medical hetereodoxies of hydropathy, homeopathy or medical herbalism is well established for the British context too.[99] The vegetarian and food reform movement urged the importance of using natural foodstuffs as the only sure foundation for good health and many hydropathists espoused the temperance cause.[100] One notable individual who took the pledge was Ralph Grindrod, a qualified doctor, active member of the Manchester and Salford Temperance Society and author of several influential temperance tracts.[101] In 1838 his long essay *Bacchus* won a prize from The New British and Foreign Temperance Society and became a well-used resource by campaigners.[102] Grindrod spent six years as a full-time temperance advocate and lecturer becoming very influential in the movement before setting up in hydropathic practice at Malvern in 1850.[103] Other hydropathists advocating the temperance cause included Archibald Hunter, who worked at Bridge of Allan along with his second wife, Annie Steedman Hunter.[104] Following her husband's death in 1894 Annie continued to treat patients using hygienic principles as well as working for the vegetarian and anti-vaccination causes.[105]

The editorship of the *Herald of Health* passed from Nichols to Charles Forward in 1886 and later to James Salisbury, promoter of vegetarian restaurants, before the title was sold to Mrs Chandos Leigh Hunt in June 1890.[106] The new owner was another active campaigner. She promoted the 'Wallace system' for total health reform through the Physical Regeneration Society, the rules of which were listed in each copy of the magazine. Dedication to the vegetarian cause was an important part of her agenda and Leigh Hunt authored recipe books, established a cookery school, a vegetarian boarding house and a bakery that eschewed the use of yeast, deemed to be injurious to health. An article in 1900 marking the end of the first decade of her editorial tenure, an anniversary which coincided with her husband Joseph Wallace's eightieth birthday, provided an opportunity to celebrate the success of their 'Wallace system'. Key to its power was its inclusive approach to 'right living' which embraced food, drink, clothes and exercise and was well publicised through the *Herald of Health*. Their system was firmly in the unorthodox camp, adopting an anti-vaccination stance and urging the avoidance of orthodox medicines while also promoting the benefits of various homeopathic remedies developed by Joseph Wallace.[107]

By the early 1900s nature cure began to emerge in Britain as a distinctive healing approach, influenced by the movements in North America and central Europe as well as the English trends in life reform discussed above. German emigrants introduced traditions of holistic approaches to America where they were taken up by a new wave of practitioners. Metcalfe noted that Kellogg's huge sanatorium at Battle Creek was based on 'nature cure' principles espoused in Germany, Sweden and Denmark and that Koch introduced German Naturheilkunde into his American practice in 1889 followed by the Kniepp method in 1891.[108] Sebastian Kneipp developed a successful practice at Worisophen which attracted an international clientele including Benedict Lust, later a leading American naturopath. *My water-cure* published in 1886, which set out the Kniepp system, had run to thirty-three German editions and been translated into several foreign languages by 1891.[109] In 1897 Lust opened his flagship sanatorium, Yungborn, in America. It was named after an institution opened by nature cure proponent Adolf Just at Jungborn in Germany the previous year. Lust's first publications, started in the 1890s were in German but by 1900 he had switched to using the English language. The *Kneipp Water Cure Monthly*, later renamed *The Naturopath and Herald of Health*, promoted a wide range of natural and drugless healing approaches including hydrotherapeutics, diet, exercise, sunbathing and massage as well as the new drugless healing methods of osteopathy and chiropractic which used physical manipulation.[110] Lust opened the first training school for naturopaths in New York in 1901 and founded the Naturopathic Society of America the following year.[111] The first decades of the twentieth century were ones of expansion for natural healing in America; in 1906 Metcalfe reported there were over two hundred and fifty institutions and more than two thousand practitioners.[112] By 1923 Lust claimed there were more than a dozen training schools, over nine thousand naturopaths and some five hundred nature cure institutions in America.[113]

In 1906 the British Association for Nature Cure was founded by Watson Macgregor Reid, an unqualified healer, with Annie Stedman

Hunter and A. T. Story, secretary of the British Phrenological Association, as vice presidents.[114] The *Nature Cure Annual* of 1907/08 shows the continuing influence of the hydropathic tradition as well as the emergence of new trends in nature cure. In addition to a photograph of a group gathered to celebrate the centenary of Preissnitz's birth, there were advertisements for Metcalfe's hydro at Richmond Hill and various publications by Archibald and Annie Hunter as well one for Orchard Leigh, owned by Bernarr Macfadden and described as 'a health home ... conducted on Physical Culture principles'.[115] Part of naturopathy's appeal was its close association with wider trends of self-improvement, including the growing physical culture movement in which Macfadden was a leading player. Stanley Lief who became one of the leaders of naturopathy in Britain in the inter-war period, trained with Macfadden in America before moving to Britain around 1914 to work for him in Brighton and later at Orchard Leigh.[116] Another practitioner who travelled to America was James Thomson who trained with Henry Lindlahr in Chicago before setting up a successful practice in Edinburgh around 1919.[117] Others gained their experience from the European tradition of nature cure. Andrew Pitcairn-Knowles, who opened the Riposo Health Hydro in Hastings in 1913, had lived much of his life in Europe and his institution specialised in the cure method developed by Johann Schroth, a contemporary of Preissnitz.[118]

Despite scattered evidence of individual practices before 1914 it was not until the inter-war period that naturopaths began to assert a more coherent identity in Britain. Milton Powell, who had also been introduced to naturopathy by Macfadden, launched a call for a national register of practitioners in 1919 and in 1921 the Nature Cure Association of Great Britain and Ireland was founded.[119] The third volume of *The health and nature cure handbook*, published in 1934 listed over one hundred and fifty practitioners and thirty treatment centres.[120] The best-known resort was Champneys at Tring in Hertfordshire, led by Stanley Lief who also ran a successful practice in London and was instrumental in launching *Health for All* magazine in 1927. Naturopaths used a wide range of natural and drugless treatments with particular emphasis given to fasting. Bathing and hydropathic methods continued to be seen as valuable natural therapeutic measures, with several homes, including Riposo, having extensive hydrotherapeutic facilities. Gordon Pitcairn-Knowles advertised Riposo as 'one of the great British centres of hydro-therapy' as well as promoting the benefits and possibilities of using the water cure at home.[121] Diet and exercise were integrated into treatment and sunbathing and an open-air life encouraged. Nature cure revitalised the radical agenda of opposition to orthodox medicine in the inter-war period. The rhetoric of naturopathy was that it stood in opposition to the fallacies of orthodox ideas and practices which treated the symptoms of disease rather than addressing the foundations of good health. Tensions between naturopaths, the state and the orthodox profession were heightened by the extension of access to state-funded health care in the inter-war period as practitioners such as osteopaths and naturopaths continued to rely on patients paying for their treatment. Many supplemented their income from outpatient fees with a range of other activities including running inpatient nature cure homes, teaching, publishing periodicals and monographs and business ventures including restaurants and health food shops.[122]

Handbooks published in the 1930s point to there being some 150 nature cure practitioners in Britain. However, many of the principles of right living fundamental to their approach had wider circulation than this indicates. By the end of the nineteenth century there was a growing consensus about the deteriorating health of working-class men and women due to poor living and working conditions. The extent of this degeneration, passed through several generations, was sufficient to undermine the strength of the nation through reduced vigour and strength of workers, soldiers and mothers. From the 1880s an emphasis on changing personal habits was increasingly endorsed by a range of societies as well as state institutions with the aim of improving health. By the late nineteenth century a growing physical culture movement disseminated ideas about fitness through magazines, including *Vim* and *Health and Strength*, and clubs and societies. Despite the focus on muscular development there was an acknowledgement that diet, exercise, fresh air and general hygiene were essential components of fitness regimes.[123] Several leading figures in the physical culture movement including Macfadden and Eustace Miles, the vegetarian athlete, were associated with the nature cure movement and promoted a wider agenda of natural living.

Gymnasiums began to open from the 1890s and by 1914 there were some 250, mainly in London and the larger industrial towns.[124] Attitudes towards physical culture for both men and women had begun to shift earlier than this. Fostered by the public schools which developed from the 1850s, the focus on team games, endurance, competition and loyalty to a male fraternity rather than the domestic family profoundly affected the nature of middle-class male culture. The ideal of masculinity that emerged gave more emphasis to self-reliance and physical fitness.[125] Despite a general decline in religion, the ideal of 'muscular Christianity' became influential, promoting the idea that healthy manliness could be obtained through discipline and physical activity.[126] These decades also saw a marked change in the physical culture of women. In the early 1850s their sporting activities were limited to archery, riding or walking and the new game of croquet. In the 1870s the *Queen* included lawn tennis, swimming, ice- and roller-skating as suitable activities for women and by the 1890s had added hunting, angling, riding, sailing, curling, golf, hockey, rowing, gymnastics and cycling to this list.[127] Facilities for sport at spas in the middle decades of the century show they were at the forefront of these trends with exercise integrated into therapeutic plans. Physical activity adapted to the capabilities of the individual patient was an integral part of the ideal regimen of the classical authors and had long been incorporated into daily routines at spas. Walking was strongly recommended by Henry Jephson at Leamington and received even greater emphasis in Preissnitz's regime. Walks on open hillsides were one of the attractions at Malvern and Ilkley, enthusiastically promoted in the accounts of Bulwer Lytton and Richard Lane.

The early hydropathic institutions were also at the forefront of the design and provision of more systematic exercise regimes, a feature particularly associated with William Macleod at Ben Rhydding. By 1852 the hydro had a large gymnasium housing the specialised equipment needed to provide the Ling System of gymnastic movements under the direction of a professional gymnast.[128] This system had been developed by Pehr Hendrik Ling in Sweden in the early decades of the nineteenth century and comprised a series of movements useful for both hygienic and therapeutic purposes. Ling distinguished four separate areas, the 'pedagogic' for healthy people, the medical, the military and the aesthetic.[129] With state support Ling opened the first gymnastic institution in Stockholm in 1812 and the system gained sufficient renown and status to continue to be taught after his death in 1839. Macleod was one of the first British medical practitioners to seriously assess its potential, Richard Metcalfe considered him to be an innovator in the use of gymnastics as a therapeutic tool adapted to the age and physical abilities of patients unable to take much walking exercise.[130] Ling's medical system as originally envisaged comprised a trained instructor working with a single patient to deliver graduated exercise tailored to the abilities and needs of the individual. Treatment options ranged from passive movements, similar to massage, in which the patient remained quiet with the bodily movements initiated by the instructor, to active movements in which the patient carried out set movements under supervision.[131] By the early 1860s a series of free movements loosely termed 'drill' and designed to exercise specific muscle groups including the abdomen, shoulders, back and chest, were encouraged at Ilkley.[132] Details were provided in *The Ben Rhydding book of gymnastics*. Walking was still encouraged, especially when enhanced by the wearing of an iron crown, weighing between three to fifty pounds, intended to improve posture. A short run of fifteen minutes a day was also recommended. However most emphasis was given to the Ben Rhydding drill which comprised marching in company, with forward and backward steps at a variety of paces including slow, double and quick, controlled by instruction from a drill leader. The basic sequence was designed to be done in a group by both male and female participants and incorporated a series of simple gymnastic movements. The booklet also outlined instructions for using the extensive equipment provided in the gymnasium which included resistance exercises with rings performed with a partner, use of a shoulder-push and dumb bells. There was also an opportunity to work on 'The Gymnastic Polymachinon' resistance apparatus which facilitated a variety of movements including rowing. This ingenious machine had been invented by a Captain Chioso and was also in use at his gymnasium in Oxford Street. The booklet concluded with a description of the rules of croquet which had recently been introduced and which now shared the green previously reserved for bowling.[133] By 1867 there was also an American Bowling Alley and a Racket Court at the hydro.[134] Similar trends are evident at other centres; Smedley's hydro had extensive outdoor 'airing' grounds by the 1860s where patrons could enjoy walking, archery and croquet. Tennis courts were later added with golf available close by. Lawn tennis, a variant of real tennis was first developed at Leamington in 1872 and in 1881 the town hosted the first of its annual tournaments.[135]

Once again, it was the problems of modern life, especially the physical effects of working environments that were perceived to lead to the requirement for more active physical therapeutic approaches. Many occupations required sitting or stooping postures to be held for long periods of time or necessitated repetitive movements. Compounded with long hours and a lack of fresh air, these conditions resulted in physical aches and pains or damage to the musculo-skeletal frame. The provision of specialised facilities for gymnastics and other exercise were also considered by James Wilson when designing his hydro, the Establishment in Malvern in 1851. Richard Lane noted plans for 'billiard-rooms and gymnastic instruments; covered walks for wet weather, and every appliance for the more delicate invalid'.[136]

The decision taken in 1911 by Harrogate council to invest in a separate hall for Mechano-Therapeutics illustrates the further uptake of these ideas in Britain. The decision was prompted by the desire to not only match but outdo facilities at continental spas where the Ling exercises and the alternative Zander system based on apparatus to train specific muscle groups were more widely available. At Harrogate it was decided to construct a universal apparatus which could be adapted to provide a wide variety of passive and active exercises for use in physical rehabilitation in the treatment of fractures, sprains and lameness. Other equipment, designed to be fully adjustable to individual height and strength, included the Velotrab designed to emulate both horse trotting as well as the newly popular sport of cycling and the 'Sano' exercise apparatus which reproduced the movements used in rowing and hill climbing.[137] The name of the latter, alluding to the popular saying 'mens sana in corpore sano' – a healthy mind in a healthy body – was indicative of the growing commercialisation of physical training equipment.

Conclusion

This chapter has examined the culture of health associated with English spas and the water cure to explore their appeal to patients and to demonstrate how treatment approaches based on regimen had wider significance and impact through links to lifestyle reform movements. Health played an important part in personal identity, embodying concerns associated with gender roles and the uneasy relationship between the individual and a rapidly changing world. In the 1830s Thomas Carlyle 'identified health with an active, vigorous life' that was of use to the wider community, his ideal man 'being whole himself, he helps create wholeness'.[138] The approach to healing at spas and hydropathics was rooted in treating the whole patient through specialist treatment but also through management of diet and daily routines. The emphasis on nature and the cultivation of good habits enjoyed during a period of respite from the world continued to be of interest to individuals in dealing with their own health and that of their families. While both orthodox and unorthodox medicine emphasised the importance of regimen to health, for some practitioners the reform of personal habits was associated with more radical agendas such as temperance and vegetarianism. A flourishing market for periodical literature provided the chief mechanism for dissemination of these ideas. Life reform and natural approaches to health maintenance and treatment in England were influenced by trends in Europe and North America. By the early twentieth century a new generation of unqualified healers promoting the full potential of the life reform message were beginning to forge a separate identity as nature cure practitioners.

Notes

1 Virginia Smith, *Clean: a history of personal hygiene and purity* (Oxford: Oxford University Press, 2007), p. 75; Klaus Bergdolt, *Wellbeing: a cultural history of healthy living*, trans. Jane Dewhurst (Cambridge: Polity Press, 2008), p. 87.

2 Charles E. Rosenberg, 'Health in the home: a tradition of print and practice', in Charles E. Rosenberg (ed.), *Right living: an Anglo-American tradition of self-help medicine and hygiene* (London: Johns Hopkins University Press, 2003), 1–20, pp. 2–3. Among the best known eighteenth-century texts on regimen were William Buchan, *Domestic medicine* (London: W. Strahan, T. Cadell, 1774), John Wesley, *Primitive physic* (London: for the author, 1747) and George Cheyne, *Essay on health and long life* (London, for the author, 1724).

3 See for example Julia Twigg, 'The vegetarian movement in England, 1847–1981 with particular reference to its ideology' (PhD thesis, University of London, 1981).

4 Smith, *Clean*, p. 267.

5 Harrison, 'Early Victorian radicals'; Twigg, 'Vegetarian movement'.

6 Harrison, 'Early Victorian radicals'; Aspinwall, 'Dr. and Mrs Low Nichols in Britain'.

7 Gleadle, 'Physiological reformers'.

8 Frawley, *Invalidism*, pp. 74–82.

9 Frawley, *Invalidism*, p. 17.

10 Roy Porter, 'Introduction' in Porter (ed.), *Medical history of waters and spas*, vii–xii, p. xii.

11 Marland and Adams, 'Hydropathy at home', pp. 509–19.

12 Price, 'Hydropathy in England', p. 279.

13 Nichols, *Woman's work in water cure;* Thomas Low Nichols, *Nichols' health manual: being also a memorial of the life and work of Mrs Mary S. Gove Nichols* (London: E. W. Allen, 1887).

14 Whorton, *Nature cures*, pp. 81–101.
15 P. S. Brown, 'Nineteenth-century American health reformers and the early nature cure movement in Britain', *Medical History*, 32 (1988), 174–94.
16 'Nature cure practitioners', in *Anon*., *The health and nature cure handbook: a complete authoritative and independent guide to nature cure and healthy living*, Vol. 3 (London: James Clarke & Co. Ltd, 1934), pp. 222–6.
17 Zweiniger-Bargielowska, *Managing the body*.
18 Roy Porter and Dorothy Porter, *In sickness and in health: the British experience 1650–1850* (London: Fourth Estate, 1988), pp. 30–8.
19 'Obituary, M.D.', *BMJ* (25 May 1878), 775–6.
20 Coventry History Centre, Glynne-Gladstone MSS, Letter from Sir John Gladstone to Thomas Gladstone, 24 February 1828, cited in Baxter, *Jephson*, p. 21.
21 Warwickshire CRO, CR 136/B/4585 and CR 4850. Letter from Dr Jephson to Colonel Newdigate, 14 August 1837, cited in Baxter, *Jephson*, p. 16.
22 John Ruskin, *Praeterita* (Orpington: G. Allen, 1900), p. 353 cited in Baxter, *Jephson*, p. 22.
23 Thomas Guthrie, *Autobiography of Thomas Guthrie and memoir* (edited by his sons D. K. Guthrie and C. J. Guthrie), Vol. 2 (London, for the authors, 1874–75), pp. 206–13, cited in Baxter, *Jephson*, p. 27.
24 Warwickshire CRO CR 1563/269, 'Leamington peripatetics' handwritten copy.
25 Baxter, *Jephson*, p. 25.
26 J. C. Jeaffreson, *A book about doctors*, Vol. 1, 2nd edn (London: Hurst and Blackett, 1861), p. 91, quoted in Baxter, *Jephson*, p. 30.
27 E. T. Cook, *Life of Ruskin*, 1912 Vol. 1, p. 213, cited in Baxter, *Jephson*, p. 27.
28 Claridge, *Hydropathy*, 5th edn.
29 Claridge, *Hydropathy*, 5th edn, p. 27.
30 Bulwer Lytton, 'Confessions of a water patient'.
31 Browne, 'Spas and sensibilities', pp. 104–6.
32 Douglas Jerrold, 'Life at the cold brandy-and-water cure', *Punch, or the London charivari*, 11 (1846), pp. 233–4 attributed by Walter Jerrold, *Douglas Jerrold and Punch* (London: Macmillan, 1910), p. 434, cited in Browne, 'Spas and sensibilities', footnote 5, p. 102.
33 Leech, *Three weeks in wet sheets*.
34 Lane, *Life at the water cure*.
35 Frawley, *Invalidism*, pp. 38–40 and 78–9.
36 Bulwer Lytton, 'Confessions of a water patient', pp. 6–7.
37 Bulwer Lytton, 'Confessions of a water patient', p. 13.
38 Bulwer Lytton, 'Confessions of a water patient', p. 7.
39 Bulwer Lytton, 'Confessions of a water patient', p. 9.
40 Lane, *Life at the water cure: facts and fancies noted down during a month at Malvern*, new edition with reprint of Edward Bulwer Lytton, 'Confessions of a water patient' (London: Henry Bohn, 1851), p. xxiii.

41 John Tosh, *A man's place: masculinity and the middle-class home in Victorian England* (Yale University Press: London, 1999), pp. 6–8.
42 Norma Clarke, 'Strenuous idleness: Thomas Carlyle and man of letters as hero', in Michael Roper and John Tosh (eds), *Manful assertions: masculinities in Britain since 1800* (Routledge: London, 1991), 25–43, pp. 29–31.
43 Clarke, 'Strenuous idleness', p. 37.
44 Bruce Haley, *The healthy body and Victorian culture* (Cambridge, MA: Harvard University Press, 1978), pp. 73–4.
45 Haley, *Healthy body*, p. 80.
46 Frawley, *Invalidism*, pp. 47–8.
47 Porter and Porter, *In sickness*, pp. 212–17.
48 Janet Oppenheim, *Shattered nerves: doctors, patients and depression in Victorian England* (New York: Oxford University Press, 1991), p. 3.
49 Roy Porter, 'Nervousness, eighteenth and nineteenth century style: from luxury to labour', in Gijswijt-Hofstra and Porter (eds), *Cultures of neurasthenia*, 31–49, p. 37.
50 Porter, 'Nervousness', p. 32, citing George Cheyne, *The English malady; or a treatise of nervous diseases* (London: G. Strahan, 1733).
51 Porter, 'Nervousness', p. 42.
52 George M. Beard, *A practical treatise on nervous exhaustion (neurasthenia): its symptoms, nature, sequences, treatment* (New York: W. Wood, 1880); George M. Beard, *American nervousness: its causes and consequences* (New York, Putnam, 1881).
53 M. Thomson, 'Neurasthenia in Britain', in Gijswijt-Hofstra and Porter (eds), *Cultures of neurasthenia*, 77–95.
54 Oppenheim, *Shattered nerves*, p. 131.
55 DRO, D3932/2, 'Rockside hydropathic establishment and residence for visitors' (c. 1904), p. 14
56 Foster, *Journal*, p. 3.
57 Foster, *Journal*, p. 6, original emphasis.
58 Foster, *Journal*, pp. 48–9.
59 Foster, *Journal*, p. 64.
60 Foster, *Journal*, pp. 69 and 75.
61 Foster, *Journal*, p. 76.
62 Bulwer Lytton, 'Confessions of a water patient', p. 15.
63 Bulwer Lytton, 'Confessions of a water patient', p. 15.
64 Foster, *Journal*, p. 18.
65 Foster, *Journal*, p. 20.
66 Tosh, *Man's place*, pp. 4–6.
67 Bulwer Lytton, 'Confessions of a water patient', p. 16.
68 Foster, *Journal*, p. 44.
69 Foster, *Journal*, p. 45.
70 Buckley, *Matlock Bank*, p. 59.
71 Foster, *Journal*, p. 44.

72 Foster, *Journal*, pp. 34 and 50.
73 Smedley, *Practical hydropathy*, 13th edn, p. 10.
74 Smedley, *Ladies' manual*, 16th edn, p. 55.
75 Smedley, *Ladies' manual*, 16th edn, title page.
76 Smedley, *Practical hydropathy*, 13th edn, p. 12.
77 Metcalfe, *Rise and progress*, p. 264.
78 Smedley, *Practical hydropathy*, 13th edn, p. 48.
79 Rosenberg, 'Health in the home', pp. 2–3.
80 Twigg, 'Vegetarian movement', p. 202.
81 Marland and Adams, 'Hydropathy at home', pp. 527–8.
82 Marland and Adams, 'Hydropathy at home', pp. 524–5.
83 Jean L. Silver-Isenstadt, *Shameless: the visionary life of Mary Gove Nichols* (Baltimore: Johns Hopkins University Press, 2002).
84 Aspinwall, 'Social Catholicism and health', pp. 263–9.
85 Nichols, *Woman's work in water cure*. This was largely a reprint of her earlier American publication, Mary S. Gove Nichols, *Experience in water-cure, a familiar exposition of the principles and results of water treatment in the care of acute and chronic disease* (New York: Fowler and Wells, 1849).
86 Nichols, *Woman's work in water cure*, p. 5.
87 Thomas Low Nichols, *How to live on sixpence a day* (London: Longman, Green, Reader and Dyer, 1871).
88 For example advertisements in *Herald of Health* (January 1879), p. ii.
89 Joanne Shattock and Michael Wolff (eds), *The Victorian periodical press: samplings and soundings* (Leicester: Leicester University Press, 1982).
90 Nichols, *Woman's work in water cure*, p. 15.
91 Nichols, *Nichols health manual*, p. 419.
92 Mrs Nichols, 'To my friends', *Herald of Health* (October, 1880), p. 401.
93 Whorton, *Nature cures*, p. 87.
94 Whorton, *Nature cures*, pp. 85–93.
95 James C. Whorton, *Crusaders for fitness: the history of American health reformers* (Princeton: Princeton University Press, 1982), pp. 107–8.
96 See for example Donegan, '*Hydropathic highway to health*' and Cayleff, *Wash and be healed*.
97 Whorton, *Nature cures*, pp. 100–1.
98 Brown, 'Early nature cure movement, pp. 183–9.
99 Harrison, 'Early Victorian radicals'; Gleadle, 'Age of physiological reformers'.
100 Twigg, 'Vegetarian movement; Durie, 'Almost twins by birth'.
101 Janet Grierson, *Temperance, therapy and trilobites: Dr. Ralph Grindrod: Victorian pioneer* (Cora Weaver: Malvern, 2001), pp. 22–4.
102 Metcalfe, *Rise and progress*, p. 93; Ralph Barnes Grindrod, *Bacchus: an essay on the nature, causes, effects and cure of intemperance* (London: J. Pasco, 1839, reprinted London, Simpkins, Marshall and Co., 1851).
103 Grierson, *Temperance*, pp. 42–7 and 71.

104 A. J. and C. E. Durie, 'Annie Steedman Hunter: a very radical reformer, *Forth Naturalist and Historian*, 26 (2003), 125–34.
105 Metcalfe, *Rise and progress*, pp. 171–5.
106 Brown, 'Early nature cure movement', p.180; *Herald of Health* (June 1890), p. 61.
107 E. J. Wood, 'A brief history of the Wallace system up to the present time', *Herald of Health* (March 1901) pp. 34–9; 'A brief history etc continued', *Herald of Health* (April 1901), pp. 52–4.
108 Metcalfe, *Rise and progress*, pp. 274–6.
109 Sebastian Kneipp, *My water-cure*, translated from the 36th German edition, 2nd edn (Kempton: Jos. Kessel, 1893), pp. xv–xviii.
110 Whorton, *Nature cures*, p. 201.
111 Whorton, *Nature cures*, pp. 192–4.
112 Metcalfe, *Rise and progress*, p. 276.
113 Whorton, *Nature cures*, pp. 204–5.
114 Brown, 'Early nature cure movement', p. 187; *Nature Cure*, 1 (1906), p. 15 quoted in Brown, 'Early nature cure movement', p. 193.
115 *Nature cure annual and health and pleasure guide 1907/08* (London: MacGregor, Reid and Shaw, 1908), p. xxxvi, inside front cover, pp.113 and xix.
116 'Obituary – Stanley Lief', *British Naturopathic Journal and Osteopathic Review*, 9 (Spring 1963), p. 252; Margaret Chambers, *The British Naturopathic Association: the first fifty years* (London: The British Naturopathic Association, n.d. but c. 1995), pp. 4–5.
117 C. Leslie Thomson, *James. C. Thomson, pioneer naturopath* 1887–1960 (Edinburgh: Kingston Clinic, 1960), reprinted from the *Kingston Chronicle*, May 1960.
118 National Osteopathic Archive, Pitcairn-Knowles File Box 5 /0205, 'Andrew Pitcairn-Knowles a chronology' and A. Pitcairn-Knowles, *The history and development of the Schroth cure* (Knowles Health Hydro: Hastings, n. d.).
119 Chambers, *British Naturopathic Association*, pp. 5–6.
120 *Health and nature cure handbook* (1934), pp. 222–6 and 188–90.
121 Gordon Pitcairn-Knowles, 'The water cure at home', *Health and nature cure handbook* (1934), pp. 107–15 and advertisement for the Knowles Health Hydro on p.31; Richard Pitcairn Knowles, *Riposo Health Hydro 1912–1962* (St Leonards on sea: Impression IT for the author, 2012).
122 This is discussed further in Adams, 'Developing naturopathy in inter-war Britain', in McHale and Gale (eds), *Routledge handbook of complementary medicine*.
123 Zweiniger-Bargielowska, *Managing the body*, pp. 3–5 and 44–50.
124 Zweiniger-Bargielowska, *Managing the body*, p. 42.
125 Tosh, *Man's place*, p. 177.
126 Donald E. Hall, 'Muscular Christianity: reading and writing the male social body', in Donald E. Hall (ed.), *Muscular Christianity: embodying the Victorian age* (Cambridge: Cambridge University Press, 1994), 3–13, pp. 7–12.

127 Kathleen E. McCrone, *Sport and the physical emancipation of English Women 1870–1914* (London: Routledge, 1988), p. 249.
128 Benson Bailey, *Ilkley, Bolton Abbey, and the pearls of Craven* (Bingley: John Harrison & Son, 1852), p. 9.
129 Arvid Kellgren, *The technic [sic] of Ling's system of manual treatment* (Edinburgh and London: Young J. Pentland, 1890), p. 2.
130 Metcalfe, *Rise and progress*, p. 103.
131 Donald Baynes, *Auxiliary methods of cure* (London: Simpkin, Marshall and Co., 1888), p. 46.
132 R. Woodrow Thomson, *Ben Rhydding: the asceplion of England* (London: Nelson & Sons, 1862), pp. 81–96.
133 Anon., *The Ben Rhydding book of gymnastics* (Ilkley: John Shuttleworth, n.d., c. 1852).
134 Thomson, *Ben Rhydding*, p. 15.
135 W. G. Gibbons, *Royal Leamington Spa: the seeds of lawn tennis* (Coventry: Jones-Sands, 1986).
136 Lane, *Life at the water cure* (1851), p. 47.
137 *Harrogate the nation's spa* (1912), p. 4.
138 Haley, *Healthy body*, p. 105.

5

Water, health and leisure

Visitors went to spas and hydropathic resorts for varied reasons; many patients travelled with relatives or friends and each individual had a unique experience, busy with different activities and treatment plans. Rest and relaxation were an integral part of therapeutic regimes, intended to offer sufficient diversion for the patient to put aside their everyday concerns and worries and to fill the hours not dedicated to treatment. Making a distinction between a health or leisure pursuit is complex, influenced by cultural context, personal motivation and norms of behaviour, further complicated by the variety of purposes and meanings that can be attributed to specific actions.[1] John Ruskin considered the objective of an activity to be important in distinguishing between work and leisure. 'Play is an exertion of body or mind, made to please ourselves, and with no determined end'. However, if cricket (for example) were 'done as an ordered form of exercise, for health's sake, it would become work directly'.[2] The same activity might be used for health maintenance, as a curative intervention, for relief of symptoms or for recreation. Thus someone walking along a graduated pathway could be completing an exercise plan as part of an individualised terrain cure to improve cardiac condition, undertaking a prescribed daily walk in the fresh air to alleviate a nervous complaint or be out for an afternoon stroll commenced without any recourse to medical advice – or indeed have some other prime motivation. With this complication in mind, this chapter examines how the treatment regimes at English watering places were related to broader trends in leisure. It examines the varied use of water for healing and pleasure and assesses how recreational pursuits available at spas compared with those in other towns.

The expansion in the therapeutic uses of water occurred in the context of changing norms in bathing for hygiene and leisure with diverse bathing cultures developing over the course of the nineteenth century. Increasing availability of clean water supplies provided by private companies and public authorities facilitated changing norms in personal hygiene practices as well as expanding opportunities for leisure activities including swimming and sea bathing. For many middle-class consumers water ceased to be an element that required significant amounts of time and effort to collect – and was accordingly used sparingly – and became a plentiful commodity delivered directly into domestic settings on a commercial basis.[3] By the end of the nineteenth century luxurious bathrooms attest to changing hygienic routines among the better off. Initiatives were also launched to ameliorate sanitary conditions for the poorer classes with the promotion of personal cleanliness seen as an integral part of the mission to improve moral habits. The increase in seaside resorts from the eighteenth century onwards popularised new activities centred on the sea and beach. Although the new fashion of 'dipping' was primarily justified on health grounds and came to be managed through the use of bathing machines and attendants, these practices overlaid earlier popular traditions of immersion. As the number of holidaymakers visiting the seaside increased, sea bathing became more closely regulated with segregated areas for male and female bathers. Changing expectations and considerations of propriety meant that by 1900 these restrictions were being relaxed, and mixed and family groups could once again bathe together in many English resorts. By the 1870s swimming pools were becoming increasingly common in many inland towns providing improved access for leisure users across the country. New legislation meant that municipal authorities could become major players in the provision of bathing facilities. The authorities at Leamington Spa adopted a policy of combining medical, Turkish and slipper baths with swimming pools in order to attract a broad-based clientele. Private hydropathic establishments and bath houses meant that extensive facilities became available in other urban centres too. On-shore bath houses providing hot and cold sea water baths were established at some seaside resorts in the eighteenth century and in the nineteenth century these became more commonplace, shifting medical bathing off the beach. Torquay and Southport were among the resorts that came to offer medical bathing facilities similar to those at many inland spas. By the inter-war period lidos providing open-air swimming and grounds for sunbathing brought some of the characteristic elements of the seaside to inland areas further eroding the differences in activities available at these resorts. Thus although medical bathing became a distinguishing feature of the mineral water and hydropathic resorts this was one aspect of broader bathing cultures that merged the boundaries between leisure, hygiene and health and became more widely available to both middle- and working-class populations.

Case studies from Malvern and Holywell in Flintshire illustrate the tensions and difficulties that arose in meeting increased demand for water in the face of competing rights of access. Holywell, one of only a few centres that survived as a centre for pilgrimage in Britain after the Reformation, experienced a significant increase in popularity at the end of the nineteenth century. Despite continuing associations with religious activities the spring also supplied commercial concerns and its situation in an industrial area meant it was vulnerable to the effects of mining. Malvern's reputation was rooted in the healing properties of its pure hill water but the nature of supply, fed by rainfall and harvested from numerous scattered springs, presented challenges of collection and storage capable of ensuring a sufficient flow to meet rising demand. The gradients of the hills, size of the catchment area, distances between pockets of population and continued use of private wells all added to the vulnerability of the public supply and meant that severe water shortages continued to be experienced into the twentieth century. Pollution and infectious disease remained a threat both to individual health and to the reputation and prosperity of the resort town.

The growing commercialisation of leisure is closely associated with increasing industrialisation, urbanisation and improved transport infrastructure.[4] From the end of the seventeenth century English spas were part of a broader growth in leisure services and commercial enterprise, primarily urban-based, that developed to satisfy the luxuries and necessities of the growing middle classes.[5] In this period the larger English spas became important centres where the wealthy gathered to relax in company with others and 'taking the waters' was framed within a culture of public consumption of luxury goods and entertainments including theatres, music and assemblies.[6] Bath became the premier provincial pre-industrial city, and by the end of the eighteenth century was about the tenth largest town in England and Wales, only challenged by London, Dublin and Edinburgh as a centre for elite cultural life.[7] By the late eighteenth century a variety of other types of urban centres, including established county towns and seaside resorts also provided a leisure infrastructure that included the balls, assemblies, parks, shops, libraries, music and theatre earlier associated with spa life.[8] This trend continued as increased urbanisation led to the more widespread dispersal of leisure amenities across the country so that by the 1880s parks, playing fields, sports grounds, libraries and theatres could be found in many towns. While spas ceased to be the only urban centres providing a good range of leisure amenities it was important they continued to match those available in most large cities and catered for changing tastes in recreation.

Bathing for health and pleasure

The development of new bathing facilities at Leamington Spa in the 1860s illustrates the diversity of mid-nineteenth-century bathing cultures. When Sir Bertie Percy indicated his wish to sell the Royal Pump Rooms the community was faced with the prospect of losing their last remaining spa facility. Although Leamington's initial growth was sparked by demand for its saline water, by the 1850s falling returns had led to the closure or conversion of most bath houses in the town. Reports in the *Leamington Spa Courier* reflect the strong local opinion that the Pump Rooms should be saved although options for refurbishment or expansion were a matter of debate and controversy.[9] A private pamphlet, 'What to do with the Royal Pump Rooms', cited a shift away from mineral waters towards hydropathic baths as well as greater availability of water for domestic use as contributing to declining demand for the local spa facilities and urged the need to cater for the growing number of tourists and residents in addition to invalids.[10] Some questioned the advisability of investing large sums in spa facilities at all as demand for baths was so low and suggested that the premises would be better redeveloped as a large and prestigious public hall to provide flexible indoor accommodation for social gatherings. Although others wished to see the Pump Rooms continue as a centre for spa activities there was debate as to how far to adopt new bathing methods such as the controversial Turkish bath. This particular scheme was opposed by some who objected to the downplaying of the natural mineral waters – which they argued underpinned the town's reputation – by placing 'the foreign appliance in the ascendant to the detriment of the native element'.[11]

The Pump Rooms, which occupied an imposing site close to the bridge joining the old and new towns, had been designed in 1814 to provide luxurious facilities for upper-class patrons visiting the town to take the waters. A large assembly hall provided pumped mineral water for drinkers along with space for relaxation. An open colonnade on three sides of the exterior gave access to the separate bathing suites for men and women which provided hot and cold baths in private cubicles along with dressing and waiting areas. The final refurbishment plans proposed substantial remodelling designed to ensure the building continued to be a specialist bathing institution while attracting a broad base of paying customers from both residents and visitors. An extension was built allowing the creation of new spaces for a Turkish bath, swimming pool and slipper baths for the poor. Mineral water was dispensed to drinkers from an alcove in the assembly room which was also used for concerts and balls.[12] This selection of facilities reflected changing cultural norms in the use of water for hygienic and leisure purposes as well as trends in its medical use. Despite these ambitious plans financial difficulties continued and the enterprise was taken into public ownership through the Local Board of Health in 1868, transferring to the Leamington Corporation in 1875.[13] These new bodies continued to pursue a similar strategy designed to harness broad-based demand. Later refurbishments added an additional swimming pool as well as upgraded medical facilities. In 1910 an annexe was built to provide comfortable surroundings in which to dispense the spa water to drinkers along with a reading room for quiet relaxation. The larger assembly room was converted into a tea lounge. A tourist guide published in 1919 emphasised the range of facilities for both recreation and treatment including 'two large tepid swimming baths', 'a handsome Turkish Bath fitted in the newest style' and the 'latest appliances known to balneology' supplemented by a 'crane and chair for cripples and invalids unable to walk'.[14] The baths for 'washing' were promoted through working men's clubs, British legion and local companies.[15]

The close interconnection between bathing for hygiene and pleasure is illustrated by the growing popularity of the Turkish bath which drew on the combined appeal of luxury, health and cleanliness. Descriptions of communal baths used in Turkey and North Africa had circulated in travel writings from the 1840s and by the 1850s prototype baths were being developed in Britain.[16] An early promoter was the diplomat and social reformer David Urquhart who worked with Dr Barter in Ireland to develop a prototype using dry hot air.[17] Urquhart opened a Turkish bath in Manchester in 1857 and within a few years more had been constructed in London and some of the northern industrial towns. Medical opinion on the bath varied and while some endorsed its value as an effective means of promoting the elimination of toxins through sweating, others objected to claims that it was a panacea for many complaints and warned of the dangers of very high temperatures for weak and elderly patients, particularly those with respiratory or cardiac problems.[18] Although hydropathists had developed a variety of mechanisms to produce an effective steam bath, including the use of lamps and boxes to speed up the sweating process, the Turkish bath offered much more than this. The treatment was designed to be leisurely and pleasurable and was conducted in a comfortable communal setting. The novelty of the experience was frequently enhanced by use of oriental architecture, an approach adopted at Leamington although, perhaps as a compromise to the traditionalists in the town, the exterior of the remodelled Pump Rooms gave no sign that a Turkish bath was hidden within it.[19]

The bathing suite comprised a series of four rooms at different temperatures, the largest and coolest of which was the frigidarium where clients relaxed after spending time in the smaller, hotter rooms being scrubbed and massaged by the shampooer. The bath does not seem to have been an instant success, closing for a time in the 1860s with consideration given to leasing it to a Dr Williams from Malvern.[20] This business failure was not unique; the Turkish suite added to the men's hot baths at Buxton in 1861 had also closed by 1865.[21] The management at Leamington persevered with the bath and by the 1870s it proved more popular. Under the supervision of George Elson and his wife, employed as shampooers, clients increased from fifteen to over fifty a week drawn from the surrounding towns of Banbury, Rugby, Coventry and Stratford-on-Avon.[22] Elson vividly describes the essentially sociable activity, noting 'of all places I know of, the Turkish bath is the most productive of volubility' and remarking of his clients, 'to hear them debating among themselves was interesting and amusing, several of them all talking at once, punctuating their remarks with roars of laughter'.[23] The baths were mainly used by men, attracting a mix of 'noble lords, many squires, numbers of professional men, military and naval, athletes and jockeys, and a few doctors'. Elson's wife attended women in the Turkish bath one day each week.[24] Although the health benefits of the Turkish bath continued to be debated among the medical fraternity clients did not need a medical prescription in order to use it.[25] Its appeal lay in its function as both a useful hygienic practice and a pleasurable recreational activity. The 1887 refurbishment of the bath continued to emphasise the importance of relaxation; with pink reflectors added to the electric lamps to enhance 'the charm of Eastern repose'.[26] Turkish baths were added to showcase bathing suites at several spas and hydros; Smedley's had one by 1882 and an elaborate suite was included in the Royal Baths built at Harrogate in 1897.[27]

Leamington's Pump Rooms also fulfilled a new municipal obligation by providing slipper baths for the poor. The association of dirt with epidemic disease led to demand from sanitary reformers for better provision of baths to encourage personal cleanliness and improve the moral habits of the lower classes. By the 1840s the growing public hygiene movement, influenced by shifts in middle-class norms of hygiene, led to calls to provide adequate bathing facilities for the poor to wash both their bodies and their clothes. Enabling legislation under the Public Baths and Washhouses Acts of 1846 and 1847 encouraged the construction of facilities by allowing parishes and town councils to fund them from local rates.[28] Take-up was patchy and in 1849 Chadwick believed there were entire streets in many districts without the use of a single bath. Although mains water began to reach working-class homes by the 1870s, water was frequently only available in the kitchen with many people taking a bath in a portable tub in front of the range. Sanitary provision in many working-class homes remained rudimentary into the twentieth century as provision of indoor baths and toilets was not made compulsory in council housing until after the First World War. Many older properties remained without baths until the 1950s.[29] In these circumstances the provision of public slipper baths continued to be a duty for municipal authorities.

Even for the middle classes the expansion in domestic water supplies was uneven and it was not until the last quarter of the nineteenth century that improved sanitation became more commonplace.[30] Prior to the introduction of piped water supplies domestic ablutions were taken using a wash stand with water poured from ewers into a basin while baths were taken in small receptacles or portable tubs perhaps supplemented by simple showers which released water from an overhead cistern. Taking a bath or shower was labour-intensive as all these methods required water to be carried into the house to the bathing area. Hot water posed a further complication with heating appliances limited to the kitchen. Specialist manufacturers began to develop baths with their own heating source from the late 1830s, at first powered by coal and later gas, but prior to the introduction of piped water to upstairs rooms these still needed filling and emptying by hand. By the 1870s it became more common to be able to take a bath with hot water piped from the kitchen or heated by gas appliance in a dedicated bathroom.[31] Correspondence in the *Builder* suggests that by the 1880s bathrooms were included in many new homes for the middle classes and within a decade many older properties had also been adapted to include them.[32] The revolution in cleanliness and personal hygiene wrought by improved heating and plumbing was further encouraged by the production of cheaper toilet soap.[33]

The transformation wrought in daily routines and attitudes towards water is illustrated by Edwin Clayhanger's musings on anticipated pleasures from the system of piped water in their new suburban villa. At the old house, attached to the family printing works,

> every drop of water on the first floor had to be carried upstairs in jugs and buckets; and every drop of it had to be carried down again. No hot water could be obtained until it had been boiled in a vessel on the fire. Hot water had the value of champagne. To take a warm hip-bath was an immense enterprise of heating, fetching, decanting, and general derangement of the entire house; and at best the bath was not hot; it always lost its virtue on the stairs and landing. And to splash – one of the most voluptuous pleasures in life – was forbidden by the code ... Splashing was immoral ... In the shop-house godliness was child's play compared to cleanliness.

In contrast the new house had

> A room solely for baths! And a huge painted zinc bath! Edwin had never seen such a thing. And a vast porcelain basin, with tiles all around it, in which you could splash! An endless supply of water on the first floor.[34]

Commentators at Cheltenham in the 1830s had suggested that the declining popularity of mineral water bathing was due in part to increased provision of hot and cold baths across the country.[35] Despite this, the numerous baths and douches that formed the basis of hydropathic treatment in the 1840s and 1850s were a novelty to most of those taking treatment, not least because of the labour required to prepare and give treatments. On his return home from Malvern Richard Lane set up a bathroom, evidence that experience of hydropathic treatment helped shape the development of new hygiene routines.[36] The more extensive provision of domestic bathrooms by the 1880s, providing facilities for hot baths and showers, coincided with the trend towards increasingly luxurious facilities at the top-end hydros. Investment in combination baths and showers incorporating massage, electrical baths and gymnasia with physical training equipment ensured that the specialist bathing institutions continued to offer patrons facilities far more extensive than those at home.

By the end of the nineteenth century elaborate bathing suites were no longer limited to the premier spas as a varied bathing culture incorporating health and leisure practices became integrated into wider social life. Municipal control at Lockwood spa offered a model that ensured existing facilities were adapted to meet changing demand and new responsibilities. Lockwood was one of a number of small Yorkshire spas that developed in the 1820s and 1830s to cater for growing numbers of mechanics and factory workers in the area.[37] In 1870 the Huddersfield Corporation renamed the facilities as Lockwood Public Baths and introduced low prices to cater for the working class. The facilities were extended several times and in 1867 provided swimming, warm, Buxton, shower, vapour, sulphurous, fumigating and shampooing baths that together attracted 30,000 bathers in a single season.[38] At nearby Slaithwaite spa, where provision for free access by the poor was in place by the 1840s, there was continuing demand from the less well off although it was reported that better-off inhabitants preferred to travel to Harrogate and Ilkley.[39]

Encouraged by Droitwich's growing reputation with both the public and the medical profession, several towns with access to strong brine sources invested in extensive bathing suites. The corporation baths at Stafford which opened in April 1893 provided facilities far exceeding their minimum obligations. The building provided a large fresh water swimming pool, private slipper baths, and a Turkish bath as well as brine baths drawn from a well first discovered while boring for the town's waterworks some sixteen years earlier.[40] Designed by the public surveyor the baths were primarily intended for the use of local people although visitors were welcomed as a way to minimise the cost to rate payers.[41] Brine baths opened at Nantwich in 1883 and by 1895 there were two separate bathing suites; the Old Baths providing a swimming pool and private bathrooms along with needle, shower, and vapour baths while the New Baths were constructed as an integral part of an upmarket hotel development situated in parkland on the outskirts of town.[42] Brine from Middlesborough was transported to Saltburn-by-the-Sea where it was available in a bathhouse close to the railway station. In 1919 the facilities available were listed as 'needle and other douches, vapour brine baths and various electric treatments'.[43]

By the end of the nineteenth century seaside resorts marketed as specialist health resorts also had extensive establishments offering medical baths to supplement the positive effect of a seaside climate and sea bathing. For example the Victoria Baths at Southport, first constructed in 1839, were rebuilt in 1871 to provide showers and private, vapour and medicated baths along with several larger plunge or swimming pools.[44] A Turkish bath was added in 1903.[45] Investors at Sidmouth sought to target a niche market of patients with cardiac problems and developed facilities specialising in providing the Nauheim cure for heart disease in the new sea water baths opened in 1895.[46] The venture was promoted in a new guide to the town with further publicity generated through the book review pages in the first edition of the *Journal of Balneology and Climatology* (*JB&C*).[47] Promotional material explained the local variation of the famous German cure; sea water was used in place of the Nauheim brine while routes for graduated exercise made use of the gentle gradients alongside the River Sid and the steep slopes of the cliffs rising on either side of the resort.[48] The Sidmouth baths were used to treat officers in the First World War and despite financial pressures and changes of ownership in the inter-war period continued to provide Nauheim baths, among other treatments, until at least 1939.[49]

Eighteenth-century sea bathing had its roots in two traditions; the elite practice of taking the waters at spas through immersion and drinking and the custom of sea bathing by working people.[50] Richard Russell, the most famous early promoter of medical sea bathing, claimed to have been drawn to try sea water only after observing ordinary people using it for treatment.[51] Sea bathing for both therapeutic and leisure purposes continued into the twentieth century although the practices associated with both these aspects changed. In the eighteenth century it was customary for men and women to be briefly immersed or 'dipped' on the same stretch of the beach, men bathing naked while females wore loose gowns. Bathing machines which transported bathers into the sea in covered wagons were introduced at several Kent resorts and at Brighton by the mid-eighteenth century. Mixed bathing continued to be the norm at most small resorts although some larger centres, including Blackpool, made provision for segregation.[52] This so-called 'promiscuous bathing' attracted increasing criticism by the early nineteenth century. Greater numbers of both sexes drawn from across the social scale, as well as the increasing popularity of active swimming rather than dipping, led to further allegations of indecent behaviour by bathers and outrage at the voyeuristic attention they sometimes attracted.[53] From the 1830s pressure mounted to address the perceived immorality of naked and mixed sea-bathing. By the 1860s municipal authorities were using by-laws to promote their preferred bathing culture. At the middle-class resorts segregated bathing from the main beaches became the norm although naked and mixed bathing continued to be practised and tolerated in many places away from resort centres.[54] By the end of the century the growing popularity of swimming and other beach attractions, including paddling, rock-pools and sandcastles, established a family-orientated culture at many seaside resorts which, along with practices at French and Belgian resorts, increased calls to relax restrictions on segregated swimming. By the 1890s mixed bathing was reintroduced in many English resorts with changing tents and cover-up bathing attire for both sexes ensuring appropriate modesty.[55]

As swimming became more popular sea water pools were developed as a way of overcoming restrictions caused by tides and currents and improving safety and accessibility. Early ventures included those at Southampton which opened in 1853.[56] Although inland resorts could not compete with the beach, the trend towards swimming pools could be emulated. One of the earliest open-air swimming pools was built in Bath where the Cleveland Pool at Bathwick opened in 1815.[57] Both indoor and open-air pools became more common in many towns from the mid-nineteenth century particularly after town councils were given the powers to fund the construction of covered pools in 1878.[58] The popularity of the sport was further encouraged by the establishment of the Amateur Swimming Association of Great Britain in 1869 and the first cross-Channel swim in 1875. A pool was included in the Pump Room development at Leamington in the 1860s and a second added in 1887 allowing one to be reserved for the use of women and children.[59] George Elson worked as a swimming teacher at Worcester teaching scholars from some of the prestigious Malvern schools before moving to Leamington to take charge of the Turkish bath.[60] The Leamington pool was used by the local swimming club who arranged a number of competitive events at the venue. The popularity of swimming flourished in the inter-war period stimulated further by the development of the lido concept. The larger lidos offered more than a pool, with diving boards and extensive terraces providing the opportunity for participation or observation of a variety of activities. They capitalised on growing interest in sunbathing and the outdoors and provided another opportunity for spas and inland places to match fashions for aquatic leisure associated with the seaside. Lidos were opened in Malvern in 1925, Cheltenham and Droitwich in 1935, Ilkley in 1936, Woodhall Spa in 1937 and Matlock in 1938. Residential urban areas also provided these facilities; by the 1930s there were around sixty open-air pools in the London area alone.[61]

Immersing the body in water became increasingly popular over the course of the nineteenth century for a variety of hygienic, leisure and therapeutic purposes. As practices changed better facilities for both therapeutic bathing and recreational swimming were provided at inland and seaside resorts as well as in many other residential towns. Although a sea dip continued to be advocated as a healthy practice for those with a robust constitution, onshore institutions providing hot and cold sea-water baths and hydropathic applications became more widely available in municipal bathhouses or private hydros. Onshore bathing facilities were established at Scarborough and Brighton by the early nineteenth century and these became more common at the seaside as the nineteenth century wore on.[62] The new baths that opened in Torquay in 1857, Westward Ho! in 1866, Ilfracombe in 1880 and Teignmouth in 1883 all provided hot and cold baths, as well as swimming pools.[63] Following redevelopment in 1922 the Torquay baths on Beacon Hill were hailed as comparable to facilities at the elite spas.[64] The medical baths at Southport and Sidmouth offered specialised treatment while Turkish baths, indoor swimming pools and lidos catered for the recreational bather in many water cure resorts. While it may appear straightforward to categorise a resort as seaside, spa or hydropathic based on their natural resources and location, this distinction was not reliable as a guide to the particular mix of bathing facilities available. While each resort offered a unique blend of amenities, collectively they demonstrate the emergence of a complex and varied bathing culture shaped by both health and leisure preferences.

The pattern of resort development in Britain differed from the rest of Europe due to earlier industrialisation and urbanisation as well as its island geography. The number of seaside resorts developed earlier and expanded faster in the British Isles and by the mid-eighteenth century widening prosperity brought increased demand from merchants, tradesmen and professional people, especially from the London area.[65] As demand trickled further down the social scale one result was greater differentiation in the resort experience and 'social tone'.[66] One route to continued appeal to the middle and upper classes was investment in health facilities. Upmarket seaside resorts at Eastbourne, Bournemouth, Torquay and Southport all continued to target invalids as an important group of consumers. In contrast to the view that leisure practices developed at the seaside came to overshadow earlier spa culture this section has shown that trends in medical bathing at the inland spas and hydropathic resorts continued to be a strong influence in shaping the provision of amenities among a wider group of health resorts.

Safeguarding water supplies

An essential requirement for any successful resort was its reputation as a healthy place with an up-to-date sanitary infrastructure and low rates of disease. Provision of a safe water supply which fulfilled demand from the residential population, visitors, medical baths and other commercial undertakings was a necessity. Despite a general trend towards better public provision of water supplies over the course of the nineteenth century individual case studies reveal the many local difficulties faced in finding enduring solutions to sanitary reform in the light of growing populations and changing trends in water consumption.[67] At Malvern, rising demand from visitors, commercial enterprises and a burgeoning residential population in scattered settlements, coupled with variable annual rainfall patterns meant that water shortages continued to be a real concern into the twentieth century. Effective measures to manage water-borne infectious disease, through the separation of clean water and sewage, often proved difficult to implement and some threat of contamination remained in many localities.[68] Fears of environmental degradation, and the need to protect natural resources while respecting private and communal rights, added to the complexity of local negotiations. These factors were also apparent at Holywell in Flintshire where rising demand from commercial enterprises, domestic consumers and religious pilgrims led to competition over access to water.

The best-known springs in the Malvern Hills, those at St Ann's and Holy Well, have a long history of varied use for domestic purposes, commercial bottling and healing.[69] The profusion of springs is fed by rainfall so that supply varies from season to season and year to year. The owners of some springs exercised monopoly rights to their water while at others there were well-established communal rights of access, for example Earl Beauchamp's fountain served the local community.[70] During the nineteenth century demand from the growing residential population and commercial enterprises led to increasing pressure on fluctuating water resources. Storage tanks and cisterns were introduced to improve the reliability of supply, an early initiative being the North Malvern tank built in 1835. Coordinated efforts to establish a public supply began at Great Malvern where the Improvement Act of 1851 gave commissioners the right to ensure the town was 'drained, cleansed, lighted, watched, regulated and otherwise improved, and effectually supplied with Sewers and Water'.[71] This legislation was designed to provide for domestic needs and watering of roads to reduce dust in summer and expressly excluded use 'for Baths, or for any manufacturing or hydropathic Purposes, or for watering Gardens, or for Fountains, or for any other ornamental or horticultural purposes'.[72] These needs continued to be fulfilled from private sources or were subject to special negotiation with the authority.

An important local consideration was the commitment to a public supply drawn from the hills, widely perceived as the foundation of the resort's reputation as a water cure centre. Early work focused on improving collection methods on the eastern side of the hills to draw water into storage tanks and mains. Supplies were reliant on annual rainfall which varied from year to year with particular pressure in the summer months when demand from visitors and residents peaked but rainfall was normally at its lowest. By 1856 stopcocks were fitted to domestic supplies and charges imposed to help moderate demand. Large storage tanks were constructed at the Wyche in 1856 and North Malvern in 1877.[73] Despite these measures water shortages still occurred in drought years. In 1864, a submission by fourteen of the town's medical practitioners set out urgent action needed to protect Malvern's viability as a water cure centre. Walter Johnson, a well-known hydropathist, argued that the fundamental problem was not insufficient annual rainfall but inadequate means for its storage and distribution. In 1881 there was another drought when water was only available for a few hours a day and sometimes not at all.[74] One option to mitigate shortages was to draw on additional private springs for short periods as not all sources were equally affected by drought. The Malvern Water Act of 1891 provided access to funds to construct an extensive reservoir at British Camp with a capacity of 44 million gallons, expected to be sufficient to meet requirements of residents in the Great Malvern area. The Malvern Link (Extension and Water) Act of 1896 addressed collection from the western catchment area for supply to communities at Malvern Link, West Malvern, Colwall and other settlements. The amalgamation of the two authorities into Malvern Urban District Council (MUDC) in 1898 brought together responsibility for the provision of water to a scattered population of some 17,000 people with the right to collect from the whole of the Malvern watershed.[75] These powers were consolidated and extended under the Malvern Water Act of 1905.[76] Fearful of disruption to their own sources, some individuals and groups fought to get protection for existing rights; the 1896 Act safeguarded flows at Royal Well and Hayslad, the 1905 Act confirmed these and added protection of flows to St Ann's Well. The spout at Hayslad was the prime supply for many of those living in Colwall, on the west of the hills, and they forced the authorities to include a clause in the Act stating that a main would be laid into the village within twelve months.[77] Nine years later the Colwall parish council opposed the 1905 legislation on the grounds that this commitment had still not been met. Despite increasing the capacity of British Camp reservoir, construction of additional storage tanks, sinking boreholes and linking additional sources into the supply there were severe water shortages in 1902 and 1904.[78] The 1905 Act confirmed the development of new waterworks at Bromsberrow, a short distance away from the hills but fed by the Malvern catchment. Relief at what was felt to be a scheme that would finally secure an adequate supply was severely undermined by a very public legal case about the safety of the town's water due to an outbreak of typhoid at Fergusson's hydro the same year.

The principal concern of a public water supply was safety but the piecemeal development of the system at Malvern, the high cost of water and periodic shortages increased its vulnerability to contamination. In June 1905 several patients and staff members fell ill at Dr Fergusson's hydro, three of whom later died. The survivors and relatives of the victims claimed damages and Fergusson in turn sued the council on the grounds that the public supply had infected his well through overflow from a drain. The case attracted nationwide media attention that adversely impacted on the number of visitors to the resort for several years, led directly to the bankruptcy of the most prestigious hydro still operating, and left the ratepayers to pick up a large bill for legal costs.[79] Evidence presented in the court cases and reported in the media highlighted the complications of water provision and the vulnerability of Malvern's supply to pollution. In the years preceding the outbreak Fergusson claimed to have drawn water from three sources; a private well in his own grounds, a pipe from Mason's Tank constructed in the 1840s and an 'unknown source'. The water from the private well was pumped into the house while water from the other two sources was stored in underground tanks and used as required. Fergusson noticed that the water in the men's plunge bath was cloudy and within a few days several patients had fallen ill. On further investigation it was discovered that a blockage in a drain owned by the public supply had caused effluent to seep into the hydro's water sources. During periods of drought the public supply had drawn on private wells to supplement resources one of which, Tudor Well, was close to Fergusson's hydro.[80] The investigation by Fosbrooke, the local Medical Office of Health, showed that the hydro's plumbing was complicated and ancient with many potential sources of contamination. He recommended turning off the 'unknown source' and the disease outbreak ceased. The council served notice on Fergusson to remedy the defective drain and these were replaced by the freehold owners who took steps to recover the costs from Fergusson the lessee. This dispute went to court with judgment going against the owners.[81]

Fergusson also faced a case brought by those who had fallen ill and when their claim for damages was successful he sued the council on the grounds that it was overflow from their drain that had led to sewage contaminating his water supply.[82] Although Fergusson won the first case in January 1908 and was awarded damages of £7,500 which was sufficient to cover compensation payable to the victims, this decision was overturned by the House of Lords the following May who found in favour of MUDC.[83] The point of law turned on whether or not there was a legal contract to supply water and the council were negligent in allowing this to become contaminated or whether Fergusson had been taking the water illegally in which case there were no grounds for a claim. During the various actions it came to light that Fergusson had been drawing on the public supply in the years prior to the 1902 drought. In that year the public supply failed and, unknown to the council, Fergusson opened a direct connection between the Tudor

Well and his hydro and continued to use this source without paying for it. The final judgment found that as 'he voluntarily took the benefit of the pipe and the water flowing from it, although he knew that he had no title to it' he had no claim in law.[84]

Despite winning the case the council were forced to levy an additional rate to meet costs of £7,000 not recoverable from Fergusson. The following year the *Malvern News*, reporting on the bankruptcy case, assessed Fergusson's losses at £23,463 comprising legal costs exceeding £14,000, and compensation for the victims and other losses of over £6,000.[85] Fergusson's son later accused the MUDC of intransigence, suggesting his father would have been willing to reach an out of court settlement that would have saved the council money and avoided unwelcome publicity.[86] However, what had been at stake was Malvern's reputation as a health resort and the competence of the public authorities to provide a safe water supply and deal effectively with an outbreak of serious epidemic disease. It was doubly frustrating as so much had been done to secure an adequate, safe and reliable public supply in the years preceding the outbreak. Fosbrooke circulated a letter to the editors of several national newspapers emphasising that the fault had been with a private water source and not the town's public supply. Despite his best efforts Fosbrooke lost his job as several on the council felt that it was his remarks that had first associated the outbreak with the public supply. The MUDC were prepared to risk adverse publicity and sacrifice individual businesses and careers in order to preserve the reputation of the resort.

The cleanliness and abundance of the Malvern spring water depended on the wider environment of the hill range. By the 1880s this was coming under increasing pressure from building, gardens and quarrying. Malvern became one of the first places to take legal action to protect the natural environment. In 1884 the first Malvern Hills Act gave a new body, the Conservators, rights to raise rates and make by-laws to protect the common lands from further encroachments.[87] Further Acts extended these powers to safeguard the hills and their water supplies for the use of residents and visitors.[88] In addition to hydropathic practice the Malvern hills were also renowned as a source for bottled water. W. and J. Burrows who ran a large enterprise from the 1850s won a prestigious prize at the International Water Exhibition at Frankfurt in 1882 and later secured several royal warrants of appointment.[89] Its chief water source was St Ann's Well from which water was pumped into tanks at the bottling plant in Great Malvern but the company also owned rights to Holy Well and in the 1880s was bottling from both sources. Schweppes also had a bottling plant in Malvern from the 1850s drawing on Holy Well and later took over the Burrows enterprise and consolidated their business at a new plant in Colwall built in the 1890s.[90] Other commercial concerns taking water from springs included the Royal Well Mineral Water Company which operated from the 1870s to 1901 and vinegar works at Colwall which operated from 1883 to 1914.[91]

In Flintshire increasing numbers of pilgrims were attracted to St Winefride's Well when it was reported that Winefrid White, a servant from Wolverhampton had recovered from an incurable disorder after bathing in the spring in 1802.[92] The cure tradition at Holywell dated back to the twelfth century and had continued on a small scale after the Reformation period. The case was investigated and endorsed by the Catholic Bishop John Milner who published a series of documents based on his investigations which led him to argue that as the healing was instantaneous it must be due to more than the normal benefits of cold bathing.[93] The well's reputation was consolidated by the cure of Sister Mary Ann Wood in 1809 and Mary White in 1830.[94] The healing cult was further encouraged by the lifting of restrictions on Catholics through the Catholic Relief Act of 1829. The established Catholic presence in the area was consolidated with the foundation of a Jesuit seminary at St Bueno in the 1840s and a Franciscan Friary in 1852.[95] Between 1862 and 1871 the local board supported improvements to the well including construction of a hospice to provide affordable accommodation for growing numbers of poor pilgrims.[96] This enterprise flourished quietly until St Winefride's popularity mushroomed following a series of miraculous cures reported in the 1890s which led to comparisons with Lourdes, the French pilgrimage site celebrated for Bernadette Soubirous's visions of Mary in 1858. The growing popularity of Lourdes was linked to Catholic resurgence after defeat in the Franco-Prussian war and the popularity of a wider Marian cult in the nineteenth century. Improved transport links, changing patterns of leisure and aggressive commercialisation all contributed to the growth in numbers of pilgrims which reached more than a million annually by 1908.[97] Under Beauclerk, several practices similar to those at Lourdes, albeit on a much smaller scale, were introduced at Holywell, including street processions with commemorative banners and candle-lit services. Churches and Catholic associations from across the country organised group visits of up to several hundred people, some attending for a day and others making a longer trip and incorporating a visit to the friary at St Pantasaph into their schedule. Many pilgrims were drawn from the working-class areas of Liverpool and other Lancashire towns and included those from Irish and Italian immigrant families.[98]

Beauclerk claimed twenty to twenty-five notable cures plus several hundred minor ones occurred in 1894.[99] Details of the cures reported in the local papers emphasised their exceptional nature and often cited witnesses to their occurrence. For example Mr Kilbride 'who had been quite blind in the right eye for eleven years, was bathing his eyes when his vision suddenly returned ... amongst those present at the time was the Bishop of Nottingham (Dr. Bagshawe), who interrogated Kilbride and satisfied himself that the sight of the eye had actually been restored'.[100] In a letter to the *Flintshire Observer* in October of that year James Williams, a local medical practitioner, confirmed that he had seen unexplained rapid 'cures' that were 'frequently so pronounced and so rapid that I can quite understand how those whose religious creed includes the dogma of the intercession of saints should attribute them to such influence'. He chose not to comment on the religious or faith aspects of the question and noted that in his opinion the cures were due to either the tonic action of the cold water or to the shock of immersion, which he believed was capable of effecting 'extraordinary cures' particularly in cases of 'hysteria, hystero-epilepsy, catalepsy, &c.' In his opinion, the tonic action alone was capable of producing 'startling' improvements in those suffering from conditions of the nervous or muscular systems, although these usually took longer to benefit.[101] At Lourdes a Bureau des Contestations Médicales was set up in 1883 to provide a mechanism for assessment and authentication of the claimed miraculous cures by medical practitioners.[102] No such organisation was set up in Wales. While the popularity of St Winefride's reflected a broader-based resurgence in Catholicism in Britain the local area was also of national importance partly due to the presence of the Jesuit college. When the vicariate of Wales was introduced by the Pope in 1895 the first incumbent was Francis Joseph Mostyn, a member of a local recusant family who had been active supporters of the well for many years.[103]

Religious use was not the only claim on the abundant stream at Holywell which also supplied water for domestic purposes and a commercial brewery as well as powering machinery used by mills and industrial enterprises. The valley was situated in an area of early industrial exploitation and was a busy, crowded place with poor provision for sanitation.[104] Over a hundred people died in the cholera epidemic of 1832. By the 1830s the area was in economic decline and a scheme to promote medical bathing was among other commercial schemes considered. A company prospectus issued in 1837 grandiosely argued the 'celebrated Well of St Winefred [*sic*] may fairly compete with the Waters of Cheltenham, Leamington, Harrogate, Buxton, Scarborough, Tunbridge, or Beulah, for the invigorative and restorative qualities of its waters'.[105] This scheme did not go ahead although the company was granted a lease to the well. In 1848 another proposal to develop a hydropathic centre was put forward spurred by the early success of Wilson and Gully. The prospectus noted 'If the report of Patients be correct the two leading Establishments at Malvern, are dividing between them nearly £30,000 as clear yearly profits'.[106] Once again the scheme came to nothing and it was a further decade until any significant improvements were made. In 1857 the well and baths were refurbished and free access granted to poor workers on Saturday afternoons.[107] Between 1867 and 1871 further investment provided better facilities for both residents and tourists for a variety of secular uses including bathing and domestic supply. A public water supply drawing on the well was established and the old open-air plunge bath was supplemented by provision of hot and cold private baths and a large covered swimming pool.[108] Despite industrial decline in the area St Winefride's stream supplied increasing commercial demands too. The expansion in the number of pilgrims from the 1890s led to a dispute over access rights. When the Jesuits' lease came up for renewal the council considered refusing this in favour of a higher rental offered by a soda-water manufacturer wishing to set up in business. Support for this proposal was fuelled by disquiet over increasing missionary activity as well as financial considerations. The Jesuits challenged the proposed scheme and a legal judgment upheld their claim on the grounds that while the local authority were entitled to use the source to provide a water supply and baths they did not have the right to lease it to a bottling company as this might endanger the public supply.[109] Competing demands on the water source were a real issue, not only due to increased use but also due to the threat of diminished flow. In 1917 mining activity led to the diversion of the underground stream as a result of which St Winefride's spring dried up completely. After considerable negotiations the spring was connected to an alternative underground source and water once again flowed down the valley, albeit not from the original spring.[110] The shrine continued to attract pilgrims with details of miraculous cures and supporting authentication recorded by the custodian of the well between 1905 and 1923.[111]

Recreation and social life

The rise of resort towns as places for pleasure and relaxation was an integral part of the fundamental processes of urbanisation and industrialisation that developed from the eighteenth century onwards and should not be seen as separate from these wider trends.[112] As centres for respite and recuperation spas have been described as 'sites of consumption that tried to pretend they had nothing to do with production' in which service industries were kept well out of sight of the areas designated for visitor use.[113] As the middle class expanded and their disposable income rose, the leisure facilities that had been limited to spas, London and a scattering of regional towns in the seventeenth century became more widely available in seaside resorts and residential towns; a trend which undermined the position of spas as the premier leisure destinations. While investors in both spas and hydropathic centres gave particular emphasis to medical facilities they also sought to adapt recreational amenities to the changing tastes of their target market of the genteel middle class. Although increasing numbers of workers had the free time and surplus income to enjoy commercialised leisure by the middle of the nineteenth century, investors and municipal authorities at water cure resorts did not target this new market. Day trippers were tolerated rather than encouraged and, as discussed in Chapter 3 the mechanism of the charitable hospital was used to regulate access by the poor.

By the early nineteenth century Cheltenham was renowned for an extensive social life, similar to that in eighteenth-century Bath, carried on in a number of prestigious public venues including the pump rooms and associated gardens at Pitville and Montpellier. Frivolity and excess flourished, based on balls, promenades, card parties, races and fox-hunting – the latest craze for the aristocracy.[114] The structure of a public social life enjoyed by 'the company' with a round of formal social engagements orchestrated by a master of ceremonies was introduced in both Cheltenham and Leamington. This model, posited on the importance of social display and performance among the social elite, served to foster feelings of community among those visiting a spa by publishing the names of new arrivals and encouraging their participation in the social round of regular events at the baths, assembly rooms and places of entertainment. However, as is well established, the popularity of this formal, orchestrated communal social life was in decline by the last quarter of the eighteenth century as increasing numbers of visitors drawn from the middling orders undermined the reality of a homogenous 'company' with shared values and norms of behaviour. These pressures, apparent in Bath as early as the 1770s, led to the elite retreating away from display in the public arena and the development of more exclusive private clubs.[115] Between the 1820s and 1840s demand for public entertainments in Leamington had weakened to the extent that in some years few concerts or balls were offered by promoters due to fears of insufficient support.[116] The trend was similar at Bristol Hot Wells.[117] The post of master of ceremonies fell into disuse with the last appointment to the position in Cheltenham made in the 1840s by which time a new air of sobriety was becoming apparent.[118] Under the influence of Francis Close, evangelical minister and active promoter of church building and educational institutions, Cheltenham became associated with charity and good works rather than gaming and festivities. Close also promoted strict Sabbath observance and opposed Sunday passenger trains until these were made compulsory by the Railway Act of 1846.[119] These trends reflected broader shifts towards self-improvement and rational forms of recreation in the early Victorian period associated with the rising influence of the middle class in shaping norms of public behaviour.

Despite these trends visitors to Cheltenham in the early 1840s could enjoy a wide range of cultural pursuits. Granville notes that there were weekly subscription balls and frequent musical events including 'chamber quartets, philharmonic meetings, and concerts without number' throughout the year supplemented with 'musical promenades' held several times a week in the summer season.[120] In addition several subscription libraries with reading rooms provided access to national and local newspapers. A similar range of social amenities developed at Leamington. R. B. Elliston, an entrepreneurial actor and theatre manager, with previous experience in Bath and London, provided a library, ball room, tea room and shop at the family-run Lower Assembly Rooms – his sons managed the library and his wife and daughter taught dancing.[121] Another notable incomer was James Bissett who transferred his museum and picture gallery from Birmingham. The gallery, which included several items obtained from Captain Cook's collection, was one of several enterprises in the town displaying artefacts and offering curiosities and exotic items for sale.[122] Bissett, who had produced a well-received and highly illustrated directory of Birmingham, authored a guide to Leamington in 1814 followed by another descriptive volume to the town and its vicinity.[123]

Many resorts developed a lively literary culture that included reading rooms, local newspapers and commercial directories. Early newspapers frequently covered a wide geographical region but as resorts expanded new publications were launched for their local market. These papers provided vital information for visitors including lists of accommodation, details of pump room opening hours, transport services, and a calendar of events as well as a forum for advertising businesses. Many published the names of visitors staying in the spa, fostering a sense of community and a lively social life. Leamington and Cheltenham both had local papers in the 1820s with other resorts following in later decades. The earliest paper to serve Leamington was the *Warwick Advertiser* founded in 1806 and several other short-lived titles appeared before the *Leamington Spa Courier* became the established local weekly paper. This successful title was started in 1828 by the printer John Fairfax who also published a series of guides and directories to the town.[124] Early newspapers in Cheltenham were the *Journal*, founded in 1824, and the *Chronicle*, later joined by the *Looker-On* in 1834 and the *Examiner* in 1839. The *Looker-On* specialised in items of interest to visitors including lists of arrivals and departures.[125] The *Harrogate Advertiser* was established in the 1830s and by the 1850s Buxton and Malvern also had their own newspapers. J. C. Bates, bookseller and printer, started the *Buxton Advertiser and List of Visitors* in 1852.[126] At Malvern two of the town's doctors promoted newspapers; Ralph Grindrod started the *Malvern Advertiser, Visitors' List and General Weekly Newspaper* in 1855 while James Gully invested in the rival *Malvern News* launched some five years later. *The Malvern Gazette* was launched in 1898.[127]

The provision of walks and gardens designed to lead to and from the various pump rooms or to show off constructed vistas were substantially extended at all inland resorts. As towns became larger there was a need to protect open spaces and improve landscaping to fulfil visitors' expectations of accessing 'nature tamed'. Indoor facilities to provide a place to stroll and sit in bad weather or accommodate concerts and other events were also constructed. Buxton was transformed from the 'bare and desolate aspect' of the late eighteenth century with the planting of tens of thousands of trees from 1811.[128] The hilly area in front of the baths was laid out in graduated terraces and accessible walks were created in Corbar Woods overlooking the town. By the 1830s guide books were celebrating the spa's romantic landscape and praising the suitable viewing points created to admire the vistas. In the late 1840s the riverside Serpentine Walks close to the bathing complex were improved and made free to visitors and the Terrace Walks further developed. Under the Buxton Improvement Company, formed in 1867, the area was redesigned to improve facilities for indoor and outdoor entertainment with the construction of a Winter Garden and boating lakes. By the 1870s roller skating and concerts were arranged in the Winter Gardens and by 1912 toboggan runs, ice skating, skiing, horse sleigh rides and curling provided recreation during the winter season.[129] Although the inland areas did not have the beach to spark an interest in natural history and invite exploration along the coastline, several spas did provide the opportunity to follow up the Victorian passion for amateur science, including geology. Ralf Grindrod's passion for fossil hunting flourished while examining rock faces exposed during the construction of railway tunnels cut through the Malvern hills and he built up a renowned collection of specimens illustrating the flora and fauna of the area which attracted attention from a number of groups including the British Association for the Promotion of Science. The hydropath was an active member of the Malvern Naturalists' Field Club and became a well-known lecturer.[130]

Even small centres like Woodhall Spa needed to provide a range of suitable activities to keep visitors amused throughout the day. On his appointment as spa physician in 1907 Lionel Calthrop was asked to review the arrangements for recreation and entertainment. While the Spa Baths included a pump room that was well supplied with papers and magazines that sufficed as 'the general rendezvous' of the small spa, Calthrop recommended a mix of investment to improve the recreational amenities. Central to his proposals was the need for a 'good band' to play three times a day – in the late morning at the Pump Room and in the afternoon and after dinner in the hotel gardens or lounge – to encourage a relaxed and cheerful ambience. In his view it was essential to provide something for people to do in the afternoons after completing their treatments and he suggested adding a putting green, clock golf and a bowling green to the existing croquet and tennis courts, and a better billiard table as part of the indoor entertainment. Facilities for children should also be improved with the provision of a playground for diabolo, skipping and other games. While the pavilion and tea house in the nearby woods provided a suitable venue to pass a rainy afternoon he considered that more evening entertainments were needed. Although Woodhall prided itself on being a quiet, rural resort the place needed to offer good quality attractions and these were best provided by combining resources. To ensure high standards at a reasonable cost he recommended collaboration with the other major hotels and clubs to develop a programme of dances, theatricals and concerts open to all spa visitors.[131]

Music had long been an important backdrop to spa life – a band accompanied water drinkers at Bath from the seventeenth century. In the nineteenth century music became more widely available, shaped by general trends in musical tastes and provision. In 1840 Granville commented favourably on the 'band, engaged purposely for the season, from London' playing at the Royal Promenade and Cheltenham Pump Room in Harrogate.[132] By the late 1880s an orchestra played regularly at several venues in the town with performances starting at 7.30 a.m. at the Pump Room and continuing until the evening. By the 1890s there were al fresco afternoon concerts in the Valley Gardens and evening recitals in the band stand on Victoria Avenue. The development of the Royal Spa included the town's first indoor concert hall and the schedule was extended to include a weekly symphony concert to supplement the more popular programmes. From 1903 the orchestra played every afternoon and evening at the new Kursaal.[133] Harrogate was not exceptional, by the 1890s 'almost everyone listened to, or at any rate heard, music at some time in the day' at Buxton too. This was mostly provided by the Pavilion orchestra playing in the band stand in the Riverside Gardens or under cover in the winter gardens.[134] These developments were part of broader expansion in musical provision across the country shaped by European influences and introduced through musical impresarios. It included growth in touring orchestras and promenade concerts that popularised opera, orchestral and band music.[135] Many performers were employed on a casual or seasonal basis finding employment at the spas and seaside resorts in the summer season and returning to London or the larger towns for the winter. By the 1870s promoters, including some local authorities, were prepared to fund municipal orchestras, although not necessarily all year round. Julian Adams' touring orchestra played at Buxton and Harrogate as well as the seaside resorts of Scarborough and Tynemouth between 1855 and 1877 when he was appointed as conductor to the first permanent resort orchestra in England at Eastbourne.[136] Several other leading seaside towns including Llandudno, Scarborough, Margate and Bournemouth had resort orchestras from time to time as did Buxton and Harrogate. Increased provision of music and concerts was popular with the residential population as well as visitors. Edward Elgar was instrumental in setting up the Malvern Concert Club in 1903 and in 1929 the first Malvern Festival was run from the refurbished Assembly Rooms recently purchased by the municipal council.[137] In the inter-war period several resort orchestras were featured in radio broadcasts with the BBC. Measures were taken to keep up with other trends in popular entertainment too, including the provision of cinemas; even the smaller resorts of Woodhall, Droitwich and Malvern gained picture houses in the 1920s.

Emphasis on fresh air and quiet recreation remained an essential component of therapeutic regimes which emphasised the need for diversion to aid recuperation. The growing emphasis on open-air activities and sports for both sexes is clearly shown in *Harrogate as a health resort*, an annual guidebook for general visitors produced by the corporation from 1898.[138] The town's oldest chalybeate wells, the Tewit and St John's, were situated on the Stray, the town's principal open space, which provided invalids and visitors free access to some two hundred acres of common land where they could stroll, cycle, ride or be driven in the open air. The resort offered '24 miles of asphalted and flagged footpaths, besides 8 miles of smooth gravel walks', suitable for walkers in all weathers but also easily accessible by the less mobile visitor in invalid carriages or the recently developed cycle bath chair. The site of the sulphur wells in the lower town, earlier called the Bog's Field, had been laid out and renamed the Valley Gardens and the lower town also offered the Crescent and Kursall Gardens. The Magnesia Pump Room in the Valley Gardens served three types of water at just 1d or 2d a glass and provided a focal point for visitors with the surrounding area laid out to gardens with plenty of seating. The 1916 brochure emphasised increased informality with visitors sitting on deck chairs taking tea and listening to the Corporation band. At the far end of the valley the gardens gave access onto Harlow Moor, which had been given to the town by the Earl of Harewood and provided the opportunity for longer walks of several miles. By 1912 photographs of women strolling through the pine woods and striding out in the open terrain of the moor were included in the brochure.[139] The 1916 edition gave greater emphasis to the surrounding countryside and to provision for sports; Birk Crag, offering spectacular views, was recommended as a short walk from the centre of the spa, and visitors had the option of two tennis clubs, three badminton clubs and three golf clubs. In addition to these public facilities the premier hotels and hydros offered private facilities to their guests. Advertisements for the Cairn, Harlow Manor and Harrogate hydros all emphasised the availability of tennis, croquet, bowling and easy access to a golf club.[140] The inter-war period saw further expansion of both public and private facilities. By 1923 seven tennis clubs offering grass and hard courts were listed and the 1929 guidebook included details of angling, boating, hockey and a rifle club in addition to suggested car tours. The Sun Pavilion and Colonnade, constructed in the Valley Gardens in 1933, was designed in response to growing interest in the therapeutic potential of sunlight; its modernist style contrasting with the late Victorian architecture of the Royal Baths and larger hydros.[141]

In his pioneering study of the rise of the English seaside published in the 1980s, John Walton argued that the growth of working-class demand and the popularity of the annual summer holiday meant that seaside resorts came to supplant the spas as the preferred English leisure destinations by 1914.[142] Further research has now shown that the pattern of resort development was more complex than this, marked by significant regional differences influenced by industrialisation and urbanisation in resort hinterlands. Towns along the Kent coast were among the first to prosper due to their proximity to London where the development of the steamer trade attracted visitors from a mix of social groups. The Lancashire resorts benefited from the wealth generated in the industrial towns and cities of the north-west with demand for holidays developing among workers in the cotton and woollen trades by 1914. The expansion of working-class demand apparent in these areas was atypical and occurred up to a generation before that in some other regions. For example the south Devon resorts, geographically remote from new industrial centres and where comprehensive railway infrastructure developed later, continued to rely on better-off groups and to emphasise their facilities for invalids.[143] This study has shown that the general expansion in resorts in the nineteenth century included notable inland centres specialising in water therapeutics. Rather than becoming overshadowed by new centres for leisure at the seaside these successful resorts continued to shape changing trends. The amenities and cultural life at the inland watering places had much in common with many seaside resorts, particularly those marketed as health resorts, while the surrounding countryside offered options for enjoying outdoor activities in the fresh air.

Many commentators in the nineteenth century decried the lack of facilities for entertainment and social life at the English spas when compared to those available at their continental rivals. Lack of patronage by the British ruling family was frequently cited as a reason why the upper classes deserted the British resorts and joined the European political elites who gravitated towards a small number of exclusive spas including Carlsbad, Vichy and Bad Homburg. However this picture of continental spas as aristocratic leisure centres is misleading. Even at the elite resorts the majority of visitors were not the crowned heads and political cadres but substantial members of the professional and business classes. The majority of the three hundred German spas as well as those in France and Italy catered for the middle classes and 'went out of their way to emphasize their "comfortable", "intimate" and "family" character as retreats concerned with health, not luxury'.[144] The second half of the nineteenth century saw a rapid expansion in the number and size of European spas, fuelled by demand from the aristocracy and the growing middle class, improved rail networks and commercial tourism. The number of visitors to French spas is estimated to have risen from less than 10,000 in 1815 to around 800,000 by 1900, the majority of whom were drawn from the middle class.[145] Mackaman has argued that the annual routine of earnest dedication to improving their health was a major influence in the formation of French bourgeois identity.[146] New resort areas became popular in this period, notably the Alps and the Italian lakes as well as seaside regions including the Normandy coast. The patterns of European development and visitor flows across the nineteenth century were influenced by broader economic trends, such as the financial crash of 1873 and the sustained boom from the 1890s, periods of warfare in the 1840s and 1870s and support for regional and national centres.[147] In the 1830s the German spas attracted many French visitors due to a ban on gambling in France. The pace of development in France accelerated after 1850, encouraged by the development of a more extensive railway network and the new administrative category of the 'ville d'eaux'.[148] Napoleon III patronised Plombières in the 1850s and Vichy was redeveloped for his visit in 1861.[149] Many French visitors continued to travel to the German spas, notably Baden-Baden, in the period up to the 1870s, but one effect of the Franco-Prussian war was greater patriotic support for the French spas.[150] In the Austria-Hungarian territories spa culture was shaped by markedly different patterns of industrialisation and urbanisation across the empire as well as strong regional and national identities. Language, ethnicity and bathing traditions grounded in pilgrimage and Turkish culture were all influential in shaping the distinctiveness of centres such as Budapest and Carlsbad.[151]

Figures available from continental resorts attest to significant numbers of British visitors to European centres. In the 1840s the German spas were most popular with the British encouraged by publications including Granville's *Spas of Germany* and Francis Head's *Bubbles from the Brunnens of Nassau*.[152] By the 1870s the French spas, including Vichy, Aix-les-Bains and Mont Dore were attracting more British visitors, partly due to the recommendations of authors such as John Macpherson and Burney Yeo.[153] It has been estimated that by 1911, one in thirty at every European watering place was British but only one in a thousand at a British spa was European.[154] The influx of British visitors helped ensure that European resorts catered to their tastes including the growing passion for sport. The first tennis match in Germany is reported to have been conducted by two Englishmen at Bad Homburg in 1874, a club was established in 1879 and the first tennis tournament hosted in the 1890s. Baden Baden, famous for its waters, casino and race track, was another spa popular with British visitors and residents where facilities for tennis were introduced and a club established by 1881.[155] Other European resort areas that attracted British visitors were the Alps, popular for mountaineering as well as treatment for tuberculosis, and the beach culture of the Côte d'Azure. The ability to travel abroad and the additional financial resource and time needed to visit European resorts was a means of expressing and maintaining cultural identities, particularly for the better off. 'Foreign travel was inherently exclusive, remaining relatively time-consuming and expensive' so that the majority of travellers were the aristocracy and wealthy middle classes.[156] Continental resorts were discussed in a range of travel literature including the Cook's handbooks, Bradshaw's guides and *Queen* magazine which dedicated several pages to travel news in each edition as well as publishing an annual *Queen Book of Travel*.[157] These sources suggest that by the end of the century the elite British spas were perceived to be catching up with their European competitors in the provision of treatments if not leisure amenities or touristic appeal. *Queen* magazine noted that facilities at the leading English resorts, including Harrogate, Buxton and Matlock were now able to compete with those at many European centres.[158] The outbreak of the First World War further disrupted the British enthusiasm for continental resorts.

Conclusion

The mix of consumers at water resorts included invalids, companions, leisure travellers and residents, individuals whose wants and desires were shaped by a mix of motives. Although medical treatment was increasingly delivered in private spaces within bathing institutions, access to a communal social life remained an important element of the resort experience. The middle decades of the nineteenth century were characterised by a move towards sobriety and rational recreation which contrasted with earlier cultures of public display, profligacy and excess. However, the provision of public areas for informal social exchange, including pump rooms, parks and winter gardens, continued to be characteristic of these resorts. Pumps for dispensing mineral water to drinkers were provided in indoor and outdoor settings and enhanced provision was made for attached reading rooms with quiet lounge areas. Band music was provided up to several times a day, often in different areas of the spa, encouraging circulation around the resorts. During the high season at least, regular programmes of entertainment were arranged, complemented by special events including horticultural shows and sporting competitions. Outdoor activities, music concerts and reading rooms continued to be preferred forms of genteel relaxation which complemented the lavish bathing institutions that reflected the burgeoning consumer culture of the late Victorian era.

By the end of the nineteenth century several spas issued separate publications aimed at the invalid and general visitor. At Bath a *Medical guide* discussed the up-to-date treatment available while *Bath as a health resort* gave more emphasis to the city's history, in particular its Roman heritage.[159] Despite their different formats and target audiences, the content of the booklets show considerable overlap demonstrating that recreation and tourist activities were of interest to patients while the baths also attracted more general visitors. In addition to a thorough description of the baths the *Medical guide* drew attention to the use of the Grand Pump Room not only by 'the sick and disabled, but ... the lovers of society and music, and the votaries of the fashion of the hour'. The adjoining Roman promenade housed a concert hall and museum displaying the Roman antiquities recovered in excavations carried out from around 1880. The Royal Victoria Park and the Sydney Gardens were noted as the largest among a number of city parks and were the venue of daily concerts in the season as well as various floral fêtes. The Assembly Rooms, Theatre Royal, Royal Literary and Scientific Institution and Art Gallery provided other diversions as did a wide range of sporting facilities. *Bath as a health resort* provided more extensive discussion of the Roman excavations and a commentary on the development of the city from medieval times – including the dazzling eighteenth century – but also included a description of the mineral springs and various bathing establishments. H. V. Morton, a popular travel writer in the inter-war period, draws out the complexity of the spa's attraction in his discussion of a visit undertaken as part of a motor tour in the mid-1920s to seek out the 'essential England'.[160] His inclusion of Bath in the itinerary attests to the city's unique place in national culture while the use of humour assumes a familiarity with the latest spa treatments among his middle-class audience that point up its multi-layered appeal.

> I had decided against a mud pack, because I did not like the picture in the handbook, which shows a nurse building up a big black mud pie on a patient's foot. I considered the whirling bath, the hydro-electric bath, the heat bath, the hot-air bath, the vapour bath, the aeration bath, and came to the conclusion that probably the best bath for a man with no real honest symptoms is the deep bath; the characteristic bath of Bath; the bath with historic and literary associations, because it is simply the scientific version of the treatment as practised by the Romans and by those of our eighteenth-century forefathers who drew the first gout dividends before investing them for us at thirty per cent.[161]

By referring to the longevity of use of the thermal waters for bathing dating back to the Romans, the extensive range of modern treatments on offer and poking fun at wealthy eighteenth-century *bon viveurs* suffering from largely self-inflicted gout, Morton draws attention to a healing approach that had stood the test of time. It was nonetheless ideally suited to meet the needs of the contemporary world for regeneration and healing, harnessing both nature and science for prophylactic and curative purposes. His preference for the classic, warm, passive immersion bath over the alarming range of modern options underlined the continuing importance of recreation and renewal in the complex and enduring appeal of water cures.

By the twentieth century local authorities were the major players in creating and maintaining both health and recreational facilities at the English resorts. These were designed to serve a variety of groups of consumers, including patients, invalids, residents and visitors. Provision was influenced by the wider availability of water with a clear trend towards greater popularity of bathing for hygienic, recreational and health purposes with Turkish baths, swimming baths and latterly lidos at several resorts. The balance between health and recreational amenities depended on a number of factors. Thus at Leamington the Pump Rooms provided for a range of health and leisure uses while at Harrogate there was significant investment in the creation of open-air spaces and parks to cater for the hundreds of patients accessing the specialist treatment facilities at the Royal Baths. Visitor attractions took a variety of guises including pilgrimage, antiquarianism and tourism. Smaller inland resorts, such at Church Stretton and Ashby de la Zouche, developed and emphasised particular local attractions to appeal to visitors, in these cases access to open hills and the attraction of an historic castle.

The growth in the number and size of both seaside and inland resorts across the nineteenth century brought greater variety in their distinctive features. It has been argued here that practices developed at spas and hydropathic resorts continued to influence wider resort cultures. John Walton has highlighted that part of the appeal of the seaside and the reason that it consolidated its position as the preferred summer holiday destination was 'greater scope for informality' especially on the beach and foreshore and its appeal for families and children. In contrast the elite spas catered for a predominantly adult clientele. Opportunities for informal social mixing continued to be available and although these no doubt provided ample opportunities for display of wealth and social position the prevailing ambience was one of respectable recreation. The social tone the spas wished to present to the public remained resolutely middle-class into the inter-war period. While spas may have ceased to be the foremost places where leisure trends were forged, they continued to have a distinctive appeal within the expanding number of destinations across the country.

The continuing importance of integrating recreation into the cure is demonstrated by a guide to spas issued by the BMA in 1951 which listed the main cultural and leisure opportunities at each centre as well as providing information on treatment options. Among the common activities noted were access to the open country, sports and outdoor diversions, music and concerts and visits to places of interest in the vicinity. The entry for Cheltenham gave particular mention to a variety of annual tournaments and festivals celebrating sport and the arts including racing, music and the West of England Kennel Club show. The entry for Bath highlighted the annual Festival of the Arts and a cricket tournament while that for Buxton emphasised the provision of a variety of 'lighter type of entertainment' including swing concerts, dancing and variety shows.[162] Despite the increasing emphasis given to medical treatment it was a subtle mix of 'health and pleasure' that continued to underpin the appeal of the spa for many visitors.

Notes

1 Bergdolt, *Wellbeing*, pp. 2–6; Peter Borsay, *A history of leisure: the British experience since 1500* (Basingstoke: Palgrave Macmillan, 2006), pp. 1–12; Susan C. Anderson and Bruce H. Tabb (eds), *Water, leisure and culture: European historical perspectives* (Oxford: Berg, 2002), pp. 1–3.

2 John Ruskin, *The crown of wild olives; works XVIII*, pp. 206–7, *cited* in Haley, *Healthy body*, p. 257.

3 Goubert, *Conquest of water;* Jenner, 'From conduit community'.

4 J. H. Plumb, *The commercialisation of leisure in eighteenth-century England* (Reading: University of Reading, 1973); J. Walvin, *Leisure and society, 1830–1950* (London: Longman, 1978); Borsay, *Leisure.*

5 P. J. Corfield, *The impact of English towns 1700–1800* (Oxford: Oxford University Press, 1982), p. 51.

6 Borsay, *English urban renaissance*, pp. 243–8.

7 Peter Borsay, 'Bath: an Enlightenment city?', in Borsay, Hirschfelder and Mohrmann (eds), *New directions in urban history*, 3–17, p. 3.

8 Jon Stobart, 'In search of a leisure hierarchy: English spa towns and their place in the eighteenth-century urban system', in Borsay, Hirschfelder and Mohrmann (eds), *New directions in urban history*, 19–40, pp. 19–22.

9 See for example, 'Local and county topics', *Leamington Spa Courier* (1 March 1862); 'The Royal Pump Room Company and baths', *Leamington Spa Courier* (1 March 1862); 'Leamington waters and baths', *Leamington Spa Courier* (29 March 1862).

10 Anon., *What to do with the Royal Pump Rooms* (Leamington Spa: James J. Barr, 1862).

11 'To the rescue!', *Leamington Spa Courier* (7 June 1862).
12 *Beck's shilling guide to Leamington* (Leamington Spa: John Beck, 1867), pp. 18–19.
13 Warwickshire CRO, CR1563/179, Leamington local board of health minutes, 17 March 1868.
14 Anon., *Pictorial and descriptive guide to Royal Leamington Spa* (London: Ward Lock and Co., 1918/19), p. 36.
15 LSAGM, M 4348.1995, Pump room and baths manager's report book, 20 February 1920.
16 William Makepeace Thackeray, *Notes of a journey from Cornhill to grand Cairo* (London: Chapman and Hall, 1846); David Urquhart, *Pillars of Hercules, or, a narrative of travels in Spain & Morocco in 1848* (London: Bentley, 1850).
17 Metcalfe, *Rise and progress*, pp. 129–41; Teresa Breathnach, 'For health and pleasure: the Turkish bath in Victorian Ireland', *Victorian Literature and* Culture, 20 (2004), 159–75; Ronan Foley, *Healing waters: therapeutic landscapes in historic and contemporary Ireland* (Farnham: Ashgate, 2010).
18 William Potter, 'The Turkish bath' [letter to the editor], *Sheffield Free Press* (22 July 1857), p. 3, quoted in Malcolm R. Shifrin, 'Victorian Turkish baths: their origin, development, and gradual decline', www.victorianturkishbath.org/, accessed 17 October 2011.
19 My thanks are due to Elizabeth Simpson, 'Bathing for health and pleasure: the Turkish bath at Leamington Spa 1860–1970', Undergraduate research scholarship scheme, University of Warwick, 2007.
20 Warwickshire CRO, CR1563/179, Leamington local board of health minutes, 7 December 1869.
21 Langham and Wells, *Baths at Buxton*, p. 84.
22 George Elson, *The last of the climbing boys* (London: J. Long, 1900), pp. 277–8.
23 Elson *Climbing boys*, pp. 271 and 277.
24 Elson *Climbing boys*, p. 267.
25 LSAGM, M 4151.1994, Medical advisory committee minutes, 24 March 1920.
26 'Re-opening of the Royal Pump Rooms and Baths at Leamington', *Lancet*, 3328 (11 June 1887), 'Medicinal Baths at Leamington Spa', *BMJ* (11 June 1887); Anon., *Leamington Spa: a history of the Pump Room bathing establishment', reprinted from The Leamington Spa Courier and the Warwickshire Standard, Saturday June 4, 1887*, p. 6.
27 DRO, D1397 B/B 29, Smedley's Hydropathic establishment, prospectus, p. 13; *Harrogate as a health resort* (1898).
28 Sheard, 'Profit is a dirty word', p. 67.
29 Agnes Campbell, Carnegie United Kingdom Trust, *Report on public baths and wash-houses in the United Kingdom* (Edinburgh: Edinburgh University Press, 1918); David J. Eveleigh, *Bogs, baths and basins: the story of domestic sanitation* (Stroud: Sutton Publishing, 2002), p. 159.
30 Eveleigh, *Bogs, baths and basins*, p. xviii.
31 Eveleigh, *Bogs, baths and basins*, pp. 73–81.

32 Eveleigh, *Bogs, baths and basins*, p. 85.
33 Smith, *Clean*, pp. 289–91.
34 Arnold Bennett, *Clayhanger* (London: Methuen, 1910), pp. 181–2.
35 Hembry, *British spas from 1815*, p. 47, citing *Cheltenham Journal* (21 June 1830).
36 Lane, *Life at the water cure* (1851), pp. 131–5.
37 Hilary Marland, *Medicine and society in Wakefield and Huddersfield, 1780–1870* (Cambridge: Cambridge University Press, 1987), pp. 230–2.
38 E. Parsons, *The Civil, ecclesiastical, literary, commercial, and miscellaneous history of Leeds, Halifax, Huddersfield, Bradford, Wakefield, Dewsbury, Otley, and the manufacturing district of Yorkshire* (Leeds: Frederick Hobson, 1834) Vol. 2, p. 395; C. P. Hobkirk, *Huddersfield: its history and natural history* (London: Simpkin, Marshall and co., 1868) p. 10, both cited in Marland, *Medicine and society*, pp. 230–4.
39 Granville, *Northern spas*, pp. 406–7; Marland, *Medicine and society*, pp. 230–3.
40 Advertisement for Stafford Corporation public baths, *Halden and son's directory of Stafford and District* (Stafford: printed for the authors, 1893), p. 58.
41 'Description of the speeches at the opening ceremony Stafford Corporation Public Baths', *Staffordshire Advertiser* (23 April 1892).
42 Ord and Garrod, *Climates and baths*, Vol. 1, pp. 567–8.
43 Luke, *Spas and health* resorts, p. 179.
44 *Slater's directory of Southport and Birkdale* (Manchester: Slater's, 1887), p. 10.
45 Stephenson's Guide to Southport (Southport: Visiter, 1903), p. 76.
46 Devon Heritage Centre, R7/7/P58, Plans of new bath house at Sidmouth.
47 'Reviews and notices of books', Neil MacVean and Leonard Williams, *The English riviera: a guide to Sidmouth* and Leonard Williams *The baths of Sidmouth*, *JB&C*, I (January 1897), p. 74.
48 A. Macindoe, *Sidmouth and the Nauheim treatment* (Sidmouth: Culverwell & Sons, 1898).
49 *Kelly's Directory of Devonshire* (London: Kelly's, 1939), p. 703.
50 John F. Travis, 'Continuity and change in English sea-bathing, 1730–1900: a case of swimming with the tide', in Stephen Fisher (ed.), *Recreation and the sea* (Exeter: Exeter University Press, 1997), 8–35, pp. 8–11.
51 Richard Russell, *A dissertation on the use of sea water in the diseases of the glands* (London: W. Owen, 1755), p. 68, quoted in Travis, 'Continuity and change', p. 11.
52 Travis, 'Continuity and change', pp. 13–14.
53 Travis, *Devon seaside*, p. 178; Travis, 'Continuity and change', p. 17.
54 Travis, 'Continuity and change', p. 20.
55 Travis, 'Continuity and change', pp. 26–8.
56 Janet Smith, *Liquid assets: the lidos and open-air swimming pools of Britain* (Swindon: English Heritage, 2005), pp. 17–19.
57 Smith, *Liquid assets*, p. 13. The pool closed in the 1970s but plans are now under way to restore it, clevelandpools.org.uk, accessed 4 September 2012.
58 Campbell, *Carnegie Report*, p. 55.
59 *Leamington Spa: a history of the Royal Pump Room bathing establishment*, p. 3.

60 Elson, *Last of the climbing boys*, pp. 260–3.
61 Smith, *Liquid assets*, pp. 26–31 and 176–83.
62 Thomas Hinderwell, *The history and antiquities of Scarborough*, 2nd edn (York: Longman, Hurst, Rees, Orme and Brown, 1811), p. 227; Edmund W. Gilbert, *Brighton: old ocean's bauble* (London: Methuen, 1954), pp. 67–75. C. A. Ellis, *An Historical Survey of Torquay*, 2nd edn (Torquay: Ellis, c. 1930), pp. 364–6.
63 Travis, *Devon seaside resorts*, p. 178.
64 Ellis, *Torquay*, pp. 364–6.
65 John K. Walton, 'The seaside resorts of Western Europe, 1750–1939', in Fisher (ed.), *Recreation and the sea*, 36–56.
66 H. J. Perkin, 'The social tone of Victorian seaside resorts in the North West', *Northern History*, 11 (1976), 180–94.
67 John Hassan, *The seaside, health and the environment in England and Wales since 1800* (London: Ashgate, 2003) provides a number of relevant case studies.
68 F. B. Smith, *The people's health* 1830–1910, 2nd edn (London: Weidenfeld and Nicolson, 1990), pp. 226–9.
69 This section draws on Cora Weaver and Bruce Osborne, *Acquae Malvernensis: a history and topography of the springs, spouts, fountains and wells of the Malverns and the development of a public water supply* (Malvern: Cora Weaver, 1994), especially Part 2, 'From springs and spouts to public main'. The authors' research includes extensive use of reports in the local press including the *Malvern Advertiser, Malvern Gazette* and *Malvern News*.
70 Weaver and Osborne, *Acquae Malvernensis*, pp. 32–3.
71 Malvern Improvement Act, 1851, preamble.
72 Malvern Improvement Act, 1851, clause XLVI.
73 Worcestershire Archive Service (WAS) BA 9196/160 (i), 'Water Supply Survey, West Midlands area' typed report prepared at request of MoH, 7 August 1948.
74 Weaver and Osborne, *Acquae Malvernensis*, pp. 178–85.
75 Malvern Water Act 1891, Malvern Link (Extension and Water Act) 1896.
76 Malvern Water Act of 1905.
77 Malvern Link (Extension and Water Act) 1896, clause 26 (i).
78 House of Commons Select Committee on Private Bills: Malvern Water Bill. Monday 26 June 1905 – petition against the bill from Colwall Parish Council.
79 Wellcome Library, GC/63/4, bound volume cutting from *Malvern News* (11 September 1909).
80 Wellcome Library, GC/63/1, Malvern typhoid case, 1907 miscellaneous items, chronological statement summer 1905.
81 Wellcome Library, GC/63/3, newspaper report of Starkey V. Fergusson, judgment for the defendant re. Malvern drainage case.
82 Wellcome Library, GC/63/4, 'Pollution of water supply by sewage', *The Times* (14 January 1908).
83 Wellcome Library, GC/63/4, news cutting, unnamed newspaper (13 January 1908).

84 WAS, BA 9196/181 (iv), Appeal John Campbell Fergusson v MUDC, May 1908, para. 296.
85 Wellcome Library, GC/63/4, news cutting, *Malvern News* (11 September 1909).
86 Wellcome Library, GC/63/3, news cutting, letter from J. N. F. Fergusson dated 28 October 1909, *Malvern News* (30 October 1909).
87 An Act for the prevention of encroachments upon the Malvern Hills, and for other purposes, 28 July 1884; Brian Smith, *A history of Malvern* (Leicester: Leicester University Press, 2nd edn, 1978), p. 248 cites W. E. Tate, 'Worcestershire field systems', *Transactions of the Worcestershire Archaeological Society*, New Series, 20 (1943), 26–31.
88 Smith, *Malvern*, p. 248. In 1925 the commissioners bought the lands of Great Malvern manor and their powers were subsequently extended by further acts.
89 *Malvern Advertiser* (29 April 1882) quoted in Weaver and Osborne, *Acquae Malvernensis*, p. 130.
90 Weaver and Osborne, *Acquae Malvernensis*, pp. 98–9 and 66.
91 Weaver and Osborne, *Acquae Malvernensis*, pp. 59 and 66.
92 Judith F. Champ, 'Bishop Milner, Holywell, and the cure tradition', in Sheils (ed.), *The Church and healing*, 153–64, pp. 153–4.
93 J. Milner, *Authentic documents relative to the miraculous case of Winefrid White etc.* (London: for the author, 1805).
94 T. W. Pritchard, *St Winefride, her holy well and the Jesuit mission, c. 650–1930* (Wrexham: Bridge Books, 2009), pp. 248–9.
95 Pritchard, *St Winefride*, pp. 293–6.
96 Pritchard, *St Winefride*, pp. 270–1 and 301–3.
97 Ruth Harris, *Lourdes: body and spirit in the secular age* (Harmondsworth: Allen Lane, 1999), pp. 3–9 and 246–9.
98 Pritchard, *St Winefride*, pp. 314–31.
99 Pritchard, *St Winefride*, p. 325.
100 *North Wales Chronicle* (Saturday 18 August 1894).
101 Flintshire archives service (FAS), P/30/1/147 Papers relating to St. Winefride's Well 1838–1938, NC/429, newscutting of letter from James Williams, *Flintshire Observer* (24 October 1894).
102 Harris, *Lourdes*, pp. 321–5; Jason Szabo, 'Seeing is believing? The form and substance of French medical debates over Lourdes', *Bulletin of the History of Medicine*, 76 (2002), 199–230.
103 Pritchard, *St Winefride*, p. 335.
104 C. N. Wright, *Scenes in North Wales* (London: T. T. & J. Tegg, 1833), p. 115.
105 FAS, P/30/1/147, 'The baths at St. Winefride's Well'.
106 FAS, D/GR/1451, Correspondence Captain Mervyn Richardson and Duke of Westminster, 1858.
107 Pritchard, *St Winefride*, pp. 266–7.
108 Pritchard, *St Winefride*, pp. 269–77.
109 Pritchard, *St Winefride*, pp. 351–9.

110 Pritchard, *St Winefride*, pp. 380–93.
111 St Winefride's museum and archives, HOWSW/2004/501 AC, Father Ryan's diary.
112 Peter Borsay and John K. Walton, 'Introduction: the resort–port relationship', in Borsay and Walton (eds), *Resorts and ports: European seaside towns since 1700* (Bristol, Buffalo, Toronto: Channel View, 2011), 1–17, p. 1.
113 David Blackbourn, 'Fashionable spa towns in nineteenth-century Europe' in Anderson and Tabb (eds), *Water, leisure and culture*, 9–21, p. 15.
114 Hart, *Cheltenham*, pp. 180–3 and 187–9.
115 Borsay, 'Bath: an Enlightenment city?', pp. 7–11.
116 Baxter, 'Social life Leamington Spa', part 1, pp. 30–4.
117 David Hussey, '"From the temple of Hygeia to the sordid devotees of Pluto". The Hotwell and Bristol: resort and port in the eighteenth century', in Borsay and Walton (eds), *Resorts and ports*, 50–65.
118 Hart, *Cheltenham*, p. 182.
119 Hart, *Cheltenham*, pp. 198–202.
120 Granville, *Midland and southern spas*, p. 322.
121 Baxter, 'Social life Leamington Spa', part I, pp. 20–1.
122 Baxter, 'Social life Leamington Spa', part 2', pp. 52–3.
123 James Bisset, *A descriptive guide to Leamington Priors* (Leamington: Merridew, 1814); James Bisset, *The origin, rise and progress of Leamington Spa* (Leamington: E. Heathcote, 1828).
124 Lyndon F. Cave, *Royal Leamington Spa: its history and development* (Chichester: Philimore, 1988), p. 78; John Fairfax, *Fairfax's new Leamington guide: including a general directory* (Leamington: John Fairfax, 1832).
125 Hart, *Cheltenham*, pp. 178 and 188.
126 Langham, *Buxton*, p. 53.
127 Smith, *Malvern*, p. 239; Grierson, *Temperance, therapy and trilobites*, pp. 125–6.
128 Langham, *Buxton*, p. 19.
129 Langham, *Buxton*, p. 80.
130 Grierson, *Temperance, therapy and trilobites*, pp. 116–24.
131 Lincolnshire Archives, Ref: 'Hawley 5: Woodhall Spa company', Lionel Calthrop, 'Recreation and entertainment', typescript note for the Directors' consideration, Directors; meeting, 9 April 1908.
132 Granville, *Northern spas*, p. 44.
133 Kenneth Young, *Music's great days in the spas and watering places* (Macmillan: London, 1968), pp. 39–40 and 52.
134 Young, *Music's great days*, p. 185.
135 Young, *Music's great days*, pp. 17–19 and 36.
136 Young, *Music's great days*, p. 36.
137 Smith, *Malvern*, pp. 255–6.
138 *Harrogate as a health resort* (1898).
139 Photograph, 'On Harlow Moor', *Harrogate as a health resort* (1912), p. 12.
140 *Harrogate as a health resort* (1916).

141 Simon Carter, *Rise and shine: sunlight, technology and health* (Oxford: Berg, 2007).
142 Walton, *English seaside resort*, pp. 5–10 and 216–18.
143 Travis, *Devon seaside resorts*.
144 Blackbourn, 'Fashionable spa towns', pp. 16–17.
145 Douglas P. Mackaman, 'Competing visions of urban grandeur: planning and developing nineteenth-century spa towns in France', in Borsay, Hirschfelder, Mohrmann (eds), *New directions in urban history*, 41–63, pp. 41 and 61.
146 Mackaman, *Leisure settings*, pp. 5–6.
147 Blackbourn, 'Fashionable spa towns', p. 20.
148 Mackaman, 'Competing visions of urban grandeur', p. 48.
149 Mackaman, 'Competing visions of urban grandeur', p. 49.
150 Mackaman, 'Competing visions of urban grandeur', p. 60.
151 Steward, Jill, 'The spa towns of the Austro-Hungarian Empire and the growth of tourist culture: 1860–1914', in Borsay, Hirschfelder, Mohrmann (eds), *New directions in urban history*, 87–125, pp. 119–20.
152 Steward, 'Representations of spa culture', p. 382, citing A. B. Granville, *Spas of Germany*, 2 vols (London: Henry Colburn, 1837) and Francis Head, *Bubbles from the Brunnens of Nassau* (London: J. Murray, 1834).
153 Steward, 'Representations of spa culture', pp. 388–9, citing John Macpherson, *The baths and wells of Europe*, 2nd edn (London: Macmillan, 1873), pp. 9–10 and I. Burney Yeo, *Health resorts and their uses* (London: Chapman and Hall, 1882), p. 159.
154 Steward, 'Representations of spa culture', p. 378.
155 Heiner Gillmeister, *Tennis: a cultural history* (Leicester University Press, 1998), pp. 235–42.
156 Steward, 'Representations of spa culture', pp. 376–7.
157 Steward, 'Representations of spa culture', pp. 392–4.
158 Steward, 'Representations of spa culture', pp. 402–3.
159 *Medical guide to the hot mineral baths of Bath* (Bath: Bath Corporation, 1901); *Bath as a health resort* (Bath: Bath Corporation, n.d. c. 1900).
160 H. V. Morton, *In search of England* (London: Methuen, 1927); M. Bartholomew, 'H. V. Morton's English utopia', in C. Lawrence and A-K. Meyer (eds), *Regenerating England: science, medicine and culture in inter-war Britain* (Amsterdam and Atlanta: Rodopi, 2000), 25–44.
161 Morton, *In search of England*, p. 143.
162 BMA, *Spa in medical practice*, pp. 65, 71 and 75.

6

National assets and national interests: spas and the state

Prior to 1914 the clientele at English spas was drawn from the middle and upper classes with limited provision of services for the poor provided through charitable organisations. The role of local authorities in providing medical bathing institutions, pump rooms, parks and gardens – all elements of the expected treatment and social facilities of watering places – had increased in many resorts. Although this publicly funded infrastructure was intended to enhance the appeal of the whole resort to visitors, these enterprises were run with an eye to commercial viability to reduce the net cost to ratepayers. Other businesses providing services to meet the needs and wants of visitors – accommodation, food, entertainment – were privately run. These included luxurious hotels and hydros, modest lodging houses, theatres, restaurants and shops. At Droitwich and Woodhall the spa facilities were also private ventures. Despite the disruption to civilian life, the wartime emergency of 1914–18 offered British spas the opportunity to capitalise on restrictions on foreign travel to attract patients to take the cure at home. It also provided an opportunity to demonstrate the effectiveness of hydrological therapies in the treatment and rehabilitation of wounded soldiers and highlight the value of the specialist expertise at spas by demonstrating their unique contribution to the national emergency. Discussions with the military authorities channelled through the Balneological and Climatological Section (B&CS) of the Royal Society of Medicine (RSM) encouraged cooperative action by spas while the pressing need for treatment for the huge numbers of casualties encouraged an exchange of ideas about therapeutic approaches with European allies. These factors meant that both civilian and military personnel were treated at British spas during the war years.

The economic crises of the 1920s and 1930s undermined the pre-war patterns of demand leading to reduced numbers of visitors and a consequent threat to the financial viability of local businesses and the prosperity of resorts. These difficult trading conditions encouraged a number of collaborative ventures to promote the British spas and introduce mechanisms to enable a broader section of the population to take advantage of their facilities. The combined cost of accommodation and treatment for a stay of several weeks was beyond the financial resources of many of those not eligible for free treatment at one of the voluntary hospitals. Although some mutual societies ran convalescent homes offering their members access to treatment, this mechanism did not address the issue of affordability for the majority of the population. The British Spa Federation (BSF) became the prime vehicle for policy discussion and development for the spas. The introduction of national schemes for health insurance across Europe from the late nineteenth century brought with it the potential for state-funded 'social cures' for the lower paid. The introduction of the National Health Insurance (NHI) scheme in 1911 and the establishment of the Ministry of Health (MoH) in 1919 provided a focus for lobbying by the BSF for the state to fund treatment for insured persons. The focus was on therapies to alleviate rheumatism, long a mainstay of much spa treatment, which came to be identified as a major cause of chronic ill health across Europe in the inter-war period.[1]

This chapter investigates the attitude of the newly formed MoH towards spa treatment in Britain and assesses the impact this had on the provision of services. The potential for increased state funding was keenly debated by members of the International Society of Medical Hydrology (ISMH) in articles published in the *Archives of Medical Hydrology* (*AMH*). This valuable source provides data on comparative policy approaches adopted across Europe on this and other issues of interest to those practising or managing spas and health resorts, including systems for taxing visitors and assessing and validating the therapeutic efficacy of mineral waters. In addition to negotiations with the MoH, managers and doctors at spas worked on a variety of other schemes to reduce costs of treatment and enhance the medical reputation of hydrological treatment. Existing ties between bathing institutions, hospitals and other charitable bodies were strengthened and new alliances developed with academic institutions to create regional networks to address the problem of rheumatism which linked local authority, voluntary and university sectors. Further investment in laboratory facilities and specialist personnel strengthened the link between research and practice considered necessary to secure funds from appeals linked to the international rheumatism campaign. On the eve of the Second World War schemes at Bath, Harrogate and Buxton were in train to secure improvements in medical facilities at hospitals and bathing institutions.

The analysis goes on to investigate how spa treatment became integrated into the National Health Service (NHS) in 1948 and the pattern of service provided into the 1970s. The introduction of the NHS fundamentally altered the market for water cures, affecting both supply and demand. The voluntary hospitals were transferred into the health service under the management of the relevant Regional Hospital Boards which became responsible for negotiating contracts with bathing institutions for the provision of treatment. Medical personnel associated with spa treatment facilities were integrated within the medical specialties of rheumatism or physical medicine, often organised on a regional basis. The relative balance between private patients and those receiving free treatment was reversed with the number of private patients dropping rapidly. New arrangements were put in place to manage referrals through the NHS. The impact of these measures is assessed through oral histories relating to Leamington Spa and other fragmentary sources available. The devolved structure of the NHS meant that policies concerning spa treatment were taken on a piecemeal basis across the country. Although some facilities continued to provide treatment until the very end of the twentieth century the model of spa treatment practised at the English spas in the inter-war period had disappeared by the 1970s. A number of factors contributing to the decline of medical hydrology within the NHS are considered, including the impact of growing financial pressures, the promise of new drug-based treatments such as cortisone and the ideal of local provision of services.[2] The trajectory of decline in medical support for water cures in Britain at the end of the twentieth century is compared to that in France and Germany and the explanations that have been put forward to explain differences in international attitudes are considered and assessed for the British context.

Spas and the state

In January 1915, just a few months into the war, members of the B&CS met to discuss the potential contribution hydrological treatment could make to the treatment of wounded soldiers suffering from stiff joints, general fatigue and nervous disorders.[3] The unprecedented numbers of servicemen suffering from orthopaedic or nervous problems had led to greater awareness of the therapeutic value of spa treatments among both the medical profession and the public. Following a request from the Army Medical Services, guidelines setting out the medical and surgical conditions suitable for hydrological treatment were issued together with a list of health resorts designed to guide referrals for treatment. Recommended resorts included all the major British spas, hydropathic resorts at Ilkley, Malvern and Matlock and selected seaside towns including Bournemouth and Weston-super-Mare.[4] The service model proposed was influenced by methods developed in France which combined hydrotherapy with heat, massage, electrical treatments and medical gymnastics in intensive regimes aimed at rehabilitation and the prevention of long-term disability.[5] Significant military and economic benefits were claimed for this 'combined physical treatment' which the French authorities suggested could reduce incapacity by some 20 per cent.[6] In addition to reducing the time taken to return soldiers to the front, effective rehabilitation also reduced compensation payable to disabled soldiers and ex-servicemen and would therefore minimise the loss of productive labour to the peacetime economy after the war.[7] The delegation sent to assess the French facilities and treatment and develop recommendations for implementation in Britain included Robert Fortescue Fox, an influential spa practitioner, medical author and founder member of the ISMH.[8] Resources everywhere were under pressure with shortages of skilled personnel compounded by staff absence due to military service. The high level of demand meant that new treatment centres were urgently needed.[9] Paradoxically, although wartime demand raised the profile of spa treatments they also underscored the limited capacity of their specialist facilities and led to the development of an alternative model of local clinics in London and other large towns. The first specialist physical treatment clinic opened in London in July 1916 to treat disabled officers. Although additional capacity was later developed at convalescent camps and military hospitals, services remained insufficient to treat all servicemen assessed as able to benefit from intensive combination treatment.

A report published in 1924 estimated that between 50,000 and 75,000 servicemen had been treated at the spas since the outbreak of war.[10] Most were suffering from chronic ailments arising from wounds or longer term conditions. At Buxton, 92 per cent of the 5,300 cases suffered from rheumatic complaints with less than one hundred cases each recorded as suffering from wounds, neurasthenia and trench fever. At Bath, 88 per cent of over 5,000 cases treated between 1914 and 1922 had rheumatic complaints. The pattern was similar at the other spas. An extensive range of treatments had been provided. At Buxton the 108,000 treatments given included immersion baths, douching, vapour baths, douche massage, ionisation, radiant heat, galvanism and faradism. Several new bathing applications were developed or adapted to treat soldiers with damaged limbs – notably the whirlpool bath designed to improve circulation and the Hubbard tank which allowed the therapist to direct treatment of several patients in a large pool while remaining outside the bath.

These wartime experiences increased awareness of the potential for central resources to be directed towards spa treatment if it were harnessed to address national health priorities. In addition to increasing demand for rehabilitation of war veterans suffering from orthopaedic and nervous complaints, new emphasis placed on the burden of rheumatism strengthened the case for investment in spa facilities.[11] A paper discussed by the B&CS in March 1919 highlighted the issues that set the agenda for lobbying by spas in the inter-war period. Key aims were the desirability of securing funding for spa treatment for the working class through NHI, some central recognition for medical hydrology through a licensing scheme for mineral waters and support for greater emphasis on the teaching of medical hydrology within the medical curriculum. Reflecting on both the distress caused by chronic illness and the economic cost of lost working time, C. W. Buckley from Buxton argued that health resorts should be developed as specialist centres to research and treat rehabilitation cases.[12] He decried lack of central funds for investment which meant British spas were run on commercial grounds for the benefit of local ratepayers and residents rather than for the greater good of the wider nation. As a result many potential patients were unable to afford spa treatment even though they did not qualify for treatment at the charitable hospitals. Buckley's vision for the future of the spas was based on state funding to support a medical model in which a team of specialists including physicians, surgeons, radiographers, bacteriologists and pathological chemists would collaborate to improve understanding and treatment of chronic disease. The need for state support to maximise the contribution of health resorts continued to be pressed throughout the inter-war period.[13]

The ideology espoused by the newly established MoH seemed in tune with the fundamental tenets of spa medicine. The principles put forward by Sir George Newman, Chief Medical Officer, in *An outline of the practice of preventive medicine*, published in 1919 emphasised his view that health was influenced by both the physical and social environment and that measures to address the burden of illness across all social classes should include both preventive and curative medicine, encouraging healthy lifestyles as well as providing better access to GP and hospital services.[14] Effective preventive medicine would improve the health of the population and reduce disease by enhancing the body's ability to heal itself. Newman's vision for the organisation of health services was centred on GP clinics to be modelled on those already in place for school medical services, venereal disease and infant and child welfare. These ideas were given greater clarity in the proposals put forward in the Dawson report in 1920, which set out a scheme for a regional network of health centres and hospitals.[15] Several aspects of these policies had similarities with the approaches towards health promotion and the alleviation of chronic illness that had been the mainstay of spa treatment for many years. In November 1923 a delegation including representatives from the ISMH and the B&CS met with Newman to press for state support for British spas. High on their agenda was the lack of a national body to assess and classify mineral waters, the ability to access funds for investment and the need to systematise the teaching of hydrology in medical schools. They urged that a permanent advisory committee, analogous to the French Commission des Eaux Minerales, was needed to survey mineral waters in Britain and the dominions, to 'give official Authorisation' to waters and to encourage research and teaching.[16] In France, where closer links between the state, elite medicine and the spas dated back to the seventeenth century, a permanent commission on mineral waters had been established by the French Academy of Medicine.[17] This had a mandate to advance scientific hydrology as well as carrying out various administrative and technical functions, including authorising the use of new mineral waters on the basis of chemical analyses carried out in the Academy's laboratories. Although the Academy did not specifically assess the therapeutic effects of mineral waters, this authorisation was felt to provide an independent scientific endorsement of the value of waters, something missing in Britain. By 1900 the Academy had authorised the exploitation of more than 1,600 springs, many of which were used for bottled water. The delegation also referred to the issue of the 'kurtax' or 'taxe de sejour', a charge levied on visitors to spas in Germany and France which provided funds for investment.[18] The British spas had no similar income source and were thus, it was argued, at a considerable disadvantage in maintaining and developing facilities. A change of policy direction had the potential to deliver economic benefits by enhancing the reputation of the British resorts and attracting more overseas visitors to the country. Newman responded negatively to all the points raised, rejecting any greater state involvement in the assessment of mineral waters and pointing out that the new medical curriculum did include provision for the teaching of physical treatments and that it was up to the committee to ensure that hydrology was included in this.[19] No substantial progress was made on any of these issues although the BSF continued to lobby on them throughout the inter-war period.[20]

As it became clear that the MoH was unwilling to publicly endorse spa therapy the strategy of the BSF shifted to pressing for hydrological treatment to be funded under NHI. The 1911 legislation provided access to medical care for lower paid workers between the ages of 16 and 70 covering 47 per cent of the adult working population in 1914 and 54 per cent in 1936. The initial earnings limit of £160 per annum was raised to £250 in 1920.[21] The scheme's main focus was funding access to GP services via the panel doctor system although it also provided limited access to hospital services. The BSF campaign was linked to the issue of rheumatism which a recent MoH report had estimated accounted for nearly one-sixth of industrial invalidity. According to official figures, over 3 million weeks of working time was lost from the insured population alone who were receiving almost £2 million in sickness benefit.[22] As spa treatment had a long-established pedigree for the treatment of gout and rheumatic disease the BSF argued that the spas were well placed to make a valuable contribution to reducing this burden. In order to achieve this finance was needed to cover the cost of accommodation and spa treatment that was beyond the financial resources of many who could potentially benefit from it. While limited free treatment was available via the spa hospitals many low-paid workers were barred from applying.

In 1925 the United Patriots' Approved Society, supported by the BSF, put forward a case for spa treatment for rheumatism to be added to the list of statutory benefits available to every insured person under the Act.[23] Their submission estimated that 17.9 per cent of the society's expenditure between 1921 and 1923 was linked to the cost of rheumatic disease. Additional treatment costs, even if expensive, would be more than offset by savings in sickness benefit while the economic burden of lost working time would also be reduced.[24] The scheme proposed to keep costs down by providing treatment on an outpatient basis with board and accommodation in specially built hostels. Despite this it was estimated that a three-week course would cost £7 19 shillings for baths, massage, electrical and all other accessory treatments including 35 shillings a week for board and accommodation. The nine major spas had identified that they had capacity to treat 1,150 patients in summer and 1,550 in winter.[25] Despite this combined approach by the BSF and a friendly society the scheme was turned down on the grounds of cost. In the Treasury's view, the potential outlay on a statutory benefit available for all insured persons was so high that it might require an additional grant or appropriation of surpluses in the valuation pool of approved societies.

Following the decision to reject a new statutory benefit, the BSF lobbied for spa treatment to be included as an additional benefit funded from surpluses held by individual societies. Evidence from MoH files suggest that opposition continued to be based on financial considerations; spa treatment simply cost too much. A major factor was the need to pay for accommodation for the duration of treatment, a cost that could be avoided if treatment were provided close to people's homes. An alternative to treatment at spas was being introduced in some towns in Europe where local clinics providing outpatient treatment were being introduced. A delegation from Britain, including Fortescue Fox and representatives of the Approved Societies and Insurance Committees visited one of these in Berlin while attending the Central International Committee on Rheumatism in the city. The treatment, which consisted of a wide range of baths, radiant heat and light was given at the end of the working day with only the more severe cases sent for inpatient treatment. Despite a lack of statistical results everyone seemed to 'to be agreed on the advantages to be derived from hydrotherapeutical treatment'.[26] A further meeting was set up with the MoH in March 1927 to debate the comparative advantages of spas and town clinics.[27] The meeting was not a success from the spas' point of view. In the course of discussion William Wilcox, one of the medical practitioners in the BSF team, commented that rheumatism 'was not a disease but a manifestation of a disease, and if the originating trouble was located and removed the rheumatism would disappear'.[28] Wilcox was referring to a view gaining ground at the time that rheumatism was the result of a local infection perhaps originating in dental problems. His comments entirely altered the opinion of the Friendly Societies present at the meeting, who withdrew support for the proposal commenting that although doctors were not agreed on effective treatments for rheumatism they did not hesitate to request the Approved Societies to launch out on heavy expenditure in one direction or another. The disagreement effectively undermined the BSF campaign and their proposals were once again turned down. Despite the failure to secure support under NHI there is evidence that some mutual societies continued to value access to spa treatment for their members. In 1927 a scheme was developed for staff from the Post Office which allowed patients to take baths and treatments at an inclusive charge of 18 shillings a week. The costs of board and accommodation were on top of this and payable by the patient. To take advantage of the scheme patients had to earn not more than £150 a year in the provinces and £160 in London.[29] In 1928 a similar scheme was negotiated for staff at the Ministry of Labour.[30]

These modest successes encouraged further lobbying and in 1929, in readiness for the next quinquennial review of NHI funds, the BSF developed a further scheme in close collaboration with the BMA and the Friendly Societies.[31] The ten spas involved in the scheme had an estimated capacity to treat two thousand patients at any time.[32] A fixed price of £9 6 shillings was proposed for a three-week course of spa treatment of which the approved society would pay 50 per cent with the patient paying the other half. Board and accommodation accounted for costs of 5 guineas with the balance covering the costs of medical advice, examination and all treatments. The accommodation was to be in special hostels which would provide an 'adequate plain diet' with treatment on an outpatient basis. Patients would be closely monitored and the physician had the option of terminating treatment for non-compliance with the regime or inappropriate behaviour. Despite attempts to reduce costs the potential expenditure was still enormous. Based on an assumption that 5 per cent of the 4 million receiving sickness benefit might be eligible, the estimated cost for 200,000 patients at £10 each came to £2 million.

Although John Hatton of the BSF was invited to the MoH to discuss the scheme it was clear that funds on this scale were simply not available.[33] In 1930 the position was further complicated by the approval given to fund rehabilitation treatment provided at the British Red Cross Clinic at Peto Place under Additional Benefit No. 16. As this benefit was limited to treatment at charitable enterprises most spa facilities, which were run as commercial concerns, were excluded despite the fact that the treatment approaches were similar. The only spa treatment that was approved for funding under NHI was for inpatient care at a hospital, such as the DRH in Buxton, which could be funded under Additional Benefit 10.[34] Not surprisingly the spas continued to press for approval to be given to other centres across the country.[35] A briefing note for the Minister prior to meeting Fred Broome of the BSF noted the MoH could not continue to resist approval of additional institutions for much longer due to these inconsistencies. However there could be no hope of general approval for an additional benefit to allow for treatment at spas as several societies were 'finding it hard to provide the existing additional benefits most in demand e.g. dental and ophthalmic'.[36] Broome recognised that 'the only ray of hope' he had taken away from the meeting was the possibility of encouraging approved societies to lobby for spa treatment to be included as an additional benefit at the next valuation round.[37] In 1936 a proposal was put forward that 'the Schedule of Additional Benefits be amended by the inclusion of Spa Treatment'.[38] By July 1939, the MoH had extended Additional Benefit 16 to treatment at the DRH as well as the Charterhouse Rheumatism Clinic, the St John Clinic and the Institute of Physical Medicine. This fragmentary evidence from the MoH files suggests that opposition to funding for spa treatment was primarily based on financial considerations. Although some viewed spa treatment as outdated, others, including several approved societies, viewed it as being as good an option as any other treatment available. The potential cost of the schemes put forward meant that a statutory benefit was out of the question while approval as an additional benefit raised the issue of inequality. The MoH, mindful of other priorities, wanted to avoid a decision 'which might have the effect of reducing the amount of money allocated by Societies for expenditure on the present benefits, or of costly benefits which only a few wealthy Societies would be able to adopt, and which would, therefore, be available to only a small proportion of insured persons'.[39]

The lack of support for spa treatment from the central state in Britain contrasts with the position in Germany discussed in Bennett-Ruete's case study of Bad Ems. The mechanism for funding spa treatment from the German social insurance scheme was established by 1900. Legislation framed by Bismarck meant that 10 per cent of the population were covered by schemes for health care by 1885 and in 1889 benefits were extended to the provision of pensions for old age and invalidity. Crucially this also provided for costs of rehabilitation where this was likely to allow an invalid to recover sufficiently to be able to earn a living, the justification being that treatment costs would be offset by savings in pension payments.[40] Thomas Maretzki emphasises the influence of naturopathic approaches in these decisions as many orthodox practitioners, including Bismarck's physican, Ernst Schweninger, used natural treatment in their practice.[41] Another significant factor was that the German schemes were administered through autonomous insurance bodies which dealt with the costs of both health care and invalidity and considered the net combined costs in assessing the benefit of treatment focused on rehabilitation. Despite this mechanism for provision of treatment for the poorer classes, Bennett-Ruete considers few workers were actually funded to take a spa cure before the war with spas preferring to target paying patients. However a reduction in the number of foreign visitors to German spas from 1914 and falling home demand due to the economic collapse in 1923 made the potential of providing 'social cures' funded through the insurance companies more attractive to spa businesses. Social benefits were extended under the Weimar Republic and negotiations between the German Spa Federation and the Insurance Funds in 1925 led to an increase in the number of workers treated.[42] This democratisation of the spas was not without its opponents and many of the agreements reached reflect similar considerations to those aired in the negotiations between the BSF and the MoH. These included concerns about the inequities of treating funded patients out of season and at off-peak hours in order to minimise disruption to private patients. After 1933, under the National Socialists, the spa cure was endorsed as part of wider campaigns to improve fitness. In addition to enabling individuals to regain their strength and become economically productive, the cure fitted with the ideals of healthy living and back-to-nature endorsed as part of campaigns to influence national identity.[43] Further amendments to legislation in 1934 consolidated the principle that spa cures could be provided for invalids if it was expected to enable them to recover the ability to earn a living. By the 1930s almost 25 per cent of all cure-goers at Bad Ems were funded by the social insurance system.[44] The situation in France was more similar to that in Britain as spa treatments were not listed among therapies reimbursed under insurance schemes. However in 1935 a technical committee appointed to look into the issue reached agreement that cheaper treatment could be provided outside the peak season at spas. The first agreement was signed with Vichy in 1938 although this was not implemented until after the war. [45]

Local initiatives and networks

The evidence from English resorts shows that sustained efforts were made by a range of actors, including municipal authorities, medical specialists and voluntary hospitals to adjust to the deteriorating market conditions of the 1920s and 1930s. Initiatives tackled a range of issues including the need for local schemes to reduce the cost of spa treatment for those on modest incomes and strengthening the reputation of medical hydrology with the wider profession. Various measures were put in place in the context of increased levels of publicity aimed at the public and medical practitioners funded by municipal authorities, railway companies, the BSF and the British Health Resorts Association (BHRA). Established mechanisms for promoting the value of spa therapy to the wider profession through articles in the medical journals continued. For example in 1922 a special issue of the *Prescriber* provided an extensive review of British health resorts.[46] Publications by the BSF and BHRA were sent to every practitioner in Britain as a way of raising awareness of spa treatment and its applications and the ways in which it could be accessed.[47]

In the post-war boom after the end of the First World War patients continued to travel to Harrogate to take the cure with the number of treatments provided increasing to over 110,000 per year in the 1920s.[48] However as the depression deepened spa takings began to fall and in 1930 the decision was taken to close the Victoria Baths and consolidate facilities at the Royal Baths complex.[49] This was remodelled between 1936 and 1939 updating treatment and leisure facilities. A covered winter gardens was developed to complement the new Sun Pavilion built in the Valley Gardens which catered for the increased popularity of sunbathing and outdoor activities. The outbreak of war in 1939 disrupted patient flows and the following year a new all-inclusive tariff was introduced as a way of sustaining demand. The scheme cost five guineas for two weeks which included three consultations with a doctor, up to twelve baths and access to the drinking wells. Patients could choose to forgo the medical consultations which reduced the price to three guineas. There was also a three-week option available.[50] The scheme was designed to offer patients a range of options within a fixed price cap. At Buxton a scheme offering an all-inclusive package including accommodation had been developed by private investors targeting patients looking for affordable services. The 100-bed Buxton clinic based in the Crescent opened in 1935 offering a three-week course of treatment at between 4 to 6 guineas weekly inclusive of bathing treatments, accommodation and board.[51]

Two issues were seen as vital to securing the reputation of medical hydrology as a separate specialty – the introduction of systematic teaching within the medical curriculum and better integration of research and clinical practice. The importance of better instruction in medical schools had been recognised since the establishment of the B&CS and some progress had been made by 1914. The Society had appointed a panel of approved lecturers available to give instruction at medical schools and to interested medical societies.[52] The Hyde lectureship had been established and the first incumbent, Fortescue Fox, delivered a series of lectures to the B&CS in 1911.[53] These were published as *The principles and practice of medical hydrology* in 1913 and further refined for students in 1924.[54] After the war the education committee of the B&CS continued to offer courses to medical schools and medical societies. A short intensive course of teaching was delivered at the University of London from 1923 to 1925 supplemented by a study trip to a spa with further lectures and demonstrations.[55] Articles in the *AMH* showed that teaching of medical hydrology was given greater emphasis in some other countries. Teaching was most systematic in Germany with courses at ten out of twenty universities, sometimes delivered as an aspect of physical therapeutics. Austria, Germany, France and the USA each had one chair of hydrotherapy with additional lectures given at some other universities. In France there was more variation across schools although Felix Garrigou had held a chair at Toulouse since its foundation in 1891. Some lectures were given in Italy, Switzerland, Holland, Belgium and Sweden. Courses were not always compulsory or examined, an exception being Columbia where the chair was held by

Simon Baruch, author of the first English language textbook *Principles and practice of hydrotherapy*.[56] Despite further lobbying for better provision within the undergraduate curriculum the only substantive progress made in the inter-war period was the appointment of Dr Geoffrey Holmes as lecturer in medical hydrology at Leeds in 1937 – the first such appointment in Britain.

In addition to a focus on undergraduate training, efforts were made to engage the wider profession in postgraduate education. A scheme of spa visits was developed based on the French *voyages d'études médicales* which had run from 1899 as a way of encouraging medical practitioners from France and elsewhere to visit spas to view treatment methods and other facilities.[57] Although the French trips were popular with British doctors the British equivalent proved less successful. A proposed trip to Strathpeffer in the Highlands in 1930 was cancelled due to lack of participants. More success was achieved by coordinating informal presentations and visits to spas with medical conferences. The Presidential address to the BMA annual conference held in Bath in 1925 made a case for the development of medical hydrology 'from a form of empiricism, based largely on tradition and superstitious belief, to a recognized branch of scientific medicine'.[58] In 1928 a delegation from the ISMH visited Buxton as did a group attending the BMA congress meeting in Manchester the following year.[59]

Despite these varied attempts to promote more systematic instruction progress was piecemeal and did not substantially improve the position of medical hydrology in the medical curriculum. In contrast in France medical hydrology became further embedded in the academic system in the inter-war period. By the 1930s professorial chairs had been established at all medical faculties providing a career structure within the specialty. This success was chiefly due to integration between medical hydrology and the other state structures promoting the commercial interests of spas.[60] In Britain the future of spa medicine became associated with two emerging disciplines both in the early stage of organisation – physical medicine and rheumatology. As David Cantor has discussed, while these offered alternative models for integration within the medical establishment both threatened to sideline the particular strengths of water treatments.[61] For rheumatologists water treatments were just one strand in a wider set of therapies that might be called on including new vaccine therapies. Research into the pathology and treatment of rheumatic disease covered a wide agenda including interest in the importance of local infection in triggering an attack. Those specialising in physical therapies endorsed a growing range of measures including hydrology, massage, light and heat for use in treating patients suffering not only from rheumatism but also other musculo-skeletal problems and chronic health issues. Hydrology was just one of several methods in their therapeutic arsenal.

Practitioners based at spas also explored opportunities to improve integration of research and clinical practice and foster links with local academic departments. At Harrogate some £4,000 was invested in a new laboratory in 1926 and a joint research committee including members from Leeds University was in place by 1935.[62] The launch of the *Harrogate Spa Medical Journal: devoted to spa research and treatment* in 1938 was intended to further foster local and regional support for the spa among medical practitioners. The publication was sponsored by the Spa Research Committee of the Harrogate Corporation, edited by A. Woodmansey, Borough Analyst and Scientific Officer and overseen by representatives of Harrogate Medical Society. Its aims were to disseminate research on the Harrogate spa treatment to local practitioners as well as the wider group of specialists in the field.[63] At Bath a small number of research initiatives were conducted at the Royal Mineral Water Hospital from 1906, some in association with colleagues from Cambridge and London.[64] However capacity for research remained rudimentary until 1934 when laboratory facilities were improved and a full-time pathologist funded. Links were strengthened with Bristol University and a research post established in 1935.[65] The International Congress on Rheumatism held in Bath and Oxford in 1938 gave international publicity to the spa's growing reputation for expertise in the field.[66]

By the 1930s there were schemes in place to upgrade facilities at the three largest mineral water hospitals in association with the international campaign against rheumatism. At Harrogate a national appeal, the Grey Cross Campaign, was launched in 1938 to raise funds to expand the Royal Bath Hospital. Publicity highlighted the enormous impact of the disease reporting that there were 50,000 new cases of chronic rheumatism and 25,000 children attacked by rheumatic fever each year within a fifty-mile radius of the hospital.[67] The appeal noted the hospital provided a national service drawing patients from thirty English counties as well as Ireland, Scotland and Wales. Despite an ongoing investment programme additional money was needed for a new nurses' home, additional ward blocks, a gynaecological department and gymnasium.[68] Among the high profile supporters of the campaign were the King, the Princess Royal, the High Sheriff of Yorkshire and Lord Horder, chairman of the Empire Rheumatism Council.[69] At Bath a successful appeal for a new 250-bed hospital was launched in 1936 and plans put in place for the Queen to lay the foundation stone in September 1939. The declaration of war put the scheme on hold.[70] In 1936 the Medical Advisory Committee at Buxton commissioned a review which also recommended launching a nationwide appeal to raise funds for a substantial expansion programme. This would increase bed numbers, provide a new orthopaedic department and improve hydrotherapy, laboratory and X-ray facilities.[71] The Duke of Devonshire was to head up the appeal and promises of several substantial donations were secured. Lord Melchett of ICI agreed to be President and pledged £200 to the proposed fund.[72] These initiatives demonstrate that the authorities at spas continued to take active steps throughout the inter-war period to maintain and improve treatment facilities at English spas based on the long-established voluntary tradition of charitable funding.

As plans for the NHS began to be formulated from the early 1940s the BSF lobbied for the place of spa treatment within the new scheme.[73] A number of proposals were put forward restating arguments about the specialist expertise available and its value in treating rheumatism and addressing cases needing rehabilitation. Some of the more ambitious schemes proposed for discussion drew on international models, the Russian example being cited in a scheme suggested in 1943 which recommended inpatient treatment for more serious cases with outpatient treatment at institutes of physiotherapy for ambulant patients.[74] By 1947 it was clear that no national policy directive would be agreed in relation to spa treatment and the BSF urged doctors and managers at each spa to take steps to secure integration within the proposed regional structure. 'The whole problem of the future of the Spas in a National Health Service is now no longer the problem of the Federation. It was the Federation which in 1944 and subsequently began its fight on behalf of the Spas. The Ministry we know is very impressed with the information given to them by the Federation, but now each Spa must work out its own solution individually with its own Regional Board and act quickly'.[75]

Minutes of the Buxton coordinating committee show they were left trying to second guess the likely policy direction to be taken by the NHS.

Working on the assumption that rheumatic services would be organised on a regional basis with a university medical school acting as a teaching and research centre they acted to strengthen clinical and research links with Stockport hospital and Manchester hospital and University.[76] In 1945 agreement was reached that facilities at Buxton would become part of the proposed regional rheumatism service centred on Manchester University with 800 beds provided at the DRH.[77] The proposal also addressed shortcomings in the provision of general medical and surgical cases and maternity services for Buxton highlighted in the survey of Hospital Services completed by the MoH in 1945.[78] Research links were to be consolidated with thirty-five beds designated for cases to be selected and managed by teams jointly appointed between the university and hospital.[79] By 1948 plans were in place for a scheme that integrated the facilities of the DRH, the local authority-run Natural and Thermal Baths and the Buxton Clinic within a proposed regional service for rheumatism. It was not envisaged that private patients would disappear as they would be able to access treatment at the baths.

Spas under the NHS

Minutes from MoH files indicate that there was little enthusiasm to include the spas within the NHS although no clear statement to this effect was ever made. In the early days of the new service there were contradictory messages about whether spa treatment would be funded or not but by August it was clear some access would continue.[80] Despite lobbying by the BSF no central agreement covering access to spa treatment was achieved and it was left to local administrators to establish systems to manage referrals for treatment, including those from outside their region.[81] Under the terms of legislation introduced in 1948 all voluntary hospitals, including those at the spas, were brought within the NHS along with a number of other organisations providing accommodation and inpatient facilities. These included Highfields Hospital in Droitwich and the Buxton Clinic. Bathing facilities owned by local authorities or the private sector remained outside the system. The voluntary spa hospitals had accepted patients from all over the country although the pattern of admissions at Harrogate, Buxton and Bath suggest that most patients were drawn from their surrounding regional areas. Under the NHS, each region was funded according to their population and was responsible for providing local services. Free inpatient treatment was made available at the hospitals in Buxton, Bath, Droitwich, Harrogate and Woodhall. Free outpatient treatment was also provided at these sites but the NHS would not contribute towards costs of travel and accommodation. Outpatient treatment only was available at Cheltenham and Leamington. In 1951 the spa practitioners group of the BMA published a booklet intended to dispel growing confusion over the services available at the various centres and the referral routes to access them. The booklet recommended spa treatment for those needing rehabilitation or convalescence after illness or injury as well as those suffering from chronic rheumatic disorders. It also noted that most spas continued to provide access to private medical consultation and treatments.[82]

Fragmentary evidence available shows that demand for inpatient spa treatment was high and across the country arrangements were soon needed to manage demand. The Birmingham Regional Hospital Board, responsible for Droitwich, produced a leaflet setting out typical arrangements. The procedure for obtaining admission was convoluted as 'Only patients who have been sent by a Consultant on the staff of a hospital can be treated so that it will be necessary for GPs to refer patients to their nearest hospital to be seen by a Consultant who will confirm or otherwise the need for spa treatment ... There are a limited number of beds for in-patients ... but these are available only for the more serious cases.'[83] For those recommended for outpatient treatment it was made clear that 'neither the Ministry of Health, the Regional Hospital Board, nor the Hospital Management Committee can accept any responsibility for payment of expenses incurred by them in respect of their residential accommodation and/or subsistence'. Publicity for the hospital in Bath stressed that patients might face a delay in admission of up to a year for women and that maximum age limits had been set at seventy for men and fifty-five for women.[84] Although outpatient treatment was introduced at the hospital to expand capacity no financial help with travel or living expenses could be offered.

Despite these restrictions there is evidence that the number of treatments provided at spas expanded in the early years of the NHS. The Leeds Region Hospital Board, responsible for the Royal Bath Hospital at Harrogate, invested in a deep pool and gymnasium to improve the facilities for treating those with rheumatism. In 1952 the White Hart Hotel was converted into patient accommodation with treatment provided at the Royal Baths. These facilities provided between 100,000 and 120,000 treatments annually, almost double the 63,000 given in 1947 and close to the peak numbers of the 1920s.[85] The number treated later rose to 150,000, a figure above the highest ever pre-war figure.[86] Although the option of private treatment was still available, patients appear to have been unwilling to pay for services which others were accessing free of charge, often in the same premises. At Harrogate the number of private patients fell from 62,000 in 1948/9 to 13,000 in 1962/3.[87] Statistics from Llandrindod Wells show the virtual disappearance of private patients; by the early 1950s only three private hydrotherapy treatments were provided compared to over a thousand given under the NHS.[88]

The reduction in income from private patients meant that NHS funding became the main source of revenue for bathing facilities and consequently any withdrawal led to financial crisis and closure. When the Royal Baths in Harrogate were given notice of termination of the NHS contract an effort was made to re-launch the baths as a private facility. This proved unsuccessful and with the exception of the Turkish baths they closed in 1969.[89] Other spa facilities also began to close. The narrative of decline was chronicled by Thomson in *Spas that heal* in 1976. The previous year had seen the closure of the Spa Treatment Centre in Bath following withdrawal of NHS funding as treatment services were transferred to the new physiotherapy and hydrotherapy departments at the United Bath Hospital.[90] At Buxton investment in hydrotherapy facilities at the DRH had also led to cancellation of the NHS contract with the resulting closure of the local authority-owned baths in 1963.[91] At these new centres treatment was provided within a hospital setting. At Droitwich the installation of a new hydrotherapy pool at Highfields Hospital led to the closure of St Andrews Baths in 1976.[92] Highfields later closed too after which patients from the Birmingham Region were sent to the Pump Rooms at Leamington for treatment. Thus by 1976 NHS-funded treatment at spas had declined considerably although was still available through the hospitals at Harrogate, Buxton and Bath and on an outpatient basis at Leamington. The 1990s brought a further round of closures of NHS facilities in the spa towns – the Leamington Pump Rooms in 1990, the Bath Hospital at Harrogate in 1994 and the DRH at Buxton in 2000.[93]

The decline in state funding for spa treatments through NHS contracts contrasts with support provided in France and Germany. In France legislation introduced in 1945 extended health insurance to all salaried employees and included spa treatments in the list of funded therapies. By 1947 the scheme reimbursed the cost of treatment and advice from a spa doctor as well as a contribution towards accommodation and travel costs. Weisz emphasises the lack of debate over the inclusion of spa treatment in the scheme and argues that this was due to the consolidation of medical hydrology within the French medical system during the inter-war years.[94] Measures were put in place to ensure that applicants were medically screened to minimise possible abuse of the system with treatment mainly approved for respiratory, digestive and arthritic complaints. The generous funding scheme led to an expansion in those taking a spa cure; 20,000 requests were dealt with in 1947 and by 1953 an estimated 120,000 curists were funded. This increase did not lead to the collapse of the private market as seems to have been the case in Britain. In Weisz's assessment it was the middle classes who benefited most and it is likely that the very poorest remained excluded from the spas. Restrictions began to be introduced by the insurance companies in the 1960s on cost grounds but no radical reduction was proposed until 1999. The second half of the twentieth century also saw a weakening of the position of hydrology within French academic medicine, a compulsory course within the medical curriculum was withdrawn in 1968 and Weisz notes a reduction in confidence in hydrological methods, encouraged by the development of new medical and surgical techniques whose effect were deemed capable of being assessed by double-blind clinical trials. The complexity of hydrological treatment regimes which might also include diet, exercise and other aspects of wider regimen meant it was deemed unrealistic to apply this method to assess their effectiveness.[95]

This comparison indicates that one important factor influencing the differential support given to spa treatments has been the structure of health care funding systems. An important distinction between the French and German social insurance-based schemes and the NHS was their separation of the function of funder and provider of services. Social insurance schemes in France and Germany were based on agreements listing approved procedures with insurance schemes passing funds to service providers for treatments given. Those providing services were not necessarily managed by public authorities. In contrast the NHS operated a system where services were organised on a regional basis with limited resources allocated to authorities responsible for decisions on funding a full range of services in their locality. Under the latter system acute services were given priority with a focus on improvements to standards in hospital care. A group of 'cinderella' services which included those based in the community and those for the chronically ill, elderly and mentally ill patients were given less priority. In the British system treatment costs and pension costs were dealt with by different parts of the welfare system with no mechanism to assess trade-offs between the two. While the NHS budget bore the cost of active rehabilitation it did not benefit directly from any savings arising from reduced pension costs for patients able to rejoin the workforce more quickly.

A definition used by the German Spa Federation in 1969 emphasised that spa treatment there was viewed as an integral part of long-term treatment.

> Spa treatment is not an alternative to clinical medicine; the spa is not simply a chemist's shop, dispensing natural remedies of the earth, climate and countryside, but rather a sensible extension of the hospital and general practice through particular methods of treatment in the course of an optimal plan of treatment.[96]

In West Germany spas continued to flourish after 1945 drawing on a range of customers that included those funded by social insurance as well as private patients. Bennett-Ruete attributes this in part to a desire to restore pre-war social and cultural institutions which was part of a broader project of national regeneration. From 1949 onwards, social guests outnumbered private patients at Bad Ems with overall numbers rising to the highest ever recorded in 1953.[97] Spa cures in Germany continue to place emphasis on the wider surroundings of the spa, on rest and recuperation as well as specific treatments.

> A cure is a remedial process characterised by a repeated (iterative) application of preponderantly natural remedies according to a plan prescribed by a doctor and which entails a change of surroundings and environment. Treatment at a spa consists of a general therapy which is systematically structured and which, besides natural remedies, also use ... physical medicine, locomotive therapy, diet, psychotherapy and also treatment with drugs, all tailored to individual needs.[98]

Although a natural thermal spring was required to achieve official designation as a *Kurort* or *Heilbad*, weight was also given to bathing facilities, parks and general surroundings, accommodation for patients and medical expertise.[99]

Evidence from oral testimony of those working at Leamington Spa indicates the complexity of comparing approaches across countries.

While the evidence from minutes and contracts might suggest that 'spa treatment' initially expanded and was later transferred to NHS facilities, evidence from oral history testimony from those working in the sector provides an insight into fundamental changes to the therapeutic approaches offered and the way these treatments were perceived by those delivering them. By 1964 the treatment in the Royal Pump Rooms was led by qualified physiotherapists from a department no longer called 'spa treatment' but 'physiotherapy'. Referrals were made directly by GPs or hospital consultants but were not overseen by a spa physician or specialist in physical medicine. Physiotherapists had responsibility for developing appropriate treatment plan for patients. The head of department commented

> I'd already come from a spa in Bath and there were some similarities in the types of – I call them old-fashioned – spa type treatments that were given, but the general trend was moving away from them really because in those days the attitude in that kind of medicine was, I'm the patient, here I am, make me better and we were moving away from that for the patient to take more responsibility themselves and to be much more active in their treatments.[100]

Among these 'spa type treatments' viewed as old-fashioned and passive were aeration baths, zotafoam for obesity and the Nauheim treatment for cardiac patients. Physiotherapy had shifted to more active regimes, and under the new management a number of the individual treatment rooms designed to provide private treatment to paying patients in comfortable surroundings were demolished and the space redesigned to provide a larger area for physiotherapy and new hydrotherapy pools in which active treatment was given. These approaches were successfully adapted to meet contemporary health concerns and at Leamington were used during the 1950s to treat patients affected by polio. The deputy physiotherapist recalls that the

> older, individualized treatments were discontinued due to cost effectiveness. ..
>
> When I went there, there was still a procedure called Vichy massage and Vortex baths. The Vichy massage was massage on a stone slab rather like a mortuary room [laughs] and jets of water sprayed on the person and massage was given. Very good for painful muscular conditions and things ... The Vichy massage went out fairly quickly for being not cost effective, because it involved one person doing the massage and at least one other person standing by to bring towels

> and – at least one or two. So we're talking about two or three people per patient so it just wasn't viable.
>
> The Vortex baths on the other hand were. These were big tubs that an individual sat in or stood in and the main advantage was stimulating circulation, so that a lot of people with poor circulation in the legs for example; MS, strokes, things like that, they could pop in one of these baths prior to going in the pool and the warm water and the massage from the jets of water relaxed their muscles, stimulated the circulation so that they were in a better condition to do the exercises in the pool.[101]

These treatments were no longer considered to be at the cutting-edge of treatment for rheumatism. One consultant general physician at Leamington had grave doubts about spa medicine which in his view was tainted with quackery and commercialism. It was, he suggested, a generational thing. One of his older colleagues had once been the spa doctor and had encouraged him to refer patients to the Pump Rooms but he was always reticent.

> I'd grown up into the development of rheumatology as a science based discipline within general medicine and physiotherapy had grown up as an empirical practice which had its roots in rehabilitation and going back even further, in the field of spa therapy dating from the eighteenth and nineteenth centuries. It was a very different scenario.[102]

However he recognised that the Pump Rooms had been an important part of the town's individual culture.

> Leamington Spa ... particularly before the Second World War ... was a place which had a population comprising a certain number of elderly retired middle class and upper middle class people, some of whom enjoyed the benefits of physiotherapy in the Pump Rooms. It [spa medicine] is part of the local economy and Leamington had its share of that ... It was a field of medicine that I viewed with extreme suspicion.[103]

This evidence suggests that treatment at Leamington was increasingly associated with physiotherapy practice and connections with medical specialists weakened. The Pump Rooms were physically separate from the hospital and as treatment techniques changed the layout and facilities of the old building became outdated and the costs of providing services increased. Patients attended treatment on an outpatient basis and there is little evidence of integration of the treatment received within broader intensive therapeutic regimes or longer-term management of individual patients as emphasised in the German model discussed by Bennett-Ruete.

Changing medical attitudes towards spa treatment are also indicated at Woodhall Spa where the coming of the NHS secured the future of hydrological treatment when it looked uncertain to survive as a commercial spa. The prosperity of the village declined in the inter-war period after the principal hotel, the Victoria, burned down in 1920 reducing the available accommodation for visitors. This situation was not resolved for over a decade until Petwood House was converted to a hotel in 1934 and the bath house and spa grounds sold to the Woodhall Spa Baths and Estate Company Limited in 1936.[104] As at other spas, some accommodation was requisitioned for military personnel during the war further reducing capacity for civilian visitors. The destruction of the Royal Hydro Hotel and its impressive winter gardens in a bombing raid brought more permanent reduction in visitor accommodation.[105] After the war the future of Woodhall as a viable spa looked bleak. However in 1948 the baths and the small thirty-bedded Alexandra Hospital were taken into the NHS as part of the Lincoln Hospitals Group and became the centre for the treatment of rheumatism for the Trent Region.[106] James Robertson recalls that with access to pathology, biochemistry and X-ray 'within a year, the treatment and management of rheumatic disease at Woodhall Spa had moved from the 19th century to the second half of the 20th'.[107] Among the new approaches given a clinical trial was the 'new wonder drug cortisone'.[108] News of this burst upon the scene in the first year of the NHS with the publication in 1949 of research results of trials at the Mayo Clinic in the USA. International acclaim for the significance of this work brought the authors a Nobel prize. Although early hopes for the drug proved to be over-optimistic with side effects and contraindications found in later research, cortisone became a powerful symbol of the potential for transformation of rheumatology treatments.[109] David Cantor asserts its importance to those working in the specialism as marking a break with previous approaches that it was hoped would consolidate their association with wider clinical medicine. Whereas rheumatology textbooks published in the 1930s stressed that 'although no dramatic results are to be expected, and treatment will inevitably be a matter of months or even years, much can be done to relieve symptoms and restore function', cortisone held out the prospect of much more positive treatment.[110] The promise of new drug therapies endorsed in clinical trials further undermined the value accorded to mineral waters. James Robertson commented that by the time of the transfer of the service from Woodhall to Lincoln in 1983 'it was accepted that the various spa waters had no curative effect at all, and it was felt that treatment could just as readily be delivered in the Lincoln Hospitals complex.'[111]

In the light of the failed attempts to secure support for spa treatment from the MoH in the inter-war period the transfer of the spa hospitals into the NHS, and the principle that free treatment became available to all, seems an unexpected success. It demonstrates that some value was accorded to them as centres of expertise. That this occurred at all was due to the existence of the voluntary hospitals and other inpatient institutions that were included in the transfer of assets into the new service. Services at spas became integrated into various regional structures of health care provision based on earlier associations with the medical specialties of physical medicine or rheumatology. Popular demand led to access to treatment expanding in the early years of the NHS but a number of factors acted to undermine this in the longer term. Chief among these was the way that spa treatment was integrated into medical and paramedical professional structures. Medical personnel became associated with hospital-based specialist centres for rheumatism with greater emphasis given to new drug-based approaches such as the use of cortisone. The provision of physical treatments, particularly massage and medical gymnastics, were increasingly delivered by physiotherapists and hydrotherapists, paramedical groups in a formative stage of development.[112] Emphasis was given to using the physical properties of water- resistance and buoyancy – with less importance attributed to natural thermal or mineral properties. A number of other physical therapies, especially medical gymnastics, massage and use of heat and light treatments, were also drawn on. Growing financial pressures within the NHS were also important. Facilities in old buildings, some built over a century earlier, to deliver water-based therapies were inappropriate for current therapeutic approaches. As the programme to improve hospital infrastructure began to be achieved new departments were constructed as part of hospital development programmes. George Kersley, looking back over events at Bath considered a mix of factors contributed to the closure of the municipally run Spa Treatment Centre in 1975. He cited the new provision for hydrotherapy in the physiotherapy department at the Royal United Hospital and the need for economy measures as well as the decline in the numbers of private patients.[113]

Conclusion

This chapter has reviewed the attitude of the central state towards spa treatment in the inter-war period and in the early years of the NHS. This section summarises important trends and suggests why the pattern of services in Britain developed as it did. Comparison with France and Germany highlights that elsewhere in Europe spa treatment did achieve more secure funding from new state-funded health care systems providing treatment for the whole population. Despite this by the end of the twentieth century more restrictions were being introduced. While firm conclusions as to why this was the case require greater comparative research the following preliminary assessment is offered. As Sigerist noted in 1942 support for spa treatment from new schemes for national health insurance played a significant part in their pattern of development in the twentieth century. In Britain new collaborative activity by the spas coordinated by the BSF sought to secure funding for spa treatment and investment in facilities from the NHI scheme introduced in 1911. Their argument focused on making a case for the potential contribution spas could make to alleviating the costly burden of chronic illness in the population, much of it associated with rheumatic disease. The main objection to funding spa treatment was cost, cited as the reason that proposals were rejected several times in the inter-war period. Existing pressure on NHI funds meant new benefits were unaffordable. Despite sustained lobbying, supported by several insurance societies, little practical support for spa treatment was secured. Evidence from MoH files indicates that while it was accepted that spas had specialist expertise and facilities, the costs of accommodation and lost working time by patients treated away from home were deemed to be prohibitive. During the First World War the limited capacity at spas was apparent and in the inter-war period this encouraged support for an alternative service model of local clinics to provide hydrological and other physical treatments on an outpatient basis. George Weisz has argued that the size of the spa sector was an important factor in their integration into state-funded health care systems. In Britain there were just fourteen members of the BSF in 1948. Of the fourteen English regions introduced under the NHS only five had working spas and of these only four had substantial capacity for inpatient treatment – Bath, Buxton, Harrogate and Droitwich. New service models based on provision in local centres of population were an alternative to investment in a few national specialist centres.

In the inter-war period the local networks, formed by municipal authorities, spa practitioners, charitable foundations, individual supporters and private enterprise, that had guided investment decisions at spas throughout the nineteenth century continued to plan for future development. These included considering options for attracting more clients from lower-income groups who were not eligible for admission to the voluntary hospitals. Although initiatives such as the Buxton Clinic and investment by the Birmingham Hospital Saturday Fund meant some increased provision was achieved for the less well off, the main hope for improving access for the poorer classes remained with the voluntary hospitals. The three large mineral water hospitals at Bath, Harrogate and Buxton all launched substantial appeals for funds in the late 1930s based on the well-established English tradition of voluntarism drawing on local, regional and national supporters. They hoped to benefit from an association with the international campaign to tackle rheumatism to attract a broad base of donors to support their development into national centres of excellence.

As planning for the introduction of the NHS took shape it became clear that spas needed to secure closer integration of their services with hospitals and universities in order to safeguard their future within a regional service. Arrangements to take voluntary hospitals into the NHS in 1948 meant that free spa treatment became available, leading to a collapse in private fees which left local authorities dependent on contracts with the NHS for funding to maintain bathing facilities. The regional structure of funding and planning within the NHS disrupted the close relationship between the local medical profession, bath house owners and bathing hospitals at individual spas. Whereas in the past representatives of these bodies had worked together and shared a common interest in the continuing popularity of the spa with visitors and patients, the creation of the NHS led to new professional networks for medical personnel with most spa physicians becoming integrated with regional services for rheumatism.

In both France and Germany systematic instruction was given in medical hydrology and closer links between spa practice and academic institutions were in place leading to better integration of research and clinical practice and a defined specialty of medical hydrology offering a medical career structure. The spa sectors were far larger too. As George Weisz has argued this meant that the need for funding for spa treatment was accepted with little questioning. The structure of health insurance funding which reimbursed approved treatments also facilitated assessment of the net costs of treatment and disability pensions. In addition there were centralised mechanisms for assessment and licensing of waters. Bennett-Ruete notes that efforts to re-establish the spas in Germany after both world wars were part of broader programmes of recovery. Sigerist notes that state-sponsored treatment for the working classes in the Soviet Union also had wider significance as an important aspect of nation-building in the aftermath of the Russian Revolution. Maretzki argues that support for spa treatment was also influenced in Germany by continuing interest in holistic approaches by many orthodox practitioners, particularly for the treatment of chronic complaints. This approach continued into the second half of the twentieth century.

In contrast, treatment under the NHS became associated with a narrower therapeutic model with few links to broader lifestyle factors. A discussion of developments at Leamington Spa highlights the complex factors influencing patterns of treatment provision. Therapeutic trends, professional careers, funding arrangements for health care and growing financial pressures all contributed to shaping policy decisions. In 1984, as threats of closure of the Leamington Pump Rooms loomed, a development proposal was put forward by a private consortium which offered an alternative model. The proposal envisaged spa treatment as comprising both health and leisure activities. The Pump Room building was to be extensively refurbished in a £5 million scheme to provide accommodation, physiotherapy and hydrotherapy facilities as well as naturopathy and beauty therapy. The facilities would also include a visitor area, cafeteria, shop and tourist information centre with leisure facilities including a jacuzzi, solarium, gymnasium, multi-gym and a bigger swimming pool. While NHS patients would continue to receive their treatment on the site it would also be open to fee-paying individuals enjoying a range of health and leisure services. The scheme failed to secure the support of Labour councillors, the minority group on the Council, who were vehemently opposed to the principle of any involvement by private enterprise and warned of plans to bar NHS patients from the Pump Rooms. There was also public opposition to the proposal to use some of the Pump Room gardens as a car park. The level of concern was such that a public enquiry was launched. Although the scheme was finally approved in 1989 the private finance partner had pulled out. Later in the year the NHS gave notice the physiotherapy department would transfer to the new district general hospital being built at Warwick. The Pump Rooms closed in 1990 following the transfer of the physiotherapy department to new premises. Opposition to the scheme was based on various concerns and principles. For some, spas were still associated with medical quackery and there was little professional incentive to support them; for others they retained an elitist image with facilities originally developed to treat those willing to pay for luxury and privacy clashing with a new culture of equity which emphasised the need for local services and basic treatment facilities for all. Despite the failure of the scheme it pointed to the new direction that the 'spa' concept would eventually take in Britain by the end of the twentieth century, forgoing the association with medical expertise that had been an integral part of its appeal since the nineteenth century and instead reasserting the appeal of individualised therapies geared towards recuperation and relaxation.

Notes

1 Cantor, 'Contradictions of specialization'; Cantor, 'Aches of industry'.
2 David Cantor, 'Cortisone and the politics of drama', in John V. Pickstone (ed.), *Medical innovations in historical perspective* (Basingstoke: Macmillan, 1992), 165–84; G. D. Kersley, *The Three R's: rheumatism, rehabilitation, research as viewed from Bath* (Bath: privately printed, c. 1980).
3 R. Fortescue Fox, 'Discussion on the value of medical baths for invalid soldiers', B&CS, *PRSM*, 8 (1915), 47–66.
4 Committee of the council of the section of balneology and climatology of the RSM, *Notes on hydrological treatment for wounded and invalid soldiers and sailors with a list of the British spas and health resorts and of the disorders which they benefit* (London: Adlard and Son, 1915).
5 'Report of committee of council: "A combined physical treatment"', B&CS, *PRSM*, 9 (1916), 45–8.
6 R. Fortescue Fox and J. Campbell McClure, 'A new combined physical treatment for wounded and disabled soldiers (heat, massage, electricity, movements)', *Lancet*, 4823 (5 February 1916), 311–12, p. 312.
7 William Gordon, 'Some observations on the treatment of disabled soldiers by the physio-therapeutic methods now being used in Paris', B&CS, *PRSM*, 9 (1916), 48–51.

8 Fortescue Fox and McClure, 'Combined physical treatment', p. 312.
9 'Physical treatment for disabled soldiers: statement and recommendations by the Committee of Council of the section of Balneology and Climatology of the RSM', *Lancet*, 4879 (3 March 1917), 348–9.
10 W. Edgecombe, 'The treatment of wounded and invalided soldiers by waters and baths. IV. Great Britain', *AMH*, 4 (1924), 140–3, p. 140.
11 Roger Cooter, *Surgery and society in peace and war: orthopaedics and the organisation of modern medicine, 1880–1948* (Basingstoke: Macmillan, 1993).
12 C. W. Buckley, 'The health resorts and the state', B&CS, *PRSM*, 12 (1919), 7–13.
13 C. W. Buckley, 'I. Great Britain', paper presented at ISMH conference 'The relation between the state, the health resort and National Health Insurance', 10 October 1928, *AMH*, 7 (1929), pp. 127–9.
14 George Newman, *An outline of the practice of preventive medicine: a memorandum addressed to the Minister of Health* (London: HMSO, 1919).
15 MoH consultative council on medical and allied services, *Interim report on the future provision of medical and allied services* (London: HMSO, 1920).
16 TNA, MH 58/159, 'Statement for the MoH from the joint committee (of the International Society of Medical Hydrology and the section of balneology of the Royal Society of Medicine) to promote the teaching of medical hydrology in England', November 1923.
17 Weisz, 'Water cures and science'.
18 Weisz, 'Spas in twentieth-century France', pp. 461–4.
19 TNA, MH 58/159, notes of meeting on 30 November 1923 between the joint committee to promote the teaching of medical hydrology in England and the MoH.
20 TNA, MH 55/1044, letter from K. R. England and W. J. Leist to Rt. Hon. Sir Godfrey Collins and the Rt. Hon. Sir Edward Hilton Young, December 1933, with attached memorandum by the BSF on Government recognition; TNA, MH/55/1044, minute sheet to Chief Medical Officer from J. A. Glover, dated 6 February 1934.
21 Anne Digby, 'The economic and medical significance of the British National Health Insurance Act', in Martin Gorsky and Sally Sheard (eds), *Financing medicine: the British experience since 1750* (Routledge: London, 2006), 182–98, p. 182. The upper age limit was reduced to sixty-five in 1928 and the lower limit adjusted to include those under sixteen already in work in 1937.
22 MoH, *Reports on public health and medical subjects*, No. 23, *The incidence of rheumatic diseases* (London: HMSO, 1924); Cantor, 'Aches of industry', p. 233.
23 Cantor, 'Contradictions of specialization', p. 138.
24 TNA, MH 55/1044, Royal Commission on NHI, statement submitted on behalf of the United Patriot's National Benefit Society, p. 9.
25 TNA, MH 55/1044, Royal Commission on NHI, statement submitted on behalf of the United Patriot's National Benefit Society, p. 4. The nine spas were Bath, Buxton, Cheltenham, Droitwich, Harrogate, Leamington, Llandrindod Wells, Strathpeffer and Woodhall Spa.

26 TNA, MH 62/35, 'Clinics for the treatment of industrial rheumatism' (London: Henry Lesser (not dated but c. December 1927).
27 TNA, MH 62/35, 'Treatment of rheumatism', letter from BSF to MoH, 11 June 1927'.
28 TNA, MH 62/35, Testimony of William Wilcox in notes of meeting 'Treatment of rheumatism', recorded as 'Extract from N.I. Gazette of 11 June 1927'.
29 TNA, LAB 2/1929, 'Spa treatment for Post Office servants', June 1927.
30 TNA, LAB 2/1929, 'Special arrangements for treatment of members of staff at British spas', issued by Ministry of Labour benevolent fund, April 1928.
31 TNA, MH 55/1044, BSF circular No. 1, *British Spa Federation: scheme for spa treatment for independent or voluntary members of friendly societies* (undated). The ten spas were Bath, Bridge of Allan, Buxton, Cheltenham, Harrogate, Leamington, Llandrindod Wells, Strathpeffer, Trefriw Wells and Woodhall Spa.
32 TNA, MH 62/35, letter from John Hatton, secretary of the BSF, to MoH, 23 February 1929.
33 TNA, MH 62/35, note of interview between the MoH and John Hatton, 18 April 1929.
34 TNA, MH 62/35, correspondence between the Independent Order of Odd Fellows, Manchester Unity Friendly Society and the MoH in September 1930.
35 TNA, MH 62/231, letter from F. J. C. Broome to the MoH, 9 October 1935.
36 TNA, MH 62/231, briefing note for Mr Neville, 9 January 1936.
37 TNA, MH 62/231, letter from F. J. C. Broome to Sir Kingsley Wood, 7 February 1936.
38 TNA, MH 62/231, letter from honorary secretary of the National Federation of Rural Approved Societies to MoH, 28 May 1936.
39 TNA, MH 62/231, letter from the MoH to John Hatton, BSF, 6 July 1939.
40 Bennett-Ruete, 'Bad Ems', pp. 95–9.
41 Maretzki and Seidler, 'Biomedicine and naturopathic healing', pp. 389–90.
42 Bennett-Ruete, 'Bad Ems', pp. 100–9.
43 Bennett-Ruete, 'Bad Ems', pp. 114–16; Michael Hau, *The cult of health and beauty in Germany: a social history, 1890–1930* (Chicago: University of Chicago Press, 2003).
44 Bennett-Ruete, 'Bad Ems', p. 118.
45 Weisz, 'Spas in twentieth-century France', pp. 477–8.
46 'British spas', *Prescriber*, 16 (1922), pp. 109–28.
47 The BSF published a number of editions of *British spas and health resorts* from 1918. The BHRA published *British health resorts: spa, seaside, inland, including the British Dominions and Colonies* in the 1930s.
48 Jennings, *Harrogate*, p. 441.
49 Jennings, *Harrogate*, p. 442.
50 *The Harrogate Cure* (Harrogate: Harrogate Corporation, 1940), p. 21.
51 Langham and Wells, *DRH*, pp. 96–7.

52 'Lectures in hydrology at the University of London and the other British Universities', *AMH*, 4 (1926), p. 149.
53 Fortescue Fox 'Lecture 3, "The medicinal spring: the teaching of medical hydrology", B&CS, *PRSM*, 4 (1911), 101–18, p. 113.
54 R. Fortescue Fox, *Medical hydrology: outlines for practitioners and students* (London: J. & A. Churchill, 1924).
55 TNA, MH 58/159. Copy of printed flyer advertising a course of lectures on medical hydrology held at the University of London and Harrogate between 9 May and 2 June 1923.
56 Domenico Barduzzi, Alois Strasser, Jean Billard *et al.*, 'The teaching of medical hydrology'; Simon Baruch, *The principles and practice of hydrotherapy* (London: Ballière and Co., 1900).
57 Weisz, 'Spas in twentieth-century France', p. 464.
58 F. G. Thomson, 'The evolution of a health resort', Presidential address to the annual meeting of the BMA, *BMJ* (25 July 1925), 153–7, p. 157.
59 Buxton Research Committee Minutes, 7 September 1928, 18 July 1929.
60 Weisz, 'Spas in twentieth-century France', pp. 459–65.
61 Cantor, 'Contradictions of specialization', pp. 136–43.
62 Royal Bath Hospital, Annual Report of the advisory committee on research into rheumatism, 1935; Royal Bath Hospital, *The national grey cross campaign* (1938), p. 10.
63 'Introductory note', *Harrogate Spa Medical Journal*, 1 (1938), pp. 2–3.
64 Rolls, *Hospital of the nation*, pp. 103–10.
65 Kersley, *Three R's*, p. 9.
66 Kersley, *Three R's*, p. 11.
67 *Grey cross campaign*, p. 8.
68 *Grey cross campaign*, pp. 10–15.
69 'Grey cross campaign against rheumatism', *Yorkshire Post* (16 May 1938), Harrogate Library, ph 362.13.
70 Kersley, *Three R's*, p. 32.
71 Buxton Library local studies collection, 'Medical advisory committee minutes, report drafted 5 February 1936'.
72 DRO, D4510/2/3, DRH, Extension appeal, finance committee meeting, 2 October 1936.
73 DRO, D4508/13/1, report on deputation of BSF to MoH, 28 June 1944.
74 DRO, D4508/13/1, memorandum by C. W. Buckley on the place of spas and spa hospitals in the NHS, 1943.
75 DRO, D4508/7/3/4, minutes of meeting of BSF with MoH, 13 March 1947.
76 DRO, D4508/13/3, minutes of visit of Dr Godber to Buxton on 7 August 1945.
77 DRO, D4508/7/3/4, Buxton co-ordinating committee, report of a sub-committee, October 1945.
78 DRO, D4508/13/3, 'A scheme for rheumatism and allied diseases at the rheumatic centre, Buxton'.

79 DRO, D4508/13/3, DRH, Report of a meeting of the finance and general purposes committee, 22 March 1946.
80 TNA, MH 77/67. Minute dated 30 June 1945 noting 'we do not intend to use the Spas generally in the National Health Service and it is only fair to tell them so'; letters from the Birmingham Regional Hospital Board, 2 July 1948 and Oxford RHB, 6 August 1948 requesting clarification of payments for spa treatment; Minute, 6 August 1948 from George Watts to Gedling, 'I am now given to understand that a fresh decision has been made, and that patients may in fact be sent to places like Droitwich for 3 weeks for treatment'.
81 DRO, D4508/13/3, 'To all members of the BSF – National Health Service Bill', memorandum from J. E. Boddington, honorary secretary to the BSF, 12 July 1947.
82 BMA, *Spa in medical practice*, pp. 29, 60 and 61–93.
83 TNA, BD 18/506, Droitwich rheumatic clinic, October 1949.
84 City of Bath Archives, printed flyer, 'Access to treatment under the NHS', Royal National Hospital for Rheumatic Diseases, September 1949.
85 Jennings, *Harrogate*, pp. 447–8.
86 J. A. Patmore, 'Harrogate and Knaresborough: a study in urban development' (MA dissertation, University of Oxford, 1959, p. 221.
87 Jennings, *Harrogate*, p. 448.
88 Powys record office, Llandrindod Wells, Bathing statistics, 1951.
89 Thomson, *Spas that heal*, p. 103; Jennings, *Harrogate*, p. 448.
90 Thomson, *Spas that heal*, pp. 50–4.
91 Langham and Wells, *Baths at Buxton Spa*, pp. 111–12.
92 Thomson, *Spas that heal*, p. 66.
93 *Bath Hospital souvenir brochure, 1826–1994* (Harrogate: Harrogate Health Care, 1994); Langham and Wells, *DRH*, p. 115.
94 Weisz, 'Spas in twentieth-century France', pp. 476–80.
95 Weisz, 'Spas in twentieth-century France', pp. 480–3.
96 Bennett-Ruete, 'Bad Ems', p. 273.
97 Bennett-Ruete, 'Bad Ems', pp. 124–5.
98 Bennett-Ruete, 'Bad Ems', p. 275.
99 Maretzki, 'Cultural variation', pp. 25–6.
100 LSAGM, Michael Bevan, '"Pulling the plug?": an oral history of spa practices and experiences at the Royal Pump Rooms, Leamington Spa, in the late twentieth century' (2007), oral testimony, Anne Golland. Thanks are due to the Wellcome Trust for funding this joint project between the Centre for the History of Medicine, University of Warwick and the LSAGM.
101 Bevan, 'Pulling the plug', oral testimony, Jack Reilly.
102 Bevan, 'Pulling the plug', oral testimony, Vivian Weinstein.
103 Bevan, 'Pulling the plug', oral testimony, Vivian Weinstein.
104 Webb, 'Woodhall Spa', pp. 41–2.
105 Marjorie Sargeant, *Echoes of Woodhall Spa: Woodhall and war* (Woodhall Spa Cottage Museum: Woodhall Spa, 2006), pp. 149–50.

106 Marjorie Sargeant, 'Dr George Armour' and 'Dr James Robertson and the healing waters', in Sergeant, *Voices of Woodhall Spa* (Woodhall Spa: Woodhall Spa cottage museum, 2007) pp. 63–74.
107 Sargeant, 'Dr James Robertson', p. 73.
108 Sargeant, 'Dr James Robertson', p. 73.
109 Cantor, 'Cortisone and the politics of drama,' pp. 166, 173 and 183–4.
110 L. S. P. Davidson, 'Rheumatoid arthritis', in W. S. C. Copeman (ed.), *Textbook of the Rheumatic Diseases* (Edinburgh, 1948) 120–42, p. 133, cited in Cantor, 'Cortisone and the politics of drama,' p. 170.
111 Sargeant, 'Dr James Robertson', p. 73.
112 Gerald Larkin, *Occupational monopoly and modern medicine* (London: Tavistock, 1983), pp. 118–24.
113 Kersley, *Three R's*, pp. 24–5.

Conclusion

Although the contemporary use of 'spas' in England focuses on leisure and beauty rather than serious curative activities this book has shown that from the early nineteenth to the mid-twentieth century water cures were accorded much greater respect by members of the medical profession, lay and unorthodox healers and patients. Water was used in multiple ways in healing practices and was applied for both health maintenance and active treatment of a range of complaints. Earlier studies by medical historians have examined spa medicine and hydropathy separately, emphasising the disputes between adherents of the two systems in the period between 1840 and 1860. This study has shown how the techniques used in both systems came to converge as water treatments were increasingly adopted by the orthodox profession. Water's powerful physiological effects were endorsed by emerging research evidence which underscored the potential of any clean water to be used in treatment applications. Clinical experience continued to be important in justifying their use. Although no consensus was reached on water's mode of action, hydrotherapy and balneology were accepted as part of orthodox therapeutics by the 1890s. Hydropathy continued to be used by unorthodox healers too and by the 1920s was incorporated within the armoury of drugless methods used by naturopaths.[1] Water cures were also promoted as suitable for use in domestic healing in health manuals aimed at the lay healer.[2]

The opportunity to integrate treatment within a wider regimen of rest and recuperation was fundamental to the perceived benefits of water cures. In 1900 F. Parkes Weber argued that patients undergoing treatment for syphilis with mercury and iodide compounds would benefit from taking this at a specialist resort where the combined effects of hydrology and climate acted to improve the general condition of the body, enabling patients to better withstand the effects of the harsh pharmaceutical treatments. At a spa 'limitation of brain work and avoidance of mental worry by care with regard to diet and by regular exercise (without fatigue) in the open air' were easily integrated into daily routines whereas often 'the patient will pay no attention to such matters as long as he remains at home and has to attend to his business; he will simply content himself by carrying out some sort of pharmaceutical treatment'. Specialist advice and skills were valued; Parkes Weber particularly endorsed the facilities and expertise at Harrogate where medical practitioners and attendants provided treatment including sulphur baths and the massage of ointment preparations into the skin. For this condition the social seclusion offered by a spa was as much an attraction as a convivial social life, offering 'freedom from the special worry of remaining at home while suffering from a secondary eruption on the face and an infectious condition of the mouth and throat'.[3] This example underscores the expertise available at water cure resorts and the ability to tailor regimes to the medical and social needs of patients. A treatment model incorporating a wider regimen continued to be endorsed into the inter-war period. In 1937 the BHRA defined a cure as

> a set course of *spa treatment* in country surroundings, with change of air and scene as well as diet and occupation. Such a course is of a definite duration, usually three weeks, and is planned and directed by the spa practitioner. The aim is to prevent or overcome invalidism by recourse to natural waters, baths and other external applications with simplicity of life and open-air pleasures ... To those elements, Waters, Climates, Methods, constantly developing with the advance of science, must also be added *Place*, the intangible *genius loci*, to which many ailing people are sensitive.[4]

The buoyant market for 'cures' in the nineteenth and twentieth centuries was fed by broad trends of rising incomes among the middle classes and is an integral part of the more general commercialisation of health and leisure in the industrial age.[5] The close interconnection between health and recreational services continued; medical uses were one aspect of more diverse bathing cultures that developed which spanned hygienic, leisure and therapeutic practices and took place in a variety of private and public settings. While facilities for invalids were an important draw at resorts many patients travelled with family or friends. All could benefit from healthful recreational and social activities.

Patmore notes the need to distinguish between the 'spa itself' and the wider 'settlement' or resort.[6] While access to natural mineral waters underpinned the development of spas in the eighteenth century, more general urban growth at some resorts later converted 'a Spa with a town, into a town with a Spa'.[7] Although the relative economic importance of bathing and drinking reduced as these urban economies expanded-as at Bath, Leamington and Cheltenham – facilities and practices associated with spa treatment continued to influence society and culture at resort towns. Preference for more rural settings is apparent in the mid-nineteenth century with the expansion in the popularity of hydropathic resorts at Malvern and Ilkley. However by the end of the century the leading spas at Bath, Buxton and Harrogate had a more urban feel mitigated by a commitment to the ideal of *rus in urbe* through the construction of parks, winter gardens and areas for recreation in the open air.

Commercial success depended on cooperation between a range of investors, land owners, entrepreneurs and charitable bodies. The ability to adapt to changing consumer demand was fundamental to a resort's financial success. Although the middle class, able to afford the cost of a stay of several weeks, were the prime market for these services, a range of initiatives sought to expand access to the poorer classes too. In the nineteenth century these centred on the charitable bathing hospitals. In the twentieth century the potential contribution of water cures to improving the nation's health was recognised by the central state; particularly their use in treating wounded soldiers and in tackling the burden of rheumatic disease. Efforts spearheaded by the BSF focused on gaining funding for spa treatment through the NHI scheme. Although this was not achieved, free treatment at English spas was made available to all under arrangements put in place on the introduction of the NHS in 1948. From the mid-nineteenth century the English spas had developed through collaboration between a network of stakeholders which included specialist medical practitioners and other workers, charitable institutions, local authorities, spa managers and private investors. These local networks, which supported the development of both treatment and recreational facilities, were undermined by the introduction of the NHS as decisions about medical treatment became the responsibility of regional boards focused on provision of a full range of health services. Investment and management decisions were no longer taken by local players with a personal interest in maintaining the facilities and services at a resort. These issues were now considered by newly appointed management boards responsible for a range of hospital and community-based services. The larger spas, particularly Buxton, Bath and Harrogate, continued to attract patients in the early years of the NHS with capacity increased to meet rising demand. In the longer term, financial pressures, the promise of new drug treatments such as cortisone, the growth of physiotherapy and the reorganisation of health and medical institutions influenced the withdrawal of funding from municipal spa facilities. This contrasts with the experience in France and Germany where a funding model based on re-imbursement of approved treatments through insurance-based health care schemes continued to fund treatment at specialist resorts into the late twentieth century.

Charting the withdrawal of NHS support for treatment disguises the continuing association of the 'spa' with recreation and recuperation and its popularity with patients. The range of options considered in the proposed redevelopment of the Pump Rooms at Leamington in the 1980s included models that brought together treatment and leisure activities. Although this project was unsuccessful, the options considered pointed to the new direction the spa was to take. Belief in the important influence of lifestyle factors including rest, diet and exercise to improve heath and manage chronic health conditions continues to be widespread. Water is recognised to be essential for life, fundamental to hygienic routines and a source of pleasure for all age groups. International demand for opportunities for leisure, relaxation and recuperation remain strong. These factors were among those that underpinned the popularity of water cures in the nineteenth and twentieth centuries. In the English context spas have shifted out of state-run medical spheres and into private leisure settings where little emphasis is given to the natural mineral or thermal properties of water or to medical expertise. However, concerns about the obesity epidemic and the increasing prevalence of chronic complaints suggest that water cures, which successfully combined the motivating factors of health and pleasure along with active engagement from patients in healthy regimens, may yet be poised for reinvention for a new generation of health seekers.

Notes

1 Adams, 'Developing naturopathy'.
2 Marland and Adams, 'Hydropathy at home'.
3 Wellcome Library, PP/FPW/B314, F. Parkes Weber, 'The use of baths, mineral waters and health resorts in the treatment of syphilis', *British Physician*, 15 June 1900, 327–8.
4 R. Fortescue Fox, 'The spa cure', in Fortescue Fox (ed.), *British health resorts: spa, seaside, inland* (London: J. & A. Churchill, 1937), p. 15. Original emphasis.
5 Borsay, Health and leisure resorts'.
6 Patmore, 'Spa towns', p. 47.
7 Granville, *Northern spas*, p. xxxix.

Select bibliography

PRIMARY SOURCES

Archives

Bath City Library
Bath General Infirmary Annual Reports

Bath Record Office
Bath Corporation records
Bath General Infirmary records

Birmingham City Library
Birmingham Hospital Saturday Fund

Buxton Library
Buxton, Medical advisory committee minutes

Derbyshire Record Office (DRO)
D1323, Buxton Borough Council and predecessors
D1323/2/9, Buxton Baths and Wells Committee minutes
D 3932/2, Rockside Hydro, Matlock Bank
D1397, Smedley's Hydro, Matlock
D 4508, Devonshire Royal Hospital and Buxton Bath Charity

Devon Heritage Centre
Plans of New Bath House at Sidmouth

Devonshire Collections, Chatsworth,
Buxton Estate Records

Flintshire Archives Service (FAS)
Papers relating to St Winefride's Well 1838–1938

Harrogate Library, local studies collection

Bath Hospital Annual Reports and related materials

E. P. L. Dixon, 'Harrogate Royal Bath Hospital and Rawson Convalescent Home'

PH615.49, Material relating to baths

Leamington Spa Art Gallery and Museum (LSAGM)

Bevan, Michael, "Pulling the Plug': an oral history archive of Leamington Spa Pump Rooms' (2007)

M 4151 1994, Medical Advisory Committee Minutes

M 4348 1995, Pump room and baths manager's report books

Lincolnshire Archives

Hawley 5: Woodhall Spa company

Manchester Archives and Local Studies

Cotton Districts Convalescent Fund (CDCF)

The National Archives (TNA)

BD 18/506 Welsh Hospital Board, spa treatment general correspondence 1948–53

BT 31/35556/267466 British Health Resorts Association

LAB 2/1929 Spa treatment for Post Office servants

MH 55/1044 Spa treatment for rheumatism: government recognition

MH 58/159 Government recognition of medical hydrology

MH 62/35 Additional benefits insured persons

MH 62/231 Additional benefits insured persons

MH 77/67 Representations of the BSF 1943–48

Census Records for England and Wales 1841–1911

National Osteopathic Archive

Pitcairn-Knowles box file

Powys Record Office,

Llandrindod Wells, Bathing statistics, 1951

St Winefride's Museum and Archives

HOWSW/2004/501 AC Father Ryan's Diary

Warwickshire County Record Office (Warwickshire CRO)

Warneford Hospital Annual Reports

CR1563 Leamington Local Board of Health

Wellcome Library

GC/63/4- bound volume re. Malvern typhoid case

PP/FPW/B314, papers of F. Parkes Weber

Worcestershire Archives Service (WAS)

Droitwich municipal records

Malvern Urban District Council (MUDC)
Royal Baths
St Andrews Baths

Official reports

Ministry of Health, *Reports on public health and medical subjects*, No. 23, *The incidence of rheumatic diseases* (London: HMSO, 1924)

Journals

Archives of Medical Hydrology (*AMH*)
British Medical Journal (*BMJ*)
British Naturopathic Journal and Osteopathic Review
Harrogate Spa Medical Journal
Journal of Balneology and Climatology (*JB&C*)
Journal of British and Foreign Health Resorts (*JBFHR*)
Lancet
Prescriber
Proceedings of the Royal Society of Medicine (*PRSM*)
Provincial Medical and Surgical journal (*PMSJ*)

Newspapers and magazines

Berrow's Worcestershire Journal
Builder
Cheltenham Examiner
Cheltenham Looker-on
Harrogate Advertiser
Health Resort
Herald of Health
Horncastle News and South Lindsey Advertiser
Illustrated London News
Leamington Spa Courier
Malvern Advertiser
Malvern Gazette
Malvern News
Nature Cure
North Wales Chronicle
Queen
Staffordshire Advertiser
The Times
Yorkshire Post

Directories and guides

Anon., *Pictorial and descriptive guide to Royal Leamington Spa* (London: Ward Lock and Co., 1918/19).
Anon., *Pictorial and descriptive guide to Woodhall Spa* (London: Ward Lock and Co., 1902).
Bath as a health resort (Bath: Bath Corporation, n.d, c. 1900).
Beck's shilling guide to Leamington (Leamington Spa: John Beck, 1867).
M. *Billing's directory and gazetteer of the county of Worcestershire* (M. Billing: Birmingham, 1855).
The Carlsbad of England: the official handbook of the Cheltenham corporation (Cheltenham: Cheltenham Corporation, c. 1925).
Derbyshire post office directory (London: Kelly, 1864).
Fairfax, John, *Fairfax's new Leamington guide: including a general directory* (Leamington: John Fairfax, 1832).
Halden and Son's directory of Stafford and district (1893).
Harrogate as a health resort (Harrogate: Harrogate Corporation, from 1898).
Kelly's directory of Devonshire (London: Kelly, 1939).
Medical guide to the hot mineral baths of Bath (Bath: Bath Corporation, 1901).
Shuttleworth's guide book to llkley and vicinity, 2nd edn (London: Hamilton, Adams & Co., Ilkley: J. Shuttleworth, n.d but c.1867); 3rd edn (Ilkley: J Shuttleworth, 1882).
Slater's directory of Southport and Birkdale (Manchester: Slaters, 1887).
Stephenson's guide to Southport (Southport: Visiter, 1903).
The Harrogate cure (Harrogate: Harrogate Corporation, 1940).

PRINTED PRIMARY SOURCES

Anon., *The Ben Rhydding book of gymnastics* (Ilkley: John Shuttleworth, n.d. c. 1852).
Anon., *Birmingham' s triumph: the Hospital Saturday Fund* (Birmingham: BHSF, 1938).
Anon., *Extracts relating to baths, wells, etc. from the Presidential address delivered before the members of the Harrogate Medical Society*, 16 November 1893 (Harrogate: R. Ackrill, 1893).
Anon., *Harrogate Cottage Hospital, its history and developments* (Harrogate: R. Ackrill, 1896), reprinted from *Harrogate Advertiser* (11 January 1896).
Anon., *The health and nature cure handbook: a complete authoritative and independent guide to nature cure and healthy living*, Vol. 3 (London: James Clarke & Co. Ltd, 1934).
Anon., *Leamington Spa: a history of the Pump Room Bathing Establishment', reprinted from The Leamington Spa Courrier and the Warwickshire Standard, Saturday June 4, 1887.*

Anon., *Memorials from Ben Rhydding: concerning the place, its people, its cures* (London: Charles Gilpin, 1852).

Anon., *Nature cure annual and health and pleasure guide 1907/08* (London: MacGregor, Reid and Shaw, 1908).

Anon., *The metropolis of the water cure: or records of a water patient in Malvern* (London: Simpkin, Marshall, and Co., 1858).

Anon., *Spas and inland resorts: health giving centres in the Midlands, the West of England and Central Wales* (London: Great Western Railway, 1923).

Anon., *Visitor's vade mecum, being an historical and descriptive sketch of Harrogate* (Harrogate: P. Palliser, 1838).

Anon., *What to do with the Royal Pump Rooms* (Leamington Spa: James J. Barr, 1862).

Anon., *Woodhall Spa: the English Kreuznach* (1886).

Bailey, Benson, *Ilkley, Bolton Abbey, and the pearls of Craven* (Bingley: John Harrison & Son, 1852).

Bainbrigge, W. H., *Remarks on the Droitwich saline springs* (Worcester: Worcester Journal office, 1871).

Barber, Francis, *The passing of the Victoria Baths: its significance, cost and consequence*, reprinted from the *Harrogate Herald*, 16 September 1931 (Harrogate: R. Ackrill, 1931).

Baruch, Simon. *The principles and practice of hydrotherapy* (London: Ballière and Co., 1900).

Baynes, Donald, *Auxiliary methods of cure* (London: Simpkin, Marshall and Co., 1888).

Beard, George M., *A practical treatise on nervous exhaustion (neurasthenia): its symptoms, nature, sequences, treatment* (New York: W. Wood, 1880).

Beard, George M., *American nervousness: its causes and consequences* (New York, Putnam, 1881).

Bennett, Arnold, *Clayhanger* (London: Methuen, 1910).

Bisset, J., *A descriptive guide to Leamington Priors* (Leamington: Merridew, 1814); 2nd edn (Coventry: J. Bisset, 1816).

Bisset, J., *The origin, rise and progress of Leamington Spa* (Leamington: E. Heathcote, 1828).

Bonacina, L. C. W., 'Climate, health and the British resorts', in BHRA, *British health resorts: spa, seaside, inland* (1939), 50–2.

Bott, W., *A description of Buxton* (Manchester: J. Harrop, 1795).

Braun, Julius, *On the curative effects of baths and waters being a handbook to the spas of Europe*, an abridged translation with notes edited by Hermann Weber (London: Smith, Elder & Co., 1875).

British Health Resorts Association (BHRA), *British health resorts: spa, seaside, inland, including the British Dominions and Colonies* (London: J. & A. Churchill, 1937) (London: BHRA, 1939).

BMA, *Astounding revelations concerning supposed massage houses or pandemoniums of vice, frequented by both sexes, being a complete exposé of the ways of professed masseurs and masseuses* (London: Skeats, 1894).
BMA, *The spa in medical practice* (London: BMA, 1951).
British Spa Federation (BSF), *British spas and health resorts* (London: E. J. Burrow, 1918).
British Spa Federation (BSF), *The spas of Great Britain* (Bath, Pitman Press, n.d. but c. 1931).
BSF, *The spas of Britain: the official handbook of the BSF* (Bath: Pitman Press, n.d. but after 1923).
Broome, F. J. C., *The Harrogate fango treatment* (Harrogate: Harrogate Corporation, n.d. but c. 1928).
Buchan, William, *Domestic medicine* (London: W. Strahan, T. Cadell, 1774).
Buckley, Joseph, *Matlock Bank as it was and is* (London: Job Caudwell, 1867).
Bulwer Lytton, Edward, 'Confessions and observations of a water patient', *New Monthly Magazine* (1845), 1–16, later republished as *Confessions of a water-patient* (London: Henry Colburn, 1845).
Burney Yeo, I., *Health resorts and their uses* (London: Chapman and Hall, 1882).
Burney Yeo, I., *The therapeutics of mineral springs and climates* (London: Cassell, 1904).
Calthrop, Lionel, *A guide to the bromo-iodine mineral water and spa baths, Woodhall Spa* (Woodhall Spa: no publisher, n.d. but c. 1912).
Calthrop, Lionel, *A guide to the spa baths, pump room and Victoria Hotel, Woodhall Spa, Lincolnshire* (Woodhall Spa: no publisher, n.d. but c. 1912).
Campbell, Agnes, Carnegie United Kingdom Trust, *Report on public baths and wash-houses in the United Kingdom* (Edinburgh: Edinburgh University Press, 1918).
Cheyne, George, *Essay on health and long life* (London, for the author, 1724).
Cheyne, George, *The English malady; or a treatise of nervous diseases* (London: G. Strahan, 1733).
Claridge, Richard T. *Hydropathy or the water cure as practised by Vincent Preissnitz* (London: James Madden, 1842), 5th edn, 1843.
Clark, James, *The sanative influence of climate with an account of the best places of resort for invalids in England, the south of Europe, etc.* (London: John Murray, 1841).
Cohen, Solomon Solis (ed.), *A system of physiologic therapeutics: a practical exposition of the methods, other than drug-giving, useful in the treatment of the sick*, Vols 1–11(London: Rebman, 1901–5).
Eardley-Wilmot, R., *On the natural mineral waters and spa of Leamington* (Leamington: W. H. Smith, 1890).
Ellis, C. A., *An historical survey of Torquay*, 2nd edn (Torquay: Ellis, c. 1930).
Elson, George, *The last of the climbing boys* (London: J. Long, 1900).
Floyer, John, *History of cold-bathing, both ancient and modern*, 5th edn (London: William and John Innys, 1722).

Fortescue Fox, R., *The principles and practice of medical hydrology: being the science of treatment by waters and baths* (London: London University Press, 1913).
Fortescue Fox, R., *Medical hydrology: outlines for practitioners and students* (London: J. & A. Churchill, 1924).
Foster, F. C., *Journal kept by F. C. Foster, whilst residing at the hydropathic establishment, Matlock Bank Derbyshire, and undergoing treatment there, from August 15th to October 25th 1860* (Bridgwater: W. H. Prosser, 1877).
Foster, M. G., *Baths and medicinal waters of Britain and Europe* (London: Simpkin Marshall, 1933).
Fowler, Sir James Kingston, *Aix-les-Bains and Mont Revard: the douche massage treatment of arthritis and fibrositis* (London: William Heinemann, 1926).
Garrod, Alfred Baring, *The essentials of materia medica, therapeutics and the pharmacopoeias* (London: Walton and Mabberly, 1855).
Garrod, Alfred Baring, *A Treatise on gout and rheumatic gout*, 3rd edn (London, Longmans, Green, 1876).
Granville, A. B., *Spas of Germany*, 2 Vols (London: Henry Colburn, 1837).
Granville, A. B., *Spas of England and principal sea-bathing places*, Vol. 1, *Northern spas*, Vol. 2, *Midland and southern spas* (London, Henry Colburn, 1841).
Grindrod, Ralph Barnes, *Bacchus: an essay on the nature, causes, effects and cure of intemperance* (London: J. Pasco, 1839, reprinted London, Simpkins, Marshall and Co., 1851).
Grindrod, R. B., *The compressed air bath: a therapeutic agent in various affections of the respiratory organs, and other diseases* (London: Simpkin, Marshall & Co, 1860).
Grindrod, R. B., *Malvern; its claims as a health resort; with notes on climate … also an exposition of the physiological and therapeutic influence of compressed air* (London: Robert Harwicke, n.d. but c. 1871).
Gully, James Manby, *The water cure in chronic disease* (London: Simpkin Marshall & Co., 1846), 2nd edn (London: Churchill, 1847), 4th edn (London: John Churchill, 1851).
Gully, James Manby, *A guide to domestic hydrotherapeia: the water cure in acute disease* (London: Simpkin Marshall, & Co; Edinburgh: A. C. Black; Malvern: H. Cross, 1863).
Guthrie, Thomas, *Autobiography of Thomas Guthrie and memoir* (edited by his sons D. K. Guthrie and C. J. Guthrie), Vol. 2 (London, for the authors, 1874–75).
Hardy, William, *Life and electricity in health and disease*, 2nd edn (Harrogate: T. Hollins Advertiser Office, 1870).
Hastings, Charles, *Illustrations of the natural history of Worcestershire* (London: Sherwood, Gilbert & Piper, 1834).
Hastings, Charles, *On the salt springs of Worcestershire: a lecture delivered before the members of the Worcestershire Natural History Society* (Worcester: Chalk and Holl, 1835).
Hawkins, E., *Medical climatology of England and Wales* (London: H. K. Lewis, 1923).
Head, Francis, *Bubbles from the brunnens of Nassau* (London: J. Murray, 1834).

Hinderwell, Thomas, *The History and Antiquities of Scarborough*, 2nd edn (York: Longman, Hurst, Rees, Orme and Brown, 1811).
Hood, Paxton, *The metropolis of the water cure or records of a water patient at Malvern* (London: Simpkin, Marshall and Co., 1858).
Hyde, Samuel, *Buxton, its Baths and Climate* (Manchester: John Heywood, 1895).
Jameson, Thomas, *A treatise on the Cheltenham waters & bilious diseases* (Ruff: Cheltenham, 1803).
Jameson, Thomas, *A treatise on the Cheltenham waters & biliary diseases*, 3rd edn (Cheltenham: J. K. and S. Griffith, 1814).
Jeaffreson, J. C., *A book about doctors*, Vol. 1, 2nd edn (London: Hurst and Blackett, 1861).
Jerrold, Walter, *Douglas Jerrold and Punch* (London: Macmillan, 1910).
Jewitt, A., *The history of Buxton; and the visitor's guide to the curiosities of the Peak* (London: published by the author, 1811).
Johnson, Edward, *The domestic practice of hydropathy* (London: Simpkin, Marshall, and Co., 1849).
Jones, John, *The Benefit of the Auncient Bathes of Buckstones* (London: William Jones, 1572).
Kellgren, Arvid, *The technic [sic] of Ling's system of manual treatment* (Edinburgh and London: Young J. Pentland, 1890).
Kersley, G. D., *The three R's: rheumatism, rehabilitation, research as viewed from Bath* (Bath: privately printed, c. 1980).
Kneipp, Sebastian, *My water-cure*, translated from his 36th German edition, 2nd edn (Kempton: Jos. Kessel, 1893).
Lane, R. J., *Life at the water cure: facts and fancies noted down during a month at Malvern* (London: Henry Bohn, 1846); new edition with reprint of Edward Bulwer Lytton, 'Confessions of a water patient' (London: Henry Bohn, 1851).
Lee, Edwin, *The mineral springs of England* (London: Whittaker and Co., 1841), republished as *The watering places of England*, 3rd edn (London: J Churchill, 1854).
Leech, John, *Three weeks in wet sheets: being the diary and doings of a moist visitor to Malvern* (London: Hamilton, Adams & Co., 1846), 4th edn (London: Hamilton, Adams, 1858)
Leichenstein, Otto, 'Balneotherapeutics' in Von Ziemssen, *Handbook of general therapeutics* Vol. 4 (1886), 243–472.
Luke, T. D., *Spas and health resorts of the British Isles* (London: A & C Black, 1919).
Lukis, J. H., The *common-sense of the water cure* (London: Robert Hardwicke, 1862).
M'Cabe, James, *Directions for drinking the Cheltenham waters* (Cheltenham: G. A. Williams, 1823).
Macindoe, A., *Sidmouth and the Nauheim Treatment* (Sidmouth: Culverwell & Sons, 1898).
Macpherson, John, *Our baths and wells: the mineral waters of the British Islands* (London: Macmillan, 1871).

Macpherson, John, *The baths and wells of Europe*, 2rd edn (London: Macmillan, 1873), 3rd edn (London: Edward Stanford, 1888).
Metcalfe, Richard, *The rise and progress of hydropathy in England and Scotland* (London: Simpkin, Marshall, Hamilton, Kent, 1906).
Milner, J., *Authentic documents relative to the miraculous case of Winefrid White etc.* (London: for the author, 1805).
Morris, J., *Dr Gully and Malvern* (Malvern: Malvern News, 1872)
Newman, George, *An outline of the practice of preventive medicine: a memorandum addressed to the Minister of Health* (London: HMSO, 1919).
Newman, George, *The rise of preventive medicine* (London: Oxford University Press, 1932).
Nichols, Mary S. Gove, *Experience in water-cure, a familiar exposition of the principles and results of water treatment in the care of acute and chronic disease* (New York: Fowler and Wells, 1849).
Nichols, Mary S. Gove, *A woman's work in water cure and sanitary education* (London: Longmans, Green, and Co., 1868).
Nichols, Thomas Low, *How to live on sixpence a day* (London: Longman, Green, Reader and Dyer, 1871).
Nichols, Thomas Low, *Nichols' health manual: being also a memorial of the life and work of Mrs Mary S. Gove Nichols* (London: E. W. Allen, 1887).
Nott, James, *The story of the water cure* (Malvern: Stevens and Co., 1900).
Oddfish, *Health and pleasure or Malvern Punch* (Malvern: J. Burns, 1863; London: Simplin Marchall, 1865).
Ord, W. M., 'Introductory remarks on the medicinal springs of Great Britain', in Ord and Garrod (eds), *Climates and baths*, 507–14.
Ord, W. M. and A. E. Garrod (eds), *The climates and baths of Great Britain*, Vol. 1, *The climates of the south of England, and the chief medicinal springs of Great Britain* (London: Macmillan, 1895).
Page, T. J., *Brief observations on the Buxton waters; with a few general directions for their use* (Bakewell: John Goodwin, 1832).
Pitcairn-Knowles, Gordon, 'The water cure at home', *Health and Nature Cure Handbook* Vol. 3, 107–15.
Pounce, Timothy, *Malvern as I found it* (London: published for the author, 1858).
Preston, Thomas, *Domestic Hydropathy; or instructions for the home practice of the water-cure, with introductory chapters on the maintenance of health and causes of disease* (Bristol: Author, 1870).
Research society of the Devonshire Hospital, *The natural thermal and chalybeate waters of Buxton: a brief account of their action and uses* (Buxton: Derbyshire Printing Co. Ltd., 1929).
Ridley, J., *The Cheltenham guide* (London: J. Ridley, 1781).
Robertson, W. H., *A guide to the use of the Buxton waters* (London: John Churchill, 1847); 19th edn (Buxton: John Cumming Bates, 1876).
Robertson, W. H. *A handbook to the peak of Derbyshire or Buxton in 1854* (London: Bradbury and Evans, 1854).

RSM, *Notes on hydrological treatment for wounded and invalid soldiers and sailors with a list of British spas and health resorts and of the disorders which they benefit* (London: Adlard and Son, 1915).
Russell, Richard, *A dissertation on the use of sea water in the diseases of the glands* (London: W. Owen, 1755).
Scudamore, Charles, *A chemical and medical report of the properties of the mineral waters of Buxton, Matlock, Cheltenham [et al]* (London, printed for the author, 1820).
Scudamore, Charles, *The analysis and medical account of the tepid springs of Buxton* (London, printed for the author, 1833).
Scudamore, Charles, *A medical visit to Gräfenberg in April and May 1843 for the purposes of investigating the merits of the water-cure treatment* (London: John Churchill, 1843).
Short, Thomas, *The natural experimental and medicinal history of the mineral waters of Derbyshire, Lincolnshire and Yorkshire* (1734).
Smedley, Caroline, *Ladies' manual of practical hydropathy*, 1st edn (London: W. S. Partridge, 1861); 16th edn (London: James Blackwood, 1878); 19th edn (London: James Blackwood, 1880).
Smedley, John, *Practical hydropathy*, 1st edn (London: John Kendrick, 1858); 4th edn (London: Job Caudwell, 1861); 11th edn (London, W. Kent and Co., 1869); 13th edn (London: W. Kent & Co., 1870); 17th edn (London, James Blackwood & Co.,1877).
Smithells, Arthur, *Report of a scientific survey of Harrogate spa waters (made in 1912–1919) for the Corporation of Harrogate* (Leeds: Chorley and Pickergill, n. d. but c. 1919).
Southall, Mary, *A description of Malvern* (London: Longman, Hurst & Co., 1822).
Steer, Henry, *The Smedleys of Matlock Bank: being a review of the religious and philanthropic labours of Mr. and Mrs. John Smedley* (London: Elliot Stock, 1897).
Thackeray, William Makepeace, *Notes of a journey from Cornhill to grand Cairo* (London: Chapman and Hall, 1846).
Thomson, C. Leslie, *James C. Thomson, pioneer naturopath* 1887–1960 (Edinburgh: Kingston Clinic, 1960), reprinted from *The Kingston Chronicle*, May 1960.
Thomson, R. Woodrow, *Ben Rhydding: the asceplion of England* (London: Nelson & Sons, 1862).
Tyrrell, Walter, *Notes of the climate of Malvern, with reference to its effect on disease*, 2nd edn (Malvern: Advertiser, 1894).
Urquhart, David, *Pillars of Hercules, or, a narrative of travels in Spain & Morocco in 1848* (London: Bentley, 1850).
Wall, John, *Experiments and observations on the Malvern waters* (London: W. Sanby, 1756).
Wall, Martin, *Medical tracts of the late John Wall of Worcester collected and republished by Martin Wall* (Oxford: Prince and Cooke, 1780).
Weber, Hermann, 'The treatment of disease by climate', in von Ziemssen, *Handbook of general therapeutics*, Vol. 4 (1886), pp. 3–239.

Weber, Hermann, *Climatotherapy* (London: Smith, Elder and Co. 1896).
Weber, Hermann and F. Parkes Weber, 'Hydrotherapy and balneotherapy', in Thomas Clifford Allbutt and Humphrey Davy Rolleston (eds), A *system of medicine by many writers* Vol. 1. (London: Macmillan, 1905), 342–81.
Weber, Hermann and F. Parkes Weber (eds), *Climatotherapy and balneotherapy: the climates and mineral water health resorts (spas) of Europe and North Africa* (London: Smith, Elder & Co., 1907).
Weir Mitchell, Silas, *Fat and blood; and how to make them* (Philadelphia, J. B. Lippincott, 1882).
Weiss, J. *The Handbook of hydropathy: for professional and domestic use: with an Appendix on the best mode of forming hydropathic* establishments (London: James Madden and Co., 1844).
Wesley, John, *Primitive physick, or an easy and natural method of curing most diseases* (London: for the author, 1747).
Williams, C. Theodore and P. Horton-Smith (eds), *The climates and baths of Great Britain,* Vol. 2, *the climate of London and the central and northern portions of England, together with those of Wales and of Ireland* (London: Macmillan and Co. 1902).
Wilson, James, *A practical treatise on the curative effects of simple and medicated vapour* (London: Churchill, 1837).
Wilson, James, *The water-cure: stomach complaints and drug diseases* (London: J. Churchill, 1842).
Wilson, James, *The water cure: a practical treatise on the cure of diseases by water, air, exercise and diet* (London: J. Churchill, 1843).
Wilson, James, *The practice of the water cure with authenticated evidence of its efficacy and safety* (London: H. Bailliere, 1844).
Wilson, James, *Principles and practice of the water cure,* 4th edn (London: J. Churchill, 1858).
Wilson, James and James Manby Gully, *The dangers of the water cure* (London, J. Churchill, 1843)
Winternitz, Wilhelm, 'Hydrotherapeutics', in von Ziemssen, *Handbook of general therapeutics* Vol. 5 (1886), 273–606.
Wood, Neville (ed.), *Health resorts of the British Islands* (London: London University Press, 1912).
Wright, C. N., *Scenes in North Wales* (London: T. T. & J. Tegg, 1833).
Ziemssen, H. von, *Handbook of general therapeutics in seven vols* (London: Smith, Elder & Co., 1885–87).

SECONDARY SOURCES

Published works

Abel-Smith, Brian, A history of the nursing profession (London: Heinemann, 1960)

Adams, Jane, 'Accommodating the poor: the role of the voluntary hospital in nineteenth-century English spas', in Cossic and Galliou (eds), *Spas in Britain and France*, 161–91.

Adams, Jane M., 'Healthy places and healthy regimens: British spas 1918–50', in Virginia Berridge and Martin Gorsky (eds), *Environment, health and history* (Basingstoke: Palgrave Macmillan, 2012), 113–32.

Adams, Jane M., 'Developing naturopathy in interwar Britain', in Nicola K. Gale and Jean V. McHale (eds), *Routledge handbook of complementary and alternative medicine: perspectives from social science and law* (Routledge: forthcoming 2015).

Addison, William, *English Spas* (London: Batsford, 1951).

Alderson, Frederick, *The inland resorts and spas of Britain* (Newton Abbot: David and Charles, 1973).

Anderson, Susan C. and Bruce H. Tabb (eds), *Water, leisure and culture: European historical perspectives* (Oxford: Berg, 2002).

Aspinwall, Bernard, 'Social Catholicism and health: Dr. and Mrs Low Nichols in Britain', in W. J. Sheils (ed.), *The Church and healing* (Oxford: Basil Blackwood, 1982), 249–70.

Barclay, Jean, *In good hands: the history of the Chartered Society of Physiotherapy 1894–1994* (Oxford: Butterworth Heinemann, 1994).

Barrow, Logie, 'Why were most medical heretics at their most confident around the 1840s? (The other side of mid-Victorian medicine)', in Roger French and Andrew Wear (eds), *British medicine in the age of reform* (London: Routledge, 1991), 165–85.

Bartholomew, M., 'H. V. Morton's English utopia', in C. Lawrence and A-K. Meyer (eds), *Regenerating England: science, medicine and culture in inter-war Britain* (Amsterdam and Atlanta: Rodopi, 2000), 25–44.

Bartripp, P. W. J., 'Hastings, Sir Charles (1794-1866)', Oxford dictionary of national biography (Oxford University Press, 2004, online edn), www.oxforddnb.com/view/article/12560, accessed 9 May 2007.

Baxter, Eric, *Dr Jephson of Leamington Spa*, Joan Lane and Robert Bearman (eds), (Warwick: Warwickshire Local History Society, 1980).

Baxter, E. G., 'The social life of visitors to Leamington Spa in the first half of the nineteenth century; part I', *Warwickshire History*, 3.1 (1975) 15–37.

Baxter, E. G., 'The social life of visitors to Leamington Spa in the first half of the nineteenth century; part II', *Warwickshire History*, 3.2 (1975) 46–70.

Beckerson, J., 'Marketing British tourism: government approaches to the stimulation of a service sector, 1880–1950', in H. Berghoff, B. Korte, R. Schneider and C.

Harvie (eds), *The making of modern tourism: the cultural history of the British experience* (Basingstoke: Palgrave Macmillan, 2002), 133–57.
Bergdolt, Klaus, *Wellbeing: a cultural history of healthy living*, trans. Jane Dewhurst (Cambridge: Polity Press, 2008).
Bivins, Roberta, *Alternative medicine? A history* (Oxford: Oxford University Press, 2007).
Blackbourn, David, '"Taking the waters": meeting places of the fashionable world', in Martin H. Geyer and Johannes Paulmann (eds), *The mechanics of internationalism: culture, society and politics from the 1840s to the First World War* (Oxford: Oxford University Press, 2001), 435–57.
Blackbourn, David, 'Fashionable spa towns in nineteenth-century Europe', in Anderson and Tabb (eds), *Water, leisure and culture*, 9–21.
Borsay, Anne, *Medicine and charity in Georgian Bath: a social history of the General Infirmary c. 1739–1830* (Aldershot: Ashgate, 1999).
Borsay, Peter, *The English urban renaissance: culture and society in the provincial town, 1660–1770* (Oxford: Oxford University Press, 1989).
Borsay, Peter, 'Health and leisure resorts 1700–1840', in P. Clark (ed.), *The Cambridge urban history of Britain*, 3 Vols, Vol. 2, *1700–1840* (Cambridge: Cambridge University Press, 2000), 775–803.
Borsay. Peter, 'Bath: an Enlightenment city?', in Borsay, Hirschfelder and Mohrmann (eds), *New directions in urban history*, 3–17.
Borsay, Peter, *The image of Georgian Bath* (Oxford: Oxford University Press, 2000).
Borsay, Peter, *A history of leisure: the British experience since 1500* (Basingstoke: Palgrave Macmillan, 2006).
Borsay, Peter, Gunter Hirschfelder and Ruth-E. Mohrmann (eds), *New directions in urban history: aspects of European art, health, tourism and leisure since the Enlightenment* (Munster: Waxmann, 2000).
Borsay, Peter and John K. Walton, 'Introduction: the resort–port relationship', in Borsay and Walton (eds), *Resorts and ports*, 1–17.
Borsay, Peter and John K. Walton (eds), *Resorts and ports: European seaside towns since 1700* (Bristol, Buffalo, Toronto: Channel View, 2011).
Bradley, James, 'Medicine on the margins? Hydropathy and orthodoxy in Britain, 1840–60', in Waltraud Ernst (ed.), *Plural medicine, tradition and modernity, 1800–2000* (London: Routledge, 2002), 19–39.
Bradley, James and Marguerite Dupree, 'Opportunity on the edge of orthodoxy: medically qualified hydropathists in the era of reform, 1840–60', *Social History of Medicine*, 14 (2001), 417–37.
Bradley, James and Marguerite Dupree, 'A shadow of orthodoxy? An epistemology of British hydropathy, 1840–1858', *Medical History*, 47 (2003), 173–94.
Bradley, James, Marguerite Dupree and Alastair Durie, 'Taking the water-cure: the hydropathic movement in Scotland, 1840–1940', *Business and Economic History*, 26 (1997), 426–37.
Breathnach, Teresa, 'For health and pleasure: the Turkish bath in Victorian Ireland', *Victorian Literature and* Culture, 20 (2004), 159–75.

Brown, P. S., 'Nineteenth-century American health reformers and the early nature cure movement in Britain', *Medical History*, 32 (1988), 174–94.

Browne, Janet, 'Spas and sensibilities: Darwin at Malvern', in Porter (ed.), *Medical history of waters and spas*, 102–13.

Bynum, W. F., *Science and the practice of medicine* (Cambridge: Cambridge University Press, 1994).

Cannadine, David, *Lords and landlords: the aristocracy and the towns, 1774–1967* (Leicester: Leicester University Press, 1980).

Cantor, David, 'The contradictions of specialization: rheumatism and the decline of the spa in inter-war Britain', in Porter (ed.), *Medical history of waters and spas*, 127–44.

Cantor, David, 'The aches of industry: philanthropy and rheumatism in inter-war Britain', in Jonathan Barry and Colin Jones (eds), *Medicine and charity before the welfare state* (London: Routledge, 1991), 225–45.

Cantor, David, 'Cortisone and the politics of drama', in John V. Pickstone (ed.), *Medical innovation in historical perspective* (Basingstoke: Macmillan, 1992), 165–84.

Cantor, David (ed.), *Reinventing Hippocrates* (Ashgate: Aldershot, 2002).

Carter, Grayson, 'The case of the Reverend James Shore', *Journal of Ecclesiastical History*, 47 (1996), 478–504.

Carter, Simon, *Rise and shine: sunlight, technology and health* (Oxford: Berg, 2007).

Cave, Lyndon F., *Royal Leamington Spa: its history and development* (Chichester: Philimore, 1988).

Cayleff, Susan E., *Wash and be healed; the water cure movement and women's health* (Philadelphia: Temple University Press, 1987).

Chambers, Margaret, *The British Naturopathic Association: the first fifty years* (London: The British Naturopathic Association, n.d. but c. 1995).

Champ, Judith F., 'Bishop Milner, Holywell, and the cure tradition', in Sheils (ed.), *Church and healing*, 153–64.

Clarke, H. G., *Royal Leamington Spa: a century's growth and development* (Leamington: Courier Press, 1947).

Clarke, Norma, 'Strenuous idleness: Thomas Carlyle and man of letters as hero', in Michael Roper and John Tosh (eds), *Manful assertions: masculinities in Britain since 1800* (Routledge: London, 1991), 25–43.

Cole, B., and R. Durack, *Railway posters from the collection of the National Railway Museum, York* (London: Lawrence King, 1992).

Coley, Noel G., 'Physicians, chemists and the analysis of mineral waters: "the most difficult part of chemistry"', in Porter (ed.), *Medical history of waters and spas*, 56–66.

Cooter, Roger (ed.), *Studies in the history of alternative medicine* (Basingstoke: Macmillan, 1988).

Cooter, Roger, *Surgery and society in peace and war: orthopaedics and the organisation of modern medicine, 1880–1948* (Basingstoke: Macmillan, 1993).

Corbin, Alain, *The lure of the sea: the discovery of the seaside in the western world 1750–1840* (London: Penguin, 1995).
Corfield, P. J., *The impact of English towns 1700–1800* (Oxford: Oxford University Press, 1982).
Corfield, P. J. with Serena Kelly, '"Giving directions to the town": the early town directories', *Urban History Yearbook* (1984), 22–34.
Cossic, Annick and Patrick Galliou (eds), *Spas in Britain and in France in the eighteenth and nineteenth centuries* (Newcastle, Cambridge Scholars Press, 2006).
Crook, Tom, '"Schools for the moral treatment of the people": public baths, liberalism and the promotion of cleanliness in Victorian Britain', *European Review of History/Revue Européenne d'Histoire*, 13 (2006), 121–47.
Cunningham, H., *Leisure in the Industrial Revolution*, c. 1780–1880 (London: Croom Helm, 1980).
Daunton, Martin J., *House and home in the Victorian city: working class housing 1850–1914* (London: Edward Arnold, 1983).
Digby, Anne, 'The economic and medical significance of the British National Health Insurance Act', in Martin Gorsky and Sally Sheard (eds), *Financing medicine: the British experience since 1750* (Routledge: London, 2006), 182–98.
Dingwall, Robert, Anne Marie Rafferty and Charles Webster, *An introduction to the social history of nursing* (London: Routledge, 1988).
Dixon, Mike and Gregory Radick, *Darwin in Ilkley* (Stroud: History Press, 2009).
Donegan, Jane B., *'Hydropathic highway to health': women and water-cure in antebellum America* (New York: Greenwood Press, 1986).
Durie, Alastair, 'Almost twins by birth: hydropathy, temperance and the Scottish churches 1840–1914', paper given to the Scottish Church History Society on 27 November 2001, www.schs.org.uk/samplepaper.htm, accessed 26 June 2006.
Durie, Alastair, 'The business of hydropathy in the north of England, c.1850–1930', *Northern History*, 39 (2002), 37–58.
Durie, Alastair, 'Medicine, health and economic development: promoting spa and seaside resorts in Scotland c. 1750–1830', *Medical History*, 47 (2003), 195–216.
Durie, Alastair, 'Unfulfilled promise: the spas of Scotland in the later nineteenth century', in Cossic and Galliou, *Spas in Britain and in France*, 433–53.
Durie, Alastair, *Water is best: the hydros and health tourism in Scotland 1840–1940* (Edinburgh: John Donald, 2009).
Durie, A. J. and C. E. Durie, 'Annie Steedman Hunter: a very radical reformer, *Forth Naturalist and Historian*, 26 (2003), 125–34.
Eveleigh, David J., *Bogs, baths and basins: the story of domestic sanitation* (Stroud: Sutton Publishing, 2002).
Fisher, Stephen (ed.), *Recreation and the sea* (Exeter: Exeter University Press, 1997).
Foley, Ronan, *Healing waters: therapeutic landscapes in historic and contemporary Ireland* (Farnham: Ashgate, 2010).
Frawley, Maria, *Invalidism and identity in nineteenth-century Britain* (London: University of Chicago Press, 2004).

Gibbons, W. G., *Royal Leamington Spa: the seeds of lawn tennis* (Coventry: Jones-Sands, 1986).
Gijswijt-Hofstra, Marijke and Roy Porter (eds), *Cultures of neurasthenia from Beard to the First World War* (Amsterdam and New York, Rodopi, 2001).
Gilbert, Edmund W., *Brighton: old ocean's bauble* (London: Methuen, 1954).
Gillmeister, Heiner, *Tennis: a cultural history* (Leicester University Press, 1998.
Gleadle, Kathryn, '"The age of physiological reformers": rethinking gender and domesticity in the age of reform', in Arthur Burns and Joanna Innes (eds), *Rethinking the age of reform: Britain 1780–1850* (Cambridge: Cambridge University Press, 2003), 200–19.
Gorsky, Martin, Martin Powell and John Mohan, 'British voluntary hospitals and the public sphere: contribution and participation before the National Health Service', in Steve Sturdy (ed.), *Medicine, health and the public sphere in Britain, 1600–2000* (London: Routledge, 2002), 123–44.
Goubert, Jean Pierre, *The conquest of water: the advent of health in the industrial age*, trans. Andrew Wilson (Princeton: Princeton University Press, 1989).
Granshaw, Lindsay, '"Fame and fortune by means of bricks and mortar": the medical profession and specialist hospitals in Britain, 1800–1948', in Lindsay Granshaw and Roy Porter (eds), *Hospitals in History* (London: Routledge, 1989), 199–220.
Grierson, Janet, *Temperance, therapy and trilobites: Dr. Ralph Grindrod: Victorian pioneer* (Cora Weaver: Malvern, 2001).
Haley, Bruce, *The healthy body and Victorian culture* (Cambridge, MA: Harvard University Press, 1978).
Hall, Donald E., 'Muscular Christianity: reading and writing the male social body', in Donald E. Hall (ed.), *Muscular Christianity: embodying the Victorian age* (Cambridge: Cambridge University Press, 1994).
Hamlin, Christopher, 'Chemistry, medicine and the legitimization of English spas, 1740–1840', in Porter (ed.), *Medical history of waters and spas*, 67–81.
Hamlin, Christopher, *Public health and social justice in the age of Chadwick: Britain, 1800–1854* (Cambridge, Cambridge University Press, 1997).
Harcup, John Winsor, *The Malvern water-cure* (Malvern: Winsor Fox Photos, 1992).
Hardy, Anne, *The epidemic streets: infectious disease and the rise of preventive medicine, 1856–1900* (Oxford: Clarendon Press, 1993).
Harley, David, 'A sword in a madman's hand: professional opposition to popular consumption in the waters literature of southern England and the Midlands, 1570–1870', in Porter (ed.), *Medical history of waters and spas*, 48–55.
Harley Warner, John, *The therapeutic perspective: medical practice, knowledge, and identity in America, 1820–1885* (Cambridge, MA: Harvard University Press, 1986).
Harris, Ruth, *Lourdes: body and spirit in the secular age* (Harmondsworth: Allen Lane, 1999).

Harrison, J. F. C., 'Early Victorian radicals and the medical fringe', in W. F. Bynum and Roy Porter (eds), *Medical fringe and medical orthodoxy* (London: Croom Helm, 1987), 198–215.
Hart, Gwen, *A history of Cheltenham* (Stroud: Alan Sutton, 1981).
Hassan, John, *The seaside, health and the environment in England and Wales since 1800* (London: Ashgate, 2003).
Hau, Michael, *The cult of health and beauty in Germany: a social history, 1890–1930* (Chicago: University of Chicago Press, 2003).
Havins, Peter J. Neville, *The spas of England* (London: Robert Hale, 1976).
Hembry, Phyllis, *The English spa 1560–1815* (London: Athlone, 1990).
Hembry, Phyllis, *British spas from 1815 to the present*, edited and completed by L. W. Cowie and E. E. Cowie (Madison, NJ: Fairleigh Dickinson University Press, 1997).
Hillier, Ken, *A history of Ashby de La Zouche* (Leicester: Jones & Co, 1998).
Hussey, David, '"From the temple of Hygeia to the sordid devotees of Pluto". The Hotwell and Bristol: resort and port in the eighteenth century', in Borsay and Walton (eds), *Resorts and ports*, 50–65.
Jancović, Vladimir, *Confronting the climate: British airs and the making of environmental medicine* (Basingstoke: Palgrave Macmillan, 2010).
Jenner, Mark S. R., 'From conduit community to commercial network? Water in London 1500–1720', in Paul Griffiths and Mark S. R. Jenner (eds), *Londinopolis* (Manchester: Manchester University Press, 2000), 250–72.
Jenner, Mark S. R. and Patrick Wallis, *Medicine and the market in England and its colonies, c.1450–c.1850* (Basingstoke: Palgrave Macmillan, 2007).
Jennings, Bernard (ed.), *A history of Harrogate and Knaresborough* (Huddersfield: Advertiser Press, 1970).
Langham, Mike, *Buxton: a people's history* (Lancaster: Carnegie Publishing Ltd, 2001).
Langham, Mike and Colin Wells, *A history of the baths at Buxton* (Leek: Churnet Valley Books, 1997).
Langham, Mike and Colin Wells, *A history of the Devonshire Royal Hospital at Buxton and the Buxton Bath Charity* (Leek: Churnet Valley Books, 2003).
Langham, Mike and Colin Wells, *The baths at Buxton Spa* (Leek: Churnet Valley Books, 2005).
Larkin, Gerald, *Occupational monopoly and modern medicine* (London: Tavistock, 1983).
Lawrence, Christopher and Mayer, Anna-K., 'Regenerating England: an introduction', in Christopher Lawrence and Anna-K. Mayer (eds), *Regenerating England: science, medicine and culture in inter-war Britain* (Amsterdam and Atlanta: Rodopi, 2000), 1–23.
Lesky, E., *The Vienna medical school of the nineteenth century* (Baltimore and London: Johns Hopkins University Press, 1976).
McCrone, Kathleen E., *Sport and the physical emancipation of English Women 1870–1914* (London: Routledge, 1988).

McIntyre, Sylvia, 'Bath: the rise of a resort town, 1660–1800', in Peter Clark (ed.), *Country towns in pre-industrial England* (Leicester: Leicester University Press, 1981), 197–249.

Mackaman, Douglas Peter, *Leisure settings: bourgeois culture, medicine, and the spa in modern France* (London: University of Chicago Press, 1998).

Mackaman, Douglas P., 'Competing visions of urban grandeur: planning and developing nineteenth-century spa towns in France', in Borsay, Hirschfelder, Mohrmann (eds), *New directions in urban history*, 41–63.

McKendrick, N., J. Brewer and J. H. Plumb, *The birth of consumer society: the commercialization of eighteenth-century England* (London: Hutchinson, 1983).

Maggs, Christopher, *The origins of general nursing* (London: Croom Helm, 1983).

Maretzki, Thomas W., 'The *kur* in West Germany as an interface between naturopathic and allopathic ideologies', *Social Science and Medicine*, 24 (1987), 1061–8.

Maretzki, Thomas W., 'Cultural variation in biomedicine: the *kur* in West Germany', *Medical Anthropology Quarterly*, 3 (1989), 22–35.

Maretzki, Thomas W. and Eduard Seidler, 'Biomedicine and naturopathic healing in West Germany: a historical and ethnomedical view of a stormy relationship', *Culture, Medicine and Psychiatry*, 9 (1985), 383–421.

Marland, Hilary, *Medicine and society in Wakefield and Huddersfield, 1780–1870* (Cambridge: Cambridge University Press, 1987).

Marland, Hilary, '"Uterine mischief": W. S. Playfair and his neurasthenic patients', in Gijswijt-Hofstra and Porter (eds), *Cultures of neurasthenia*, 117–39.

Marland, Hilary and Jane Adams, 'Hydropathy at home: the water cure and domestic healing in mid-nineteenth-century Britain', *Bulletin of the History of Medicine*, 83 (2009), 499–529.

Morris, C. (ed.), *The journeys of Celia Fiennes* (London: Cresset Press, 1949).

Morton, H. V., *In search of England* (London: Methuen, 1927).

Neale, R. S., *Bath: a social history 1680–1850* (London: Routledge and Kegan Paul, 1981).

Oppenheim, Janet, *Shattered nerves: doctors, patients and depression in Victorian England* (New York, Oxford University Press, 1991).

Patmore, J. A., 'The spa towns of Britain', in R. P. Beckinsale and J. M. Houston (eds), *Urbanization and its problems: essays in honour of E. W. Gilbert* (Oxford: Basil Blackwood, 1968), 47–69.

Perkin, H. J., 'The social tone of Victorian seaside resorts in the North West', *Northern History*, 11 (1976), 180–94.

Pickstone, John V., *Medicine and industrial society: a history of hospital development in Manchester and its region, 1752–1946* (Manchester: Manchester University Press, 1985).

Pimlott, J. A. R., *The Englishman's holiday: a social history* (London: Faber and Faber, 1947).

Pitcairn Knowles, Richard, *Riposo Health Hydro 1912–1962* (St Leonards on sea: Impression IT for the author, 2012).

Plumb, J. H., *The commercialisation of leisure in eighteenth-century England* (Reading: University of Reading, 1973).

Porter, Roy (ed.), *The medical history of waters and spas, Medical History*, Supp. No. 10 (London: Wellcome Institute for the History of Medicine, 1990).

Porter, Roy, 'Introduction', in Porter (ed.), *Medical history of waters and spas*, vii–xii.

Porter, Roy, 'Nervousness, eighteenth and nineteenth century style: from luxury to labour', in Gijswijt-Hofstra and Porter (eds), *Cultures of neurasthenia*, 31–49.

Porter, Roy and Dorothy Porter, *In sickness and in health: the British experience 1650–1850* (London: Fourth Estate, 1988).

Porter, Roy and G. S. Rousseau, *Gout: the patrician malady* (London: Yale University Press, 1998).

Price, Robin, 'Hydropathy in England 1840–70', *Medical History*, 25 (1981), 269–80.

Pritchard, T. W., *St Winefride, her holy well and the Jesuit mission, c.650–1930* (Wrexham: Bridge Books, 2009).

Rees, Kelvin, 'Water as a commodity: hydropathy in Matlock', in Cooter (ed.), *Alternative medicine*, 28–45.

Roberts, Richard, 'Leasehold estates and municipal enterprise: landowners, local government and the development of Bournemouth, c. 1850–1914', in David Cannadine (ed.), *Patricians, power and politics in nineteenth-century towns* (Leicester: Leicester University Press, 1982), 175–218.

Rolls, Roger, *The hospital of the nation: the story of spa medicine and the mineral water hospital at Bath* (Bath: Bird, 1988).

Rosenberg, Charles, E., 'Health in the home: a tradition of print and practice', in Rosenberg (ed.), *Right living*, 1–20.

Rosenberg, Charles, E. (ed.), *Right living: an Anglo-American tradition of self-help medicine and hygiene* (London: Johns Hopkins University Press, 2003).

Rupke, N. A. (ed.), *Medical geography in historical perspective, Medical History*, Supplement No. 20 (London: Wellcome Institute for the History of Medicine, 2000).

Sargeant, Marjorie, *Echoes of Woodhall Spa: Woodhall and war* (Woodhall Spa Cottage Museum: Woodhall Spa, 2006).

Sargeant, Marjorie, *Woodhall Spa and the world 1885–1890* (Woodhall Spa: Woodhall Spa Cottage Museum, 2006).

Sargeant, Marjorie, *Voices of Woodhall Spa*' (Woodhall Spa: Woodhall Spa Cottage Museum, 2007).

Shattock, Joanne and Michael Wolff (eds), *The Victorian Periodical Press: Samplings and soundings* (Leicester: Leicester University Press, 1982).

Sheard, Sally, 'Profit is a dirty word: the development of public baths and wash-houses in Britain 1847–1915', *Social History of Medicine*, 13 (2000), 63–85.

Sigerist, Henry E., 'American spas in historical perspective', *Bulletin of the History of Medicine*, 11 (1942), 133–47.

Silver-Isenstadt, Jean L., *Shameless: the visionary life of Mary Gove Nichols* (Baltimore: Johns Hopkins University Press, 2002).

Smith, Brian, *A history of Malvern* (Leicester: Leicester University Press, 1964), 2nd edn 1978.

Smith, F. B., *The people's health 1830–1910*, 2nd edn (London: Weidenfeld and Nicolson, 1990).

Smith, Janet, *Liquid assets: the lidos and open-air swimming pools of Britain* (Swindon: English Heritage, 2005).

Smith, Leonard D., 'Behind closed doors: lunatic asylum keepers, 1800–1860', *Social History of Medicine*, 1 (1988) 301–27.

Smith, R. A. L., *Bath* (London: Batsford, 1944).

Smith, Virginia, *Clean: a history of personal hygiene and purity* (Oxford: Oxford University Press, 2007).

Steward, Jill, 'The spa towns of the Austro-Hungarian Empire and the growth of tourist culture: 1860–1914', in Borsay, Hirschfelder and Mohrmann (eds), *New directions in urban history*, 87–125.

Steward, Jill, 'The culture of the water-cure in nineteenth-century Austria, 1800–1914', in Anderson and Tabb (eds), *Water, leisure and culture*, 23–35.

Steward, Jill, 'Representations of spa culture in the nineteenth-century British media: publicity, the press and the *ville d'eaux* (1800–1914)', in Cossic and Galliou, *Spas in Britain and France*, 375–410.

Stobart, Jon, 'In search of a leisure hierarchy: English spa towns and their place in the eighteenth-century urban system', in Borsay, Hirschfelder and Mohrmann (eds), *New directions in urban history*, 19–40.

Strang, Veronica, *The meaning of water* (Oxford: Berg, 2004).

Sweet, Rosemary, *The writing of urban histories in eighteenth-century England* (Oxford: Clarendon Press, 1997).

Szabo, Jason, 'Seeing is believing? The form and substance of French medical debates over Lourdes', *Bulletin of the History of Medicine*, 76 (2002), 199–230.

Thompson, F. M. L., *The rise of respectable society: a social history of Victorian Britain, 1830–1900* (London: Fontana, 1988).

Thomson, M., 'Neurasthenia in Britain', in Gijswijt-Hofstra and Porter (eds), *Cultures of neurasthenia*, 77–95.

Thomson, William A. R., *Spas that heal* (London: Adam and Charles Black, 1978).

Tosh, John, *A man's place: masculinity and the middle-class home in Victorian England* (Yale University Press: London, 1999).

Travis, John F., *The rise of the Devon seaside resorts 1750–1900* (Exeter: University of Exeter Press, 1993).

Travis, John F., 'Continuity and change in English sea-bathing, 1730–1900: a case of swimming with the tide', in Stephen Fisher (ed.), *Recreation and the sea* (Exeter: Exeter University Press, 1997), 8–35.

Turner, E. S., *Taking the cure* (London: Michael Joseph, 1967).

Walton, John K., *The English seaside resort: a social history 1750–1914* (Leicester: Leicester University Press, 1983).

Walton, John K., 'The seaside resorts of Western Europe, 1750–1939', in Fisher (ed.), *Recreation and the sea*, 36–56.

Walton, John K., *The British seaside: holidays and resorts in the twentieth century* (Manchester: Manchester University Press, 2000).
Walton, John K., 'Spas and seaside cultures in the age of the railway: Britain and France compared', in Cossic and Galliou, *Spas in Britain and France*, 475–498.
Walvin, J., *Leisure and Society, 1830–1950* (London: Longman, 1978).
Ward, S. V., *Selling places: the marketing and promotion of towns and cities 1850–2000* (New York: Routledge, 1998).
Weaver, Cora, *The healing baths of Droitwich Spa* (Malvern: Cora Weaver, 1999).
Weaver, Cora and Bruce Osborne, *Acquae Malvernensis: a history and topography of the springs, spouts, fountains and wells of the Malverns and the development of a public water supply* (Malvern: Cora Weaver, 1994).
Weisz, George, 'Water cures and science: the French Academy of medicine and mineral waters in the nineteenth century', *Bulletin of the History of Medicine*, 64 (1990), 393–416.
Weisz, George, 'Spas, mineral waters and hydrological science in twentieth-century France', *Isis*, 92 (2001) 451–83.
Whorton, James C., *Crusaders for fitness: the history of American health reformers* (Princeton: Princeton University Press, 1982).
Whorton, James C., *Nature cures: the history of alternative medicine in America* (Oxford: Oxford University Press, 2002).
Wicksteed, Jane H., *The growth of a profession, being the history of the Chartered Society of Physiotherapy 1894–1948* (London: Edward Arnold, 1948).
Winter, Alison, 'Harriet Martineau and the reform of the invalid in Victorian Britain', *Historical Journal*, 38 (1995), 597–616.
Woodward, John, *To do the sick no harm: a study of the British voluntary hospital system to 1875* (London: Routledge and Kegan Paul, 1974).
Young, Kenneth, *Music's great days in the spas and watering places* (Macmillan: London, 1968).
Zweiniger-Bargielowska, Ina, *Managing the body: beauty, health, and fitness in Britain, 1880–1939* (Oxford: Oxford University Press, 2010).

Unpublished theses

Adams, Jane, 'The mixed economy for medical services in Herefordshire, c.1770–1850' (PhD dissertation, University of Warwick, 2004).
Bennett-Ruete, Jackie L., 'A social history of Bad Ems; spa culture and the welfare state in Germany' (PhD dissertation, University of Warwick, 1988).
Kinder, Susan, 'The struggle for legitimacy in Victorian alternative medicine: the case of hydropathy and mesmerism' (PhD dissertation, University of London, 2005).
Nolte, Annette, 'The ebb and flow of hydropathy: the water-cure movement in Europe and America' (PhD dissertation, University of Texas at Arlington, 2001).

Patmore, J. A., 'Harrogate and Knaresborough: a study in urban development' (MA dissertation, University of Oxford, 1959).
Root, Sheryl, 'The healing touch: spiritual healing in England, c.1870–1955' (PhD dissertation, University of Warwick, 2005).
Smith, V. S., 'Cleanliness: the development of ideas and practice in Britain 1770–1850' (PhD dissertation, London School of Economics, 1985).
Twigg, Julia, 'The vegetarian movement in England, 1847–1981 with particular reference to its ideology' (PhD dissertation, University of London, 1981).
Webb, Helen Mary, 'Woodhall Spa: functional aspects of an inland resort town' (BA dissertation, University of Durham, 1978).

Internet sources

clevelandpools.org.uk. Website of Cleveland pool, Bath.
www.ismh-direct.net. Website of the International Society of Medical Hydrology.
www.nelsonsnaturalworld.com. Website of A. Nelson and Co. Ltd.
www.victorianturkishbath.org, Malcolm R. Shifrin, 'Victorian Turkish baths: their origin, development, and gradual decline'.
www.visitbuxton.co.uk. Website of Visit Buxton.

Index

EU authorised representative for GPSR:
Easy Access System Europe, Mustamäe tee 50,
10621 Tallinn, Estonia
gpsr.requests@easproject.com

www.ingramcontent.com/pod-product-compliance
Ingram Content Group UK Ltd.
Pitfield, Milton Keynes, MK11 3LW, UK
UKHW011005120926
8556IPUK00027B/95
9780719095696